Mechanisms and Machine Science

Volume 39

Series editor

Marco Ceccarelli
LARM: Laboratory of Robotics and Mechatronics
DICeM; University of Cassino and South Latium
Via Di Biasio 43, 03043 Cassino (Fr), Italy
ceccarelli@unicas.it

More information about this series at http://www.springer.com/series/8779

Philippe Wenger · Christine Chevallereau
Doina Pisla · Hannes Bleuler
Aleksandar Rodić
Editors

New Trends in Medical and Service Robots

Human Centered Analysis, Control and Design

Springer

Editors
Philippe Wenger
Ecole Centrale de Nantes 1
Institut de Recherche en Communications et Cybernétique de Nantes
Nantes Cedex 03
France

Christine Chevallereau
Ecole Centrale de Nantes 1
Institut de Recherche en Communications et Cybernétique de Nantes
Nantes Cedex 03
France

Doina Pisla
Research Center for Industrial Robots Simulation and Testing
Technical University of Cluj-Napoca
Cluj-Napoca
Romania

Hannes Bleuler
IMT—LSRO1
EPFL
Lausanne
Switzerland

Aleksandar Rodić
Robotics Laboratory
Mihajlo Pupin Institute
Belgrade
Serbia

ISSN 2211-0984 ISSN 2211-0992 (electronic)
Mechanisms and Machine Science
ISBN 978-3-319-30673-5 ISBN 978-3-319-30674-2 (eBook)
DOI 10.1007/978-3-319-30674-2

Library of Congress Control Number: 2016934190

Printed on acid-free paper

This Springer imprint is published by Springer Nature
The registered company is Springer International Publishing AG Switzerland

Preface

Research in medical and service robotics has been continuously growing over the past decade as a logical response to the increasing needs of our evolving society. Research in medical and service robotics covers a large field of domains such as clinical robotics (surgery and diagnosis), robotics for rehabilitation and assistance (exoskeleton and prostheses), service robotics (humanoid and wheeled robots, autonomous surveying and rescue robots), and cognitive robotics, among others. These fields of research require a multidisciplinary approach ranging from mechanism theory and biomechanics to life and social sciences. One of the most important common features in medical and service robotics is probably the strong, intimate link with human. In many cases, human is even placed at the center of important issues involved in the analysis, design, and control of medical and service robots. This is particularly true in elderly and assistive robotics, where the interactions with human must be treated with respect to both physical and cognitive aspects. The place of human has been pointed out during the fourth workshop on Medical and Service Robotics, MeSRob'2015, held at IRCCyN in Nantes, France. In addition to classical scientific presentations, several keynotes have been given to illustrate the increasing need of robotics for elderly people.

This book collects 22 papers that were all presented during MeSRob'2015 and selected on the basis of a peer-review process. They cover classical issues in medical and service robotics but also more rarely discussed questions such as legal aspects. We are grateful to the sponsors of this workshop (IFToMM, CEA-LIST, BA-Systèmes, CNRS, Région-Pays-de-la-Loire), the authors and reviewers, and the scientific and organizing committees.

MeSRob is now a well-established workshop. The fifth edition will take place in Graz, Austria. We are confident that MesSRob will become more and more attractive.

Philippe Wenger
Christine Chevallereau
Doina Pisla
Hannes Bleuler
Aleksandar Rodić

Contents

Effect of Non-passive Operator on Enhanced Wave-Based Teleoperator for Robotic-Assisted Surgery: First Case Study

Jing Guo, Chao Liu and Philippe Poignet

Abstract Minimally invasive surgery (MIS) has been advanced by new medical/surgical robotic technologies, aiming to achieve less invasiveness, smaller or even no scar procedures. Miniaturized surgical robot presents promising alternative to better benefit MIS, but considerable constraints including cables for power and communication may degrade its performance. Wireless communication posses great potential to be utilized, however time delay is inevitably introduced which challenges the design of teleoperation system from both stability and transparency point of view. Wave variable based teleoperation provides stable force reflecting teleoperation with arbitrary time delay, but with both compromised position and force tracking performances. Recently we proposed a wave variable compensated structure to improve the position and tracking performance together with energy reservoir based regulators for stability purpose (Guo et al. In: Proceeding European Control Conference (ECC), Linz, pp. 1980–1985 (2015), [23]), but with assumption of passive operator and environment. In this paper, several experiments are conduced to evaluate the passivity of operator using the enhanced wave variable compensated structure, and to study the influence of non-passive behavior conducted by operator to the performance of teleoperation and overall system stability. This first case study shows that non-passive behaviors of operator (such as rigid grasp and trajectory tracking tasks) can inject extra energy into system and may cause stability issues for whole system.

Keywords Bilateral teleoperation · Time delay · Robotic-assisted surgery · Telesurgery · Non-passive operator

---

J. Guo (✉) · C. Liu · P. Poignet
LIRMM, University of Montpellier - CNRS, Montpellier, France
e-mail: jguo@lirmm.fr

C. Liu
e-mail: liu@lirmm.fr

P. Poignet
e-mail: poignet@lirmm.fr

P. Wenger et al. (eds.), *New Trends in Medical and Service Robots*,
Mechanisms and Machine Science 39, DOI 10.1007/978-3-319-30674-2_1

1 Introduction

Minimally invasive surgery (MIS) has promoted the surgical procedures in past decades over traditional open surgery by significantly improving patients benefits such as less invasiveness, smaller scars and less recovery time, as explained in literatures [1–3]. Recent research effort is moving towards further reduce the surgical procedure invasiveness and decrease the number and size of visible incisions, as which is also presented in [4]. Targeted to achieve single incision or scar-less procedures, laparo-endoscopic single site surgery (LESS) and natural orifice transluminal endoscopic surgery (NOTES) have attracted growing interests [5–7]. It is mentioned that NOTES shows promising approach over LESS due to it potentially eliminates abdominal incisions during diagnosis and treatment of abdominal pathologies [8]. But it is also observed that several main drawbacks existing such as anatomical constraints and method of guiding flexible tools to reach abdomen [1].

In view of the limitation of current NOTES platform, Tortora [9] proposed a modular magnetic NOTES platform for NOTES procedures, which contains a trans-abdominal magnetic frame for robotic modular anchoring, dedicated miniaturized surgical tools and a magnetically-actuated retraction system. The surgical platform can be established inside human body by delivering several miniaturized robotic tools, and then operate dedicated clinical tasks without leaving scars on body surface. However, it is noticed that cables for power supply and communication may degrade the performance of the aforementioned platform in following aspects: cables may decrease the degree-of-freedom of robotic devices; cables make limited workspace more crowded and may even intertwine together during procedures.

In order to reduce the risks caused by cables for modular magnetic NOTES platform, it is considered to use wireless communication to replace communication cables. In [10] some preliminary work has been presented that Zigbee was identified as one of potential alternative solutions, and some time delay evaluation experiments were also conducted which shown that the time delay caused by Zigbee communication was almost constant to 135 ms (round trip time delay with 32 bytes data transmission) in our set-ups.

Currently, master-slave teleoperation configuration is widely used for robotic-assisted surgery, by which the surgeon can easily manipulate the robot for dedicated clinical operations in remote site. But most developed teleoperated surgical robotic systems do not poss the force feedback to operator which brings possible difficulties to surgeon compared with traditional open surgery [11]. And time delay existing during communication increases the challenges from both perspectives of stability and performance of force reflecting bilateral teleoperation system [12].

Wave variable based teleoperation structure was proposed to provide useful framework for stabilizing bilateral teleoperation system with arbitrary communication delay [13]. However, this conservative condition based method can only provide compromised position and force tracking performance. Various structures and methods [14–19] based on wave variable teleoperation have been proposed to improve position and/or force tracking performance with consideration of passivity condition.

But it is noticed that all the wave variable based teleoperation structures proposed so far in literatures only consider to passivate the delayed communication channels, with assumption of passive operator and environment.

Very recently, we proposed a new wave-based teleoperator with wave variable compensated structure [23]. Experiments of [24] show that enhanced position and force tracking can be stably achieved over traditional wave variable structure, with the help of energy reservoir based regulators to adjust the compensating terms. In these works, both operator and environment were assumed to be passive.

For human operator, non-passivity may occur in various cases, such as in posture-maintenance (i.e. rigid grasp) tasks or trajectory following tasks [20–22]. In general, the non-passive operator may be a source of energy injection in teleoperation system and in some cases it may violate the system passivity condition or even cause stability issues for teleoperation system.

In this paper, we investigated the effect of non-passive behavior of the operator on enhanced wave variable compensated structure. As the operator may not always perform passively, which means that energy may be injected into system thus makes teleoperation system unstable. We carried out several experiments and the results indicate that human operator could be non-passive and degraded tracking performance or even unstable system can be observed as the consequence.

The rest of this paper is organized as follow. Section 2 provides the fundamental knowledge of wave variable based teleoperation structure. The wave variable compensated structure proposed in [23] is briefly presented in Sect. 3. In Sect. 4, the experiment studies are presented with result analysis. Some conclusion and perspective are provided in Sect. 5.

2 Traditional Wave Variable Structure

A force reflecting bilateral teleoperation structure can be treated as a chain of 2-port system in which the master, slave and communication channel can be modeled as two port system, and the operator and environment are considered as a single port [23]. Then the passivity of a 2-port system can be defined as: Eq. (1):

$$\int_0^T P_{out} dt \leq \int_0^T P_{in} dt + E_{store}(0) \tag{1}$$

where $E_{store}(0)$ denotes the initial energy stored.

Based on passivity condition, the traditional wave variable teleoperation structure was proposed in [13] as illustrated in Fig. 1. The information exchanged between delayed communication are modified as wave variables, instead of velocity and force, the forward and backward wave variables u_m, v_s are constructed as:

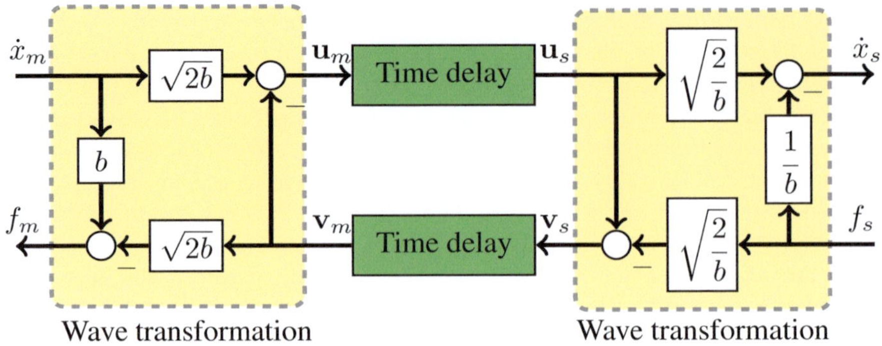

Fig. 1 Traditional wave variable teleoperation structure

$$u_m(t) = \frac{1}{\sqrt{2b}}(f_m(t) + b\dot{x}_m(t)) \tag{2}$$

$$v_s(t) = \frac{1}{\sqrt{2b}}(-f_s(t) + b\dot{x}_s(t)) \tag{3}$$

With the assumption that the communication delay is constant as T, then the wave variables u_s, v_m are similarly derived as:

$$u_s(t) = \frac{1}{\sqrt{2b}}(f_s(t) + b\dot{x}_s(t)) = u_m(t - T) \tag{4}$$

$$v_m(t) = \frac{1}{\sqrt{2b}}(-f_m(t) + b\dot{x}_m(t)) = v_s(t - T) \tag{5}$$

From Eqs. (2–5), force and velocity on both master and slave side can be derived respectively as:

$$f_m(t) = \frac{b}{\sqrt{2b}}(u_m(t) - v_m(t)) \tag{6}$$

$$\dot{x}_m(t) = \frac{1}{\sqrt{2b}}(u_m(t) + v_m(t)) \tag{7}$$

$$f_s(t) = \frac{b}{\sqrt{2b}}(u_s(t) - v_s(t)) \tag{8}$$

$$\dot{x}_s(t) = \frac{1}{\sqrt{2b}}(u_s(t) + v_s(t)) \tag{9}$$

The passivity of delayed communication channel can be guaranteed using wave variable structure as below:

$$\begin{aligned} E(t) = & \frac{1}{2}\int_0^t (f_m(t)\dot{x}_m(t) - f_s(t)\dot{x}_s(t))dt \\ = & \frac{1}{2}\int_0^t (u_m^T u_m - v_m^T v_m - u_s^T u_s + v_s^T v_s)dt \\ = & \frac{1}{2}\int_{t-T}^t u_m^T u_m dt + \frac{1}{2}\int_{t-T}^t v_s^T v_s dt \geq 0 \end{aligned} \quad (10)$$

which means that time delay induced energy is always stored in the communication channel.

But, it is noticed that this method is far conservative to achieve a good position and force tracking performance since:

$$f_m(t) = f_s(t-T) + b(\dot{x_m}(t) - \dot{x}_s(t-T)) \quad (11)$$

$$\dot{x}_s(t) = \dot{x}_m(t-T) + \frac{1}{b}(f_m(t-T) - f_s(t)) \quad (12)$$

And the last two terms in Eqs. (11–12) represent disturbing bias which degrade the tracking performance. Wave impedance b can somehow be used to tune the tracking performance, but still it is hard to achieve both good position and force tracking performance at the same time by solely tuning b.

3 Wave Variable Compensated Structure and Energy Reservoir Based Regulator

3.1 Wave Variable Compensated Structure

In previous work [23], we proposed a modified wave variable based teleoperation structure to achieve enhanced position and force tracking performance. As in Fig. 2, two compensated terms Δu and Δu are utilized to compensate wave variables (details can be found in [23]).

The proposed structure can achieve enhanced force and position tracking performance as:

$$f_m(t) = f_s(t-T) \qquad \dot{x}_s(t) = \dot{x}_m(t-T) \quad (13)$$

with the compensated wave variable terms Δu and Δv as following:

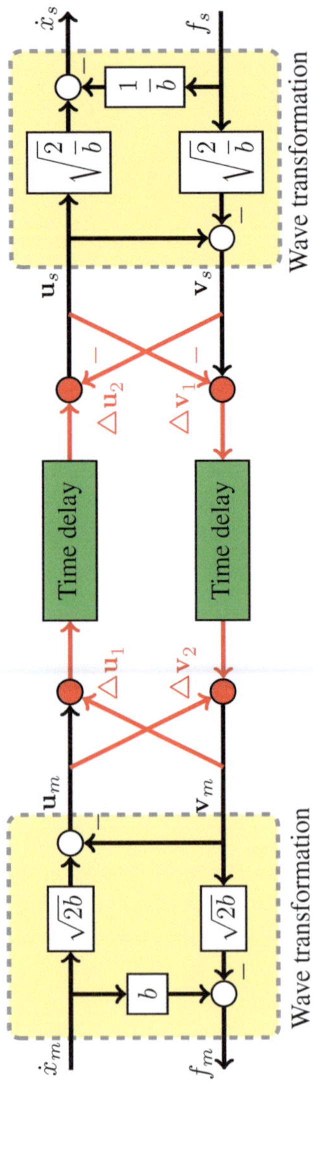

Fig. 2 Wave variable compensated structure

$$\Delta u = v_m(t-T) - v_s(t) \tag{14}$$

$$\Delta v = u_m(t) - u_s(t-T) \tag{15}$$

But it is noticed that the compensated terms may somehow inject extra energy, which can destroy the passivity condition of system, thus further cause instability issue of whole teleoperation system.

3.2 Energy Reservoir Based Regulator

In order to stabilize the proposed wave variable compensated approach, an energy reservoir based regulator method is employed to provide stable tracking performance. In [23], we defined two energy reservoirs both on master and slave side to track the net energy introduced before and after compensation, and used a regulator to limit injected wave variable compensation. However, this method was still based on conservative passivity condition, which may degrade the compensation performance, thus conflict with desired tracking performance.

In [24], another energy reservoir definition was proposed, with consideration of master and slave system together. In which, the energy reservoirs are defined as below to track the net energy dissipated by slave and master system:

$$E_s(t) = \int_0^t (u_m^2(t-T)) - v_s^2(t)dt \tag{16}$$

$$E_m(t) = \int_0^t (v_s^2(t-T) - u_m^2(t))dt \tag{17}$$

Then adjust the compensated wave variables as following:

$$\Delta u = \alpha\left[1 - e^{-\beta E_s(t)}\right](v_m(t-T) - v_s(t)) \tag{18}$$

$$\Delta v = \alpha\left[1 - e^{-\beta E_m(t)}\right](u_m(t) - u_s(t-T)) \tag{19}$$

where α and β are positive parameters to determine the speed of regulation and the size of energy reservoirs respectively. During teleoperation, the energy reservoirs should be non-empty ($E_s(t) \geq 0$ and $E_m(t) \geq 0$), and the compensating terms (Δu and Δv) can be choked off when master or slave system become non-passive, which guarantees the system to be always passive.

3.3 Non-passive Operator

The aforementioned energy reservoir based regulators assume that the master and slave system are passive, and use the energy dissipated by master and slave system to adjust compensated terms. However, non-passive behaviors of operator are not considered. Recent research effort [20–22] indicated that during some teleoperation tasks (i.e. rigid grasp, trajectory tracking), some operators performed in non-passive way, which means that extra energy was introduced into teleoperation system and may cause unexpected non-passive or even unstable performance.

From Eqs. (16–17), it is clear that the energy reservoirs are tracking the net energy dissipated by slave and master side. If the operator is performing non-passive tasks, the energy will decrease during tasks, sometimes may reach 0. It means that the compensated wave variable cannot be choked off, instead excess compensation may happen which causes system unstable.

4 Experimental Studies on Effect of Non-passive Operator

In order to analyze the effect of non-passive behavior of operation on enhanced wave-based teleoperator, experiments were conducted with two Omega 7 robotic devices (one as master and one as slave), a Nano 17 force sensor (ATI, Industrial Automation) was attached to slave robot by a 3D printed adapter to evaluate the contact force. Time delay is set as 200 ms using UDP communication. A phantom (which is made by extra soft PVC (80 % soft PVC + 20 % softener) and medium density PVC (70 % soft + 30 % hard PVC)) is used for contact experiment to mimic the human tissue environment. Figure 3 shows the experiment setup.

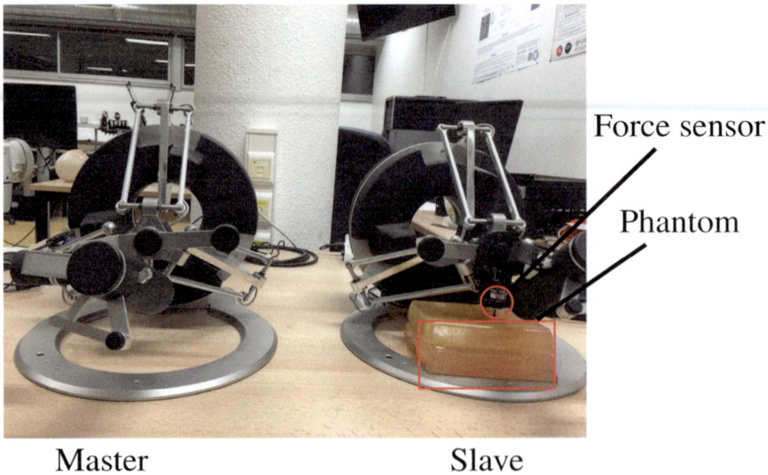

Fig. 3 Experiment setup with two Omega 7 devices

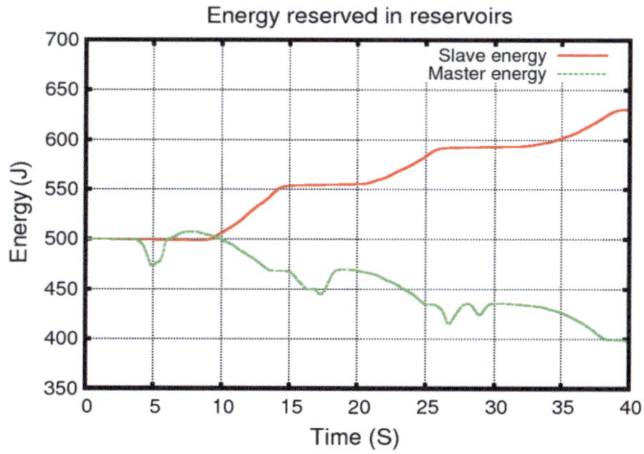

Fig. 4 Energy reserved in reservoirs on master and slave side with initial energy reservoir as 500 (in contact)

4.1 Energy Reserved in Reservoir with Non-passive Operator

The first experiment records the energy reserved in reservoir by master and slave sides as calculated in Eqs. (16–17). Due to safety consideration, initial energy reservoir values of master and slave side are set to 500. A 29-year-old male operator manipulates the master robot to move following sine wave trajectory,and accordingly the slave is moved from free space to contact phantom. The energy reserved in reservoir by both master and slave sides are shown in Fig. 4, where it is clear to see that the slave side, even when contacting phantom, behaves passively and dissipates energy all the time. But for the master side, it can be seen that the dissipated power is negative and therefore the overall energy keeps decreasing, which means that the behavior of operator is non-passive and injects extra energy into system.

4.2 Effect of Non-passive Operator on Enhanced Wave Variable Compensated Structure

In previous sections, it is highlighted that the main objective of enhanced wave variable compensated structure is to achieve enhanced position and force tracking performances for delayed bilateral teleoperation system as illustrated in Eq. (13). In order to demonstrate the effect of non-passive operator on proposed structure, another experiment was conducted with lower initial energy reservoir value of 50.

In Fig. 5, energy reserved in reservoirs by both master and slave sides are recorded. Firstly it is noticed that master side is not passive most of the time, as energy reserved in reservoir by the master side (in green line) is mostly below the initial value (50), and even decreases to close 0 at 26 s. Also it is worth mentioning that even when the experiment is running in free motion, the noise of force sensor causes the energy reserved in reservoir on slave side decrease slightly, but not so significant.

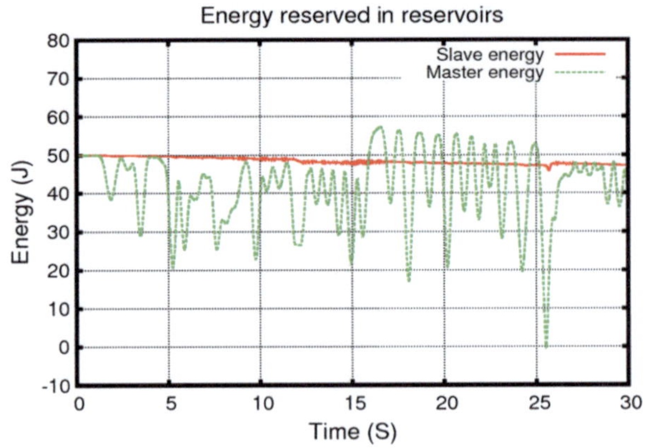

Fig. 5 Energy reserved in reservoirs on master and slave side with initial energy reservoir as 50 (free motion)

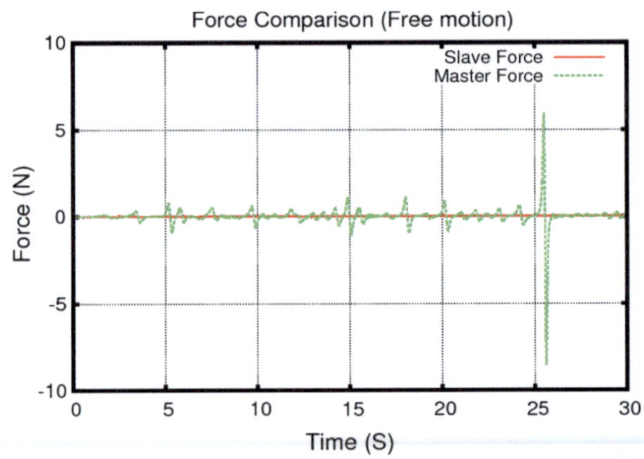

Fig. 6 Force tracking performance with initial energy reservoir as 50 (free motion)

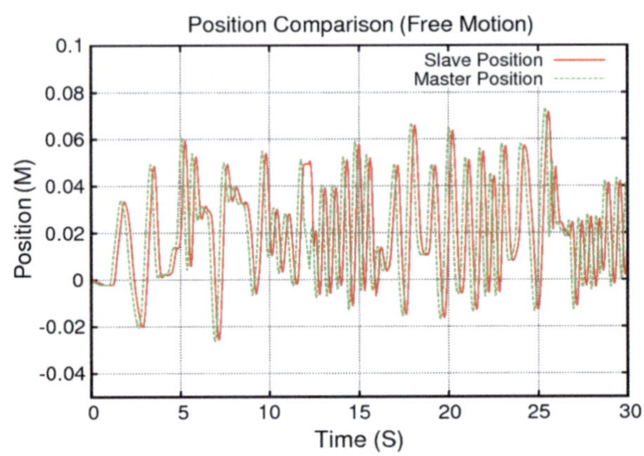

Fig. 7 Position tracking performance with initial energy reservoir as 50 (free motion)

Figures 6 and 7 show the effect of non-passive operator on force and position tracking performance during free motion teleoperation task. It is seen in Fig. 6 that the feedback force is chattering and quite different from the measured force from slave side which is non mean noise signal caused by force sensor. What needs to be emphasized is at 26 s, the feedback force jumps to +6N and quickly drops to −8N, which is because the master side energy drops to around 0. Certainly, when operator feels the obvious change of force he/she stops non-passive operation till the system becomes stable.

For position tracking performance, Fig. 7 shows that the slave tracks well as the master moves. This is because in free motion the energy dissipated by slave side decreases only slightly due to the noise of force sensor but not significant enough to influence the performance of position tracking.

In order to compare the performance of previous experiment with initial energy reservoir of 50, another experiment was conducted with higher initial energy reservoir of 500 with the same experimental configuration. In Fig. 8, it is shown that the slave side keeps passive during experiment; although some fluctuation of energy

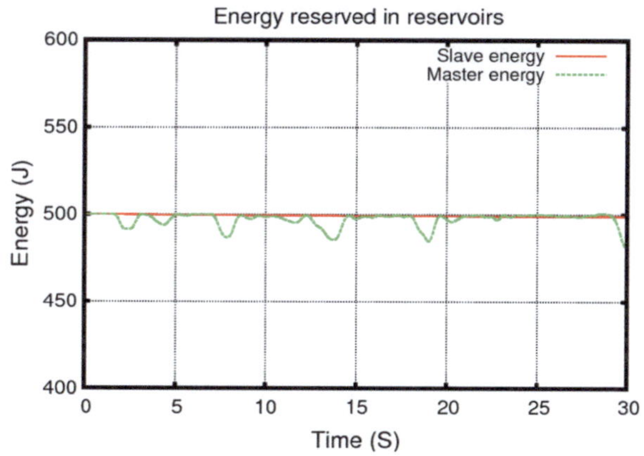

Fig. 8 Energy reserved in reservoirs on master and slave side with initial energy reservoir as 500 (free motion)

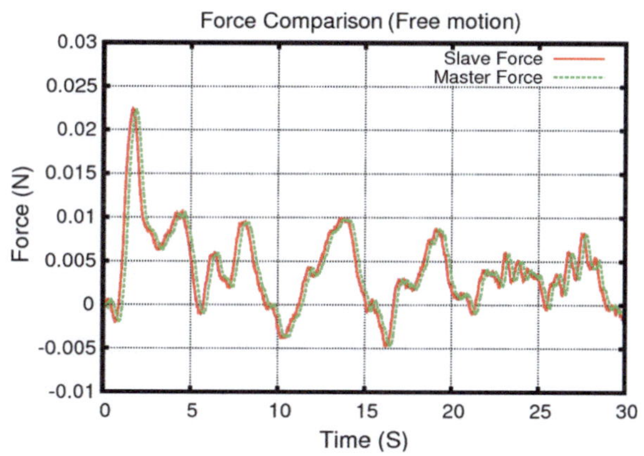

Fig. 9 Force tracking performance with initial energy reservoir as 500 (free motion)

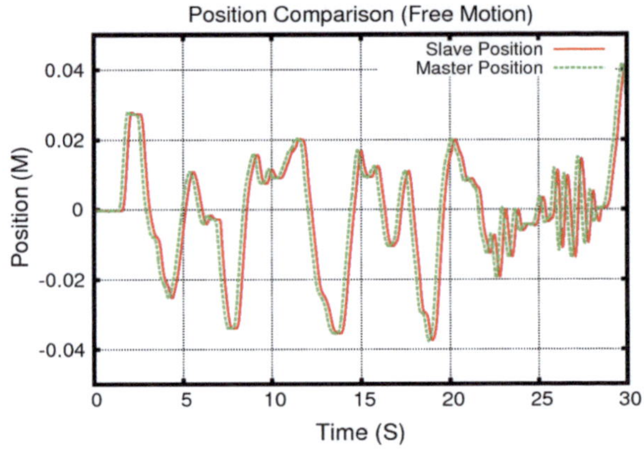

Fig. 10 Position tracking performance with initial energy reservoir as 500 (free motion)

reserved in master side can be noticed, mostly the master side can be considered asymptotic passive.

Figures 9 and 10 provide the force tracking and position tracking performance during free motion with initial energy reservoir of 500. And it is noticed that stable and enhanced tracking performance are achieved thanks to new configuration of energy reservoir. Therefore, through these two experiments it is shown that bigger initial value of the energy reservoir helps to handle non-passive operator motion and consequently the tracking performances. For sure, the initial value cannot be arbitrary large either, which may make the utilization of energy reservoir to be useless.

5 Conclusion and Perspective

In our recent works, an enhanced wave variable compensated teleoperation structure [23, 24] was proposed, in order to guarantee stable tracking performance, energy reservoir based regulators were used to adjust the injected energy by wave variable compensation. This structure can achieve enhanced position and force tracking under aforementioned configuration for normal surgical procedures, but not sufficient for some challenging situations in which non-passive operator and/or environment need to be taken into account. To study the effect of non-passive operation on the performance and stability of the enhanced wave variable compensated structure, some experiments were carried out which indicated that the behavior of operator was not always passive and may inject extra energy into whole teleoperation system, thus degrade or destroy the stability of system. One possible solution is to increase the initial value of the energy reservoir to help handle occasional non-passive behaviors, but it won't work if non-passivity continues over long period.

This work shows that non-passive operator may exist in real teleoperation tasks and can potentially cause stability issues. This issue should be taken into consideration by researchers in future design of new teleoperation structure or methods especially for telesurgery.

References

1. Salerno, M., Tognarelli, S., Quaglia, C., Dario, P., Menciassi, A.: Anchoring frame for intra-addominal surgery. Int. J. Rob. Res. **32**, 360–370 (2013)
2. Wortman, T.D., Strabala, K.W., Lehman, A.C., Farritor, S.M., Oleynikov, D.: Laparoscopic single site surgery using a miltifunctional miniature in vivo robot. Int. J. Med. Rob. Comput. Assist. Surg. **7**, 17–21 (2011)
3. Champagne, B., Stulberg, J.J., Fan, Z., Delaney, C.P.: The feasibility of laparoscopic colectomy in urgent and emergent settings. Surg. Endosc. **23**, 1791–1796 (2009)
4. Bergeles, C., Yang, G., Z.: From passive tool holders to microsurgeons: safer, smaller, smarter surgical robots. IEEE Trans. Biomed. Eng. **61**, 1565–1576 (2014)
5. Tacchino, R., Greco, F., Matera, D.: Single-incision Laparoscopic-cholecystectomy: surgery without a visible scar. Surg. Endosc. **23**, 896–899 (2009)
6. Lirici, M.M.: Single site Laparoscopic surgery: an intermediate step toward no(visible) scar surgery or the next gold standard in minimally invasive surgery? Minim. Invasive Surg. Ther. Allied Technol. **21**, 1–7 (2012)
7. Asakuma, M., Perretta, S., Allemann, P., et al.: Chanllenges and lessons learned from NOTES cholecystectomy initial experience: a stepwise approach from the laboratory to clinical application. J. hepato-Biliary-Pancreat. Surg. **16**, 249–254 (2009)
8. Nagy, Z., M. Fluckiger, Oung, R., et al.: Assembling reconfigurable endoluminal surgical systems: opportunities and challenges. Int. J. Biomech. Biomed. Rob. **1**, 2–16 (2009)
9. Tortora, G., Salerno, M., Ranzani, T., Tognarelli, S., Dario, P., Menciassi, A.: A modular magnetic platform for natural orifice transluminal endoscopic surgery. In: Proceedings of Engineering in Medicine and Biology Society (EMBC), 35th Annual International Conference of the IEEE, Osaka, pp. 6265–6268 (2013)
10. Guo, J., Liu, C., Poignet, P.: Scaled position-force tracking for wireless teleoperation of miniaturized surgical robotic system. In: Proceedings of Engineering in Medicine and Biology Society (EMBC), 36th Annual International Conference of the IEEE, Chicago, pp. 361–365 (2014)
11. Taylor, R.H., Dan, S.: Medical robotics in computer-integrated surgery. IEEE Trans. Rob. Auto. **19**, 765–780 (2003)
12. Lawrence, D.A.: Stability and transparency in bilateral teleoperation. IEEE Trans. Rob. Auto. **9**, 624–637 (1993)
13. Niemeyer, G., Slotine, J.J.: Stable adaptive teleoperation. IEEE J. Ocean. Eng. **16**, 152–162 (1991)
14. Kawashima, K., Tadano, K., Sankaranarayan, G., Hannoford, B.: Bilateral teleoperation with time delay using modified wave variable. In: Proceeding IEEE/RSJ International Conference on Intelligent Robots and Systems (IROS), Nice, pp. 424–429 (2008)
15. Kawashima, K., Tadano, Wang, G., K., Sankaranarayan, G., Hannoford, B.: Bilateral teleoperation with time delay using modified wave variable based controller. In: Proceeding IEEE International Conference of Robotics and Automation (ICRA), Kobe, pp. 4326–4331 (2009)
16. Ye, Y., Liu, P.X.: Improved haptic feedback fidelity in wave-variable-based teleoperation orientated to telemedical application. IEEE Trans. Instrimentation Measur. **58**, 2847–2855 (2009)
17. Ye, Y., Liu, P.X.: Improved trajectory tracking in wave-variable-based teleoperation. IEEE/ASME Trans. Mechatron. **15**, 321–326 (2010)
18. Bate, L., Cook, C.D., Li, Z.: Reducing wave-based teleopertor reflections for unknown environments. IEEE Trans. Ind. Electron. **58**, 392–397 (2011)
19. Li, H., Kawashima, K., Li, H., Kawashima, K.: Achieving stable tracking in wave-variable-based teleoperation. IEEE/ASME Trans. Mechatron. **19**, 1574–1582 (2014)

20. Jazayeri, A., Tavakoli, M.: Revisiting Llewellyn's absolute stability criterion for bilateral teleoperation systems under non-passive operator or environment. In: Proceeding IEEE/RSJ International Conference on Intelligent Robots and Systems (IROS), Algarve, pp. 70–75 (2012)
21. Jazayeri, A., Dyck, M., Tavakoli, M.: Stability analysis of teleoperation systems under strictly passive and non-passive operator. In: Proceeding World Haptic Conference, IEEE, Daejeon, pp. 695–700 (2013)
22. Jazayeri, A., Tavakoli, M.: Bilateral teleoperation system stability with non-passive and strictly passive operator or environment. Control Eng. Pract. **40**, 45–60 (2015)
23. Guo, J., Liu, C., Poignet, P.: Stable and enhanced position-force tracking for bilateral teleoperation with time delay. In: Proceeding European Control Conference (ECC), IEEE, Linz, pp. 1980–1985 (2015)
24. Guo, J., Liu, C., Poignet, P.: Enhanced position-force tracking of time-delayed teleoperation for robotic-assisted surgery. In: Proceedings of Engineering in Medicine and Biology Society (EMBC), 37th Annual International Conference of IEEE, Milano, pp. 4894–4897 (2015)

Singularity Analysis of a Novel Minimally-Invasive-Surgery Hybrid Robot Using Geometric Algebra

Tanio K. Tanev

Abstract The paper presents an analysis of the singularities of a novel type of medical robot for minimally invasive surgery (MIS) using the language of the geometric algebra. The analysis focuses on the parallel manipulator, which is the key component of the robot. The proposed new parallel manipulator provides a remote centre of motion located at the incision point of the patient's body. The aim of the paper is to derive the geometric condition for singularity in terms of geometric algebra and thus to reveal the singular configurations in order to avoid them during the surgical procedure. The obtained geometric condition for singularity leads further to the derivation of the algebraic formulation of the singularity surface which is graphically presented.

Keywords Singularity · Parallel robot · Kinematics · Minimally invasive surgery · Geometric algebra

1 Introduction

Surgical robots enhance the capability of surgeons and allow the development of new operating procedures in the treatment of diseases. These techniques are less invasive and more precise, which leads to better clinical outcome, reduced hospital stay and decreased trauma for the patients. At the end of 20th century, the traditional open surgery evolved to minimally invasive surgery and further to robotised minimally invasive surgery. In the innovative minimally invasive surgery, long surgical instruments are inserted into the human body through small incisions (less than 10 mm in diameter) on the abdomen. The surgeon holds and manoeuvres the instruments thus operating remotely through them. The next logical step of development of the minimally invasive technique was to replace the surgeon's hands with robot arms guided by surgeons, who monitor remotely the internal movements of the instruments through video images delivered by an endoscopic camera.

T.K. Tanev (✉)
Institute of Systems Engineering and Robotics, Bulgarian Academy of Sciences,
Acad. G. Bonchev Str., B1.1, 1113 Sofia, Bulgaria
e-mail: tanev_tk@hotmail.com

P. Wenger et al. (eds.), *New Trends in Medical and Service Robots*,
Mechanisms and Machine Science 39, DOI 10.1007/978-3-319-30674-2_2

From kinematics point of view, the small abdominal incision restricts the motion of the instrument and acts as a pivoting point. Thus, only four degrees of freedom are possible, three rotations around three intersecting axes in the pivoting point and a translation along the longitudinal axis of the surgical tool. The term Remote Centre-of-Motion (RCM) [23] is used to describe this specific movement. RCM is a point where one or more rotations are centred and located outside the mechanism itself. Robots for minimally invasive surgery utilize several types of mechanisms which can enforce RCM. Zeus medical system applies an isocentre-based RCM mechanism [11], while da Vinci surgical system [5] and BlueDRAGON [18] use parallelograms for RMC mechanism. The spherical mechanism is preferably a RCM mechanism in many proposed devices for minimally invasive surgery [15, 24]. Parallel manipulators with spherical linkages have also been proposed especially for laparoscopic surgery [10, 13]. Some other parallel and hybrid manipulators have been suggested for application in laparoscopy [17, 19]. Obviously, the general type of parallel manipulators used in the robot-assisted minimally invasive surgery need to provide programmable RCM [2]. The mechanical RCMs are considered to be more suitable for the robot-assisted minimally invasive surgery due to the fewer degrees of freedom, the simpler control system and safer manipulation.

The singular configurations in parallel manipulators should be avoided during the robot motion since in such configurations the manipulator may have undesired behaviour and compromised performance. This is especially important for medical robots as such undesired behaviour could endanger both the outcome of the surgical procedure and the safety of the patient. That is why the singularities in parallel medical manipulators need to be well analysed and established and therefore should be avoided during surgical manipulations. Many researchers have studied the singularities of parallel manipulators using different mathematical tools. Geometric methods are applied by many researchers [6, 14, 25]. Some "non-traditional" methods, such as Grassmann geometry [16], Grassmann-Cayley algebra [1, 9] and geometric algebra [20, 22], have been used for singularity analysis of parallel manipulators.

This paper utilizes geometric algebra to geometrically characterize the singularities of a novel hybrid robot, especially the parallel manipulator of the robot. The proposed hybrid robot consists of a parallel manipulator and an additional translational joint attached to the moving platform. This robot, which was first proposed in [21], possesses the ability of the spherical linkage to provide remote centre of motion and overcomes some drawbacks of the parallel spherical manipulators, such as a possible clogging and a bulky structure.

2 Robot Design and Kinematics

The considered minimally-invasive-surgery hybrid robot consists of a parallel manipulator and an additional translational joint attached to the moving platform [21]. The novel parallel manipulator, which is a key component of the considered hybrid robot,

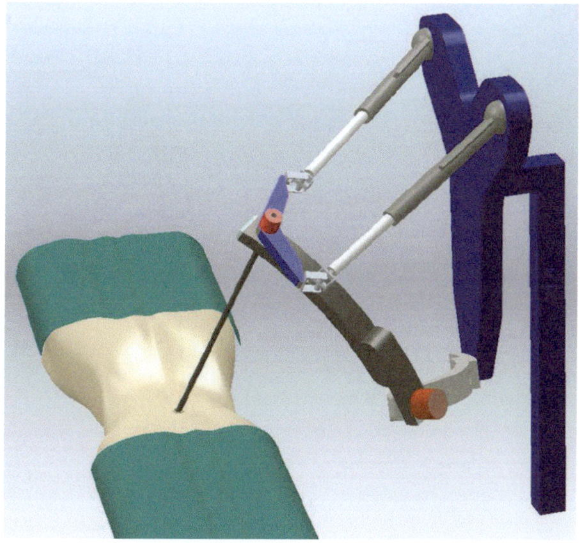

Fig. 1 A CAD model of the robot for minimally invasive surgery

has three limbs (legs) and 2SPU1RRR structure. A CAD model of the considered hybrid robot is shown in Fig. 1.

Two limbs (A_1B_1 and A_2B_2) have an identical SPU (spherical-prismatic-universal) joints structure and the third one (A_3B_3) is a RRR (R stands for revolute) spherical linkage, i.e. the axes of all three revolute joints (R) of this limb intersect in a single point (Fig. 2). An additional prismatic joint is attached to the moving platform, which provides a translation along the longitudinal axis of the surgical instrument (end-effector). The parallel manipulator provides RCM of the end-effector and the RCM is at the incision point of the patient's body. Thus, the parallel mechanism has three degrees of freedom and the hybrid robot has four degrees of freedom in total.

Each limb has one driven joint, respectively. The prismatic joints of the SPU limbs and the second (middle) revolute joint of the RRR limb are driven. In addition to these three active joints for the parallel mechanism, an active prismatic joint allowing translation of the end-effector along the line OB_3 is added. The axis of the revolute joint (at A_3), attached to the base platform, is perpendicular to the plane of the base platform ($A_1A_2A_3$) and the axis of the revolute joint (at B_3), attached to the moving platform, is perpendicular to the plane of the moving platform ($B_1B_2B_3$). The origins of the reference (base) coordinate system OXYZ and the coordinate systems $\{1\}$, $\{2\}$ and $\{3\}$ coincide with the intersection point of the three axes of the revolute joints of the spherical RRR limb. The Z_i-axes ($i = 1, 2, 3$) are along the axes of the three revolute joints, respectively. The $O_4X_4Y_4Z_4$ coordinate system is attached to the moving platform and Z_4-axis is along the direction of translation of the last prismatic joint.

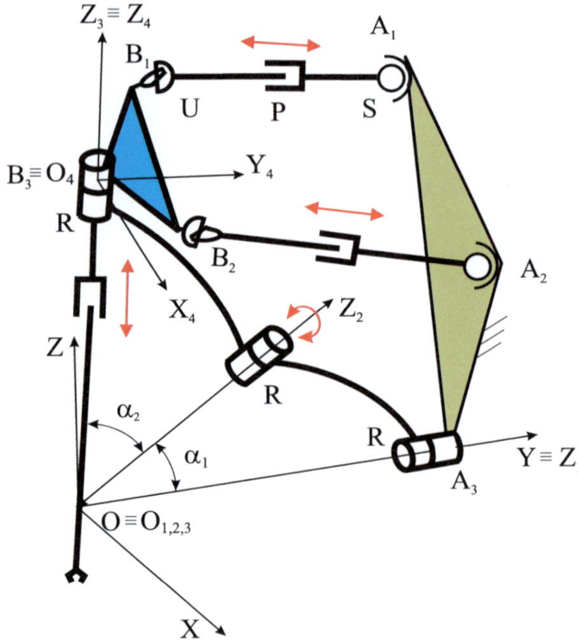

Fig. 2 Kinematic scheme of the robot

2.1 *Robot Kinematics*

The kinematics of the robot is presented very briefly here, as a more detailed description is given in [21]. The kinematic modelling of the parallel mechanism is parametrized by the three angles of rotation (θ_1, θ_2 and θ_3) about the three Z_i ($i = 1, 2, 3$) axes. Using the D-H (Denavit-Hartenberg) notations, the transformation of the coordinate systems can be written as a product of the following rotation (R) and translation (T) matrices

$$\mathbf{Q}_i = R(\alpha_{i-1})T(a_{i-1})R(\theta_i)T(d_i). \tag{1}$$

The D-H parameters are given in Table 1, where α_1, α_2, d_4 are constant design parameters and θ_1, θ_2, θ_3 are joint variables (α_i is angle between Z_i and Z_{i+1} axes measured about X_i, $i = 1, 2$, i.e., α_1 and α_2 are angles between joint axes of the RRR spherical linkage and are determined by the design of the links of this linkage; $d_4 = \|\mathbf{OO}_4\|$).

Then, the transformation matrix for the considered robot manipulator can be written as follows

$$\mathbf{Q} = \mathbf{Q}_1\mathbf{Q}_2\mathbf{Q}_3\mathbf{Q}_4. \tag{2}$$

For the forward position problem, the following constrained equations can be written :

$$L_i = \|\mathbf{OA}_i - \mathbf{OB}_i\|, \; i = 1, 2, \tag{3}$$

Table 1 D-H parameters

i	α_{i-1}	a_{i-1}	d_i	θ_i
1	$-\pi/2$	0	0	θ_1
2	α_1	0	0	θ_2
3	α_2	0	0	θ_3
4	0	0	d_4	0

where $\|...\|$ denotes the Euclidean norm; $\mathbf{OB}_i = \mathbf{Q} \cdot (\mathbf{O}_4\mathbf{B}_i)$; $\mathbf{O}_4\mathbf{B}_i$ is a vector given in the $O_4X_4Y_4Z_4$ coordinate system. The vectors $\mathbf{OA}_i$ and $\mathbf{O}_4\mathbf{B}_i$ are determined by the design of the manipulator.

The two leg lengths (L_1 and L_2) and the angle θ_2 are the given parameters for the forward problem of the parallel mechanism. Expanding Eq. 3, we get the following two equations for the unknown variables θ_1 and θ_3

$$p_{i1}c_1c_3 + p_{i2}c_1s_3 + p_{i3}s_1c_3 + p_{i4}s_1s_3 + p_{i5}c_1 + p_{i6}s_1 + p_{i7}c_3 + p_{i8}s_3 + p_{i9} = 0, \quad (4)$$

where $c_i = \cos\theta_i$, $s_i = \sin\theta_i$ (i = 1, 2); $p_{i1}, p_{i2}, \ldots, p_{i9}$ (i = 1, 2) are coefficients which are determined by the design and input parameters.

Applying tangent-half formulas in Eq. 4 and eliminating one of the two unknowns, an eight-order polynomial in one unknown is obtained [21].

3 Singularity Analysis of a General Parallel Robot with Limited Mobility Using Geometric Algebra

The geometric algebra approach for singularity analysis of parallel manipulators with limited mobility has been developed and presented by the author in two previous papers [20, 22]. A brief recollection of the approach is given here. Firstly, a very concise introduction to the geometric algebra is presented in this section, since extensive treatments can be found in [3, 4, 7].

3.1 Concise basics of the geometric algebra

Clifford algebra was created in the 19th century. In the second half of the 20th century this algebra has been rediscovered and further developed into a unified language named geometric algebra by Hestenes [7], Lasenby and Doran [3], Dorst, Fontijne and Mann [4], and some other authors. In geometric algebra, a single basic kind of multiplication called *geometric product* between two vectors is defined. The geometric product of two vectors **a** and **b** can be decomposed into symmetric and antisymmetric parts [7]. i.e.

$$\mathbf{ab} = \mathbf{a} \cdot \mathbf{b} + \mathbf{a} \wedge \mathbf{b}, \tag{5}$$

where $\mathbf{a} \cdot \mathbf{b}$ is the *inner product* and $\mathbf{a} \wedge \mathbf{b}$ is the *outer product* of the two vectors.

The inner product $\mathbf{a} \cdot \mathbf{b}$ is a scalar-valued (grade 0). The result of the other product $\mathbf{a} \wedge \mathbf{b}$ is an entity called *bivector* (grade 2). Higher-grade elements can be constructed by introducing more vectors. The outer product of k vectors $\mathbf{a}_1, \mathbf{a}_2, \ldots, \mathbf{a}_k$ generates a new entity $\mathbf{a}_1 \wedge \mathbf{a}_2 \wedge \ldots \wedge \mathbf{a}_k$ called a k blade. The integer k is named grade. The geometric algebra G_n contains nonzero blades of maximum grade n which are called pseudoscalars of G_n. The unit pseudoscalar of G_3 of 3-D Euclidean metric space with the standard orthonormal basis $\{\mathbf{e}_1, \mathbf{e}_2, \mathbf{e}_3\}$ could be written as

$$I_3 = \mathbf{e}_1 \wedge \mathbf{e}_2 \wedge \mathbf{e}_3 = \mathbf{e}_1\mathbf{e}_2\mathbf{e}_3. \tag{6}$$

The inverse of the unit pseudoscalar of G_3 is

$$I_3^{-1} = \mathbf{e}_3 \wedge \mathbf{e}_2 \wedge \mathbf{e}_1 = -\mathbf{e}_1 \wedge \mathbf{e}_2 \wedge \mathbf{e}_3. \tag{7}$$

The idea for a unit pseudoscalar and its inverse can be extended for an n-dimensional Euclidean metric space. The inverse of the unit pseudoscalar is used for obtaining the dual of a blade, which will be applied in the next sections.

An addition between elements of different grades results in an entity called a *multivector*. Inner and outer products are dual to one another and the following identities could be written [8]

$$(\mathbf{a} \cdot \mathbf{M})I_n = \mathbf{a} \wedge (\mathbf{M}I_n), \tag{8}$$

$$(\mathbf{a} \wedge \mathbf{M})I_n = \mathbf{a} \cdot (\mathbf{M}I_n), \tag{9}$$

where $\mathbf{a}$ is a vector; $\mathbf{M}$ is multivector and I_n is the unit pseudoscalar of n-dimensional space.

3.2 *Geometric Algebra Approach to Singularity of Parallel Manipulators with Limited Mobility*

We need to represent screws and joint screws in terms of the geometric algebra. Any oriented line $\mathbf{l}$ is uniquely determined by giving its direction $\mathbf{u}$ and its moment, thus, in the geometric algebra of 3-D vector space with the basis $\mathbf{e}_1, \mathbf{e}_2, \mathbf{e}_3$ it can be written as [7]

$$\mathbf{l} = \mathbf{u} + \mathbf{r} \wedge \mathbf{u}, \tag{10}$$

where $\mathbf{r} = r_x\mathbf{e}_1 + r_y\mathbf{e}_2 + r_z\mathbf{e}_3$ is the position vector of a point on the line; $\mathbf{u} = u_x\mathbf{e}_1 + u_y\mathbf{e}_2 + u_z\mathbf{e}_3$ is a vector along the line.

Thus, in the geometric algebra of the 3-D vector space G_3, a line is expressed as a multivector composed from a vector part plus a bivector. An extension of the equation of the line (Eq. (10)), i.e. adding the moment corresponding to the pitch, leads to the equation of a general screw:

$$\mathbf{s} = \mathbf{u} + \mathbf{r} \wedge \mathbf{u} + h\mathbf{u}I_3 \equiv v_1\mathbf{e}_1 + v_2\mathbf{e}_2 + v_3\mathbf{e}_3 + b_1\mathbf{e}_2 \wedge \mathbf{e}_3 + b_2\mathbf{e}_3 \wedge \mathbf{e}_1 + b_3\mathbf{e}_1 \wedge \mathbf{e}_2, \tag{11}$$

where $v_i(i = 1, 2, 3)$ and $b_i(i = 1, 2, 3)$ are scalar coefficients; $I_3 = \mathbf{e}_1\mathbf{e}_2\mathbf{e}_3$ is the unit pseudoscalar of G_3; h is the pitch of the screw.

The joint screw of a rotational joint is a line (screw with a zero pitch) and it is given by Eq. (10), while the joint screw of a prismatic joint can be written as follows

$$\mathbf{s} = \mathbf{w}I_3 \equiv w_1\mathbf{e}_2 \wedge \mathbf{e}_3 + w_2\mathbf{e}_3 \wedge \mathbf{e}_1 + w_3\mathbf{e}_1 \wedge \mathbf{e}_2, \tag{12}$$

where $\mathbf{w} = w_1\mathbf{e}_1 + w_2\mathbf{e}_2 + w_3\mathbf{e}_3$ is a unit vector along the translation direction of the prismatic joint.

In Eq. (11), the screw is expressed as a multivector in G_3. It could also be expressed as a vector in the geometric algebra G_6. In the geometric algebra of 6-D vector space with the basis $\mathbf{e}_1, \mathbf{e}_2, \mathbf{e}_3, \mathbf{e}_4, \mathbf{e}_5, \mathbf{e}_6$, a screw can be written as a vector (grade 1), i.e.,

$$\mathbf{S} = v_1\mathbf{e}_1 + v_2\mathbf{e}_2 + v_3\mathbf{e}_3 + b_1\mathbf{e}_4 + b_2\mathbf{e}_5 + b_3\mathbf{e}_6, \tag{13}$$

where the coefficients are the same as in Eq. (11).

In this paper, the screws written in G_3 and G_6 are distinguished by the following notations: a lower case letter (**s**, **l**) denotes a screw written as a multivector in G_3 of 3-D space; an upper case letter (**S**, **L**) denotes a screw written as a vector in G_6 of 6-D space; letters with a tilde mark ($\tilde{\mathbf{s}}, \tilde{\mathbf{S}}$) denote the elliptic polars of the screws (**s** and **S**), given in G_3 and G_6 , respectively.

The relationship between twists of freedom and the wrenches of constraint, as well as the duality in geometric algebra, are employed for the development of the geometric algebra approach to singularity analysis of parallel manipulators with limited mobility. The twists of non-freedom (wrenches of non-constraint) and wrenches of constraint (twists of freedom) are elliptic polars; twists of freedom (wrenches of constraint) and twists of non-freedom (wrenches of non-constraint) are orthogonal complements which together span a six space [12]. In terms of the geometric algebra, the operation of transformation of a screw (Eq. (11)) into an elliptic polar screw can be written as

$$\mathbf{s} = I_3\langle \mathbf{s}\rangle_1 + I_3^{-1}\langle \mathbf{s}\rangle_2 \equiv b_1\mathbf{e}_1 + b_2\mathbf{e}_2 + b_3\mathbf{e}_3 + v_1\mathbf{e}_2 \wedge \mathbf{e}_3 + v_2\mathbf{e}_3 \wedge \mathbf{e}_1 + v_3\mathbf{e}_1 \wedge \mathbf{e}_2, \tag{14}$$

where $\langle \mathbf{s}\rangle_k$ denotes the k-vector part of **s**; I_3^{-1} is the inverse of the unit pseudoscalar I_3 for the geometric algebra G_3.

In case of a parallel manipulator with fewer than six degrees of freedom, some legs may not possess full mobility. A leg with full mobility and a leg with less than six dof could be treated in a similar way. In that case, we suppose that the remaining degrees of freedom are represented by dummy joints (or driven but locked joints) and the associated with them dummy screws. Taking the outer product of five screws of the jth leg, written in G_6, gives the following 5-blade

$$^{j}\mathbf{A}_k = {}^{j}\mathbf{S}_1 \wedge {}^{j}\mathbf{S}_2 \wedge \ldots \wedge {}^{j}\mathbf{S}_{k-1} \wedge {}^{j}\mathbf{S}_{k+1} \wedge \ldots \wedge {}^{j}\mathbf{S}_6, \tag{15}$$

where the subscript k denotes the active joint of the jth leg.

The 5-blade from Eq. (15) involves five screws (out of six with the exception of the $^{j}\mathbf{S}_k$ screw). The kth joint is active. In a non-degenerate space, the dual of a blade represents the orthogonal complement of the subspace represented by the blade. The dual of the above 5-blade $^{j}\mathbf{A}_k$ is given by the following formula

$$^{j}\mathbf{D}_k = {}^{j}\mathbf{A}_k I_6^{-1}, \tag{16}$$

where $I_6 = \mathbf{e}_1\mathbf{e}_2\mathbf{e}_3\mathbf{e}_4 e_5\mathbf{e}_6$ is the unit pseudoscalar of the G_6 and I_6^{-1} is its inverse.

Suppose that the parallel manipulator has n legs and m ($m = 6 - q$) degrees of freedom. We assume that the remaining q degrees of freedom are represented by dummy joints (or driven but locked joints) and the associated with them dummy screws. Thus, in non-singular configuration the driven joints and the geometry (or the dummy joints) of the manipulator sustain a general wrench applied to the moving platform. Therefore, the singular configuration can occur when all dual $^{j}\mathbf{D}_k$ or reciprocal $^{j}\mathbf{R}_k$ ($^{j}\mathbf{R}_k = {}^{j}\tilde{\mathbf{D}}_k$) screws, representing active and dummy joints, are linearly dependent. Using the language of the geometric algebra, the condition of singularity for the parallel manipulator with less than six degrees of freedom (but with dummy joints) can be expressed as

$$\mathbf{D}_{a_1} \wedge \ldots \wedge \mathbf{D}_{a_k} \wedge \mathbf{D}_{d_1} \wedge \ldots \wedge \mathbf{D}_{d_r} = 0, \tag{17}$$

where $k + r = 6$; k is the number of the active joints and r is the number of the dummy joints; $\mathbf{D}_{a_i}$ is a dual vector (grade 1-blade) associated to the ith active joint and $\mathbf{D}_{d_i}$ is a dual vector (grade 1-blade) associated to the ith dummy joint.

Equation (17) involves dummy screws, and therefore, they need to be eliminated. Applying some identities of the geometric algebra [8] and manipulating certain blades from Eq. (17) the dummy screws could be eliminated. Thus, the new equation resulting from Eq. (17) after elimination of the dummy screws will contain only passive joint screws, which was shown in [20, 22]. This process of elimination is explained in more details in the next section.

The effectiveness and advantages of the proposed approach for singularity analysis are summarized next. The approach allows manipulating the components of the equation for singularity in a basis-free manner and thus, establishing and interpreting the singular configurations. This property of the approach could be considered an advantage over the screw Jacobian approach, for example. This advantage is especially useful for parallel manipulators with limited mobility, which is shown in the next section. Although the proposed method utilizes the idea of dummy joints in case of parallel manipulators with limited mobility, there is no need to use a particular dummy joint since the dummy screws are represented only by the space of non-freedom. In addition, the approach can establish the singularities for parallel manipulators with both full and limited mobility as well as distinguish different types of singularities such as constraint ones. A further benefit which arises from the established geometrical condition for singularity is that the algebraic formulation can be obtained from the geometrical condition. This algebraic equation is equivalent to the determinant of the 6×6 screw Jacobian of the manipulator.

4 Singularity Analysis of the Minimally-Invasive-Surgery Parallel Manipulator

In this section, the singularity analysis of the novel robot for minimally invasive surgery is presented. Here, the parallel manipulator, which is the essential part of the robot, is the main subject of the analysis.

4.1 Geometric Condition for Singularity

The two SPU legs (leg 1 and leg 2) of the parallel manipulator have full mobility and therefore, have only dual vectors $\mathbf{D}_1$ and $\mathbf{D}_2$, respectively, associated with the active joints. The third (RRR) leg has one dual vector ($\mathbf{D}_3$) associated with the active joint (middle R joint) and three dual vectors ($\mathbf{D}_4$, $\mathbf{D}_5$ and $\mathbf{D}_6$) associated with the three dummy joints. The dual vectors for the two SPU legs can be written as follows

$$\mathbf{D}_j \equiv^j \mathbf{D}_k = ({}^j\mathbf{S}_1 \wedge^j \mathbf{S}_2 \wedge^j \mathbf{S}_3 \wedge^j \mathbf{S}_5 \wedge^j \mathbf{S}_6) I_6^{-1},\ (j = 1, 2), \tag{18}$$

where the fourth P (prismatic) joint is active and is not included in the formula.

These dual vectors $\mathbf{D}_1$ and $\mathbf{D}_2$ are lines (zero pitch screws) and their elliptic polars $\mathbf{R}_1$ ($\mathbf{R}_1 = \tilde{\mathbf{D}}_1$) and $\mathbf{R}_2$ ($\mathbf{R}_2 = \tilde{\mathbf{D}}_2$) are lines along the SPU legs, respectively.

The dual vectors (one vector associated with the middle R joint and three vectors associated with the dummy joints) for the third RRR leg are as follows

$$\mathbf{D}_3 \equiv^3 \mathbf{D}_a = ({}^3\mathbf{S}_1 \wedge^3 \mathbf{S}_3 \wedge^3 \mathbf{S}_{d_1} \wedge^3 \mathbf{S}_{d_2} \wedge^3 \mathbf{S}_{d_3}) I_6^{-1}, \tag{19}$$

$$\mathbf{D}_4 \equiv^3 \mathbf{D}_{d_1} = ({}^3\mathbf{S}_1 \wedge^3 \mathbf{S}_2 \wedge^3 \mathbf{S}_3 \wedge^3 \mathbf{S}_{d_2} \wedge^3 \mathbf{S}_{d_3}) I_6^{-1}, \tag{20}$$

$$\mathbf{D}_5 \equiv^3 \mathbf{D}_{d_2} = ({}^3\mathbf{S}_1 \wedge^3 \mathbf{S}_2 \wedge^3 \mathbf{S}_3 \wedge^3 \mathbf{S}_{d_1} \wedge^3 \mathbf{S}_{d_3}) I_6^{-1}, \tag{21}$$

$$\mathbf{D}_6 \equiv^3 \mathbf{D}_{d_3} = (^3\mathbf{S}_1 \wedge^3 \mathbf{S}_2 \wedge^3 \mathbf{S}_3 \wedge^3 \mathbf{S}_{d_1} \wedge^3 \mathbf{S}_{d_2})I_6^{-1}, \tag{22}$$

where $^3\mathbf{S}_i$, $(i = 1, 2, 3)$ are joint screws of the R-joints ($^3\mathbf{S}_1$ is a joint screw of the R-joint attached to the base platform, while $^3\mathbf{S}_3$ is a joint screw of the R-joint attached to the moving platform) and $^3\mathbf{S}_{d_i}$, $(i = 1, 2, 3)$ are screws of the dummy joints.

The condition for singularity (Eq. (17)) becomes

$$\mathbf{D}_1 \wedge \mathbf{D}_2 \wedge \mathbf{D}_3 \wedge \mathbf{D}_4 \wedge \mathbf{D}_5 \wedge \mathbf{D}_6 = 0. \tag{23}$$

The process of the elimination of the dummy vectors is explained below, where some identities (Eqs. (8) and (9)) of the geometric algebra are used. Let us consider the blade composed by the two dual vectors $\mathbf{D}_3$ and $\mathbf{D}_4$

$$\begin{aligned} \mathbf{D}_3 \wedge \mathbf{D}_4 = -\mathbf{D}_4 \wedge \mathbf{D}_3 &= -\mathbf{D}_4 \wedge [(^3\mathbf{S}_1 \wedge^3 \mathbf{S}_3 \wedge^3 \mathbf{S}_{d_1} \wedge^3 \mathbf{S}_{d_2} \wedge^3 \mathbf{S}_{d_3})I_6^{-1}] \\ &= -[\mathbf{D}_4 \cdot (^3\mathbf{S}_1 \wedge^3 \mathbf{S}_3 \wedge^3 \mathbf{S}_{d_1} \wedge^3 \mathbf{S}_{d_2} \wedge^3 \mathbf{S}_{d_3})]I_6^{-1} \\ &= -(\mathbf{D}_4 \cdot^3 \mathbf{S}_{d_1})(^3\mathbf{S}_1 \wedge^3 \mathbf{S}_3 \wedge^3 \mathbf{S}_{d_2} \wedge^3 \mathbf{S}_{d_3})I_6^{-1} \\ &= -c_1(^3\mathbf{S}_1 \wedge^3 \mathbf{S}_3 \wedge^3 \mathbf{S}_{d_2} \wedge^3 \mathbf{S}_{d_3})I_6^{-1} \end{aligned} \tag{24}$$

where $c_1 = \mathbf{D}_4 \cdot^3 \mathbf{S}_{d_1} \equiv^3 \mathbf{D}_{d_1} \cdot^3 \mathbf{S}_{d_1} \neq 0$ is a scalar, while referring to Eq. (20) it can be seen that the following inner products are zero: $\mathbf{D}_4 \cdot^3 \mathbf{S}_i = 0, (i = 1, 2, 3)$ and $\mathbf{D}_4 \cdot^3 \mathbf{S}_{d_i} = 0, (i = 2, 3)$.

Similarly, the above elimination procedure can be applied for the remaining outer products involving dummy vectors and the final result can be written as the following 4-blade

$$\mathbf{D}_3 \wedge \mathbf{D}_4 \wedge \mathbf{D}_5 \wedge \mathbf{D}_6 = -c_1c_2c_3(^3\mathbf{S}_1 \wedge^3 \mathbf{S}_3)I_6^{-1}, \tag{25}$$

where $c_1 =^3 \mathbf{D}_{d_1} \cdot^3 \mathbf{S}_{d_1}$, $c_2 =^3 \mathbf{D}_{d_2} \cdot^3 \mathbf{S}_{d_2}$, $c_3 =^3 \mathbf{D}_{d_3} \cdot^3 \mathbf{S}_{d_3}$; $c_i (i = 1, 2, 3)$ are scalars.

Thus, the condition for the singularity (Eq. (23)) becomes

$$\mathbf{D}_1 \wedge \mathbf{D}_2 \wedge (^3\mathbf{S}_1 \wedge^3 \mathbf{S}_3)I_6^{-1} = 0. \tag{26}$$

Keeping in mind Eq. (18), it could be seen that only passive joint screws are involved in the components of Eq. (26) and besides that all of the passive joint screws. Applying the identities of the geometric algebra, Eq. (26) further becomes

$$\mathbf{D}_1 \wedge [\mathbf{D}_2 \cdot (^3\mathbf{S}_1 \wedge^3 \mathbf{S}_3)]I_6^{-1} = \mathbf{D}_1 \wedge (\mathbf{V}I_6^{-1}) = (\mathbf{D}_1 \cdot \mathbf{V})I_6^{-1} = 0. \tag{27}$$

The inner product between a vector and a bivector (Eq. (27)) produces the vector $\mathbf{V} = \mathbf{D}_2 \cdot (^3\mathbf{S}_1 \wedge^3 \mathbf{S}_3)$. Therefore, $\mathbf{V}$ is perpendicular to $\mathbf{D}_2$ in 6-D space and $\mathbf{V}$ belongs to the bivector space $^3\mathbf{S}_1 \wedge^3 \mathbf{S}_3$. Since the screws $^3\mathbf{S}_1$ and $^3\mathbf{S}_3$ are lines passing through the origin of the coordinate system, i.e., the secondary parts of these screws are zero, therefore the vector $\mathbf{V}$ represents a line passing through the origin, too (Fig. 3). Thus, the line $\mathbf{V}$ lies in the plane defined by the lines $^3\mathbf{S}_1$ and $^3\mathbf{S}_3$.

The fact that the vectors $\mathbf{V}$ and $\mathbf{D}_2$ are mutually perpendicular in 6-D space implies that the elliptic polar $\mathbf{R}_2$ (line) of the screw $\mathbf{D}_2$ ($\mathbf{R}_2 = \tilde{\mathbf{D}}_2$) and the line $\mathbf{V}$ should intersect at a common point, i.e., the screws $\mathbf{V}$ and $\mathbf{R}_2$ are reciprocal (Fig. 3). From Eq. (27) it can be concluded that the manipulator is in singular configuration when the inner product of vectors $\mathbf{D}_1$ and $\mathbf{V}$ is zero ($\mathbf{D}_1 \cdot \mathbf{V} = 0$). This means that the elliptic polar $\mathbf{R}_1$ (line) of the screw $\mathbf{D}_1$ ($\mathbf{R}_1 = \tilde{\mathbf{D}}_1$) and the line $\mathbf{V}$ should intersect, i.e., the screws $\mathbf{V}$ and $\mathbf{R}_1$ are reciprocal (Fig. 3). Thus, the geometric condition for singularity could be stated as: the considered parallel manipulator is in singular configuration if the vector (line) $\mathbf{V}$ intersects both lines ($\mathbf{R}_1$ and $\mathbf{R}_2$) which are along the SPU legs, respectively. This condition could be restated as: the parallel manipulator is in singular configuration if the intersection points of the two lines along the SPU legs with the plane, defined by the axes of the first and the third revolute joints, and the pivoting point (the intersection point of axes of the three R-joints) lie in a single line (Fig. 4). The uncontrollable motion in this singular configuration is a pure rotation about the line $\mathbf{V}$ (Figs. 3 and 4). The intersection at infinity is included, too. For example, in a special case (a special geometry of the robot) the tree lines $\mathbf{R}_1$, $\mathbf{R}_2$ and $\mathbf{V}$ could be parallel and in this case they intersect at infinity.

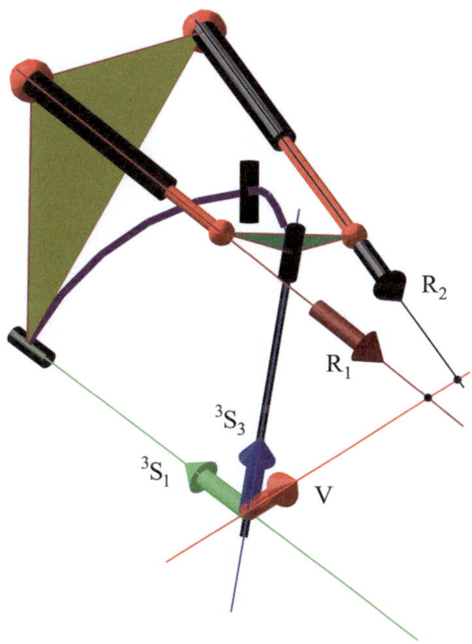

Fig. 3 A singular configuration of the robot

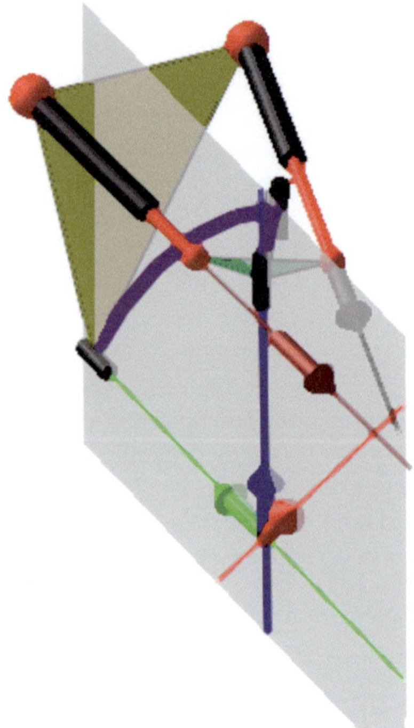

Fig. 4 A singular configuration of the robot and the plane defined by two joint axes ${}^3\mathbf{S}_1$ and ${}^3\mathbf{S}_3$

4.2 Singularity Surface

Algebraic formulation of the singular condition can be obtained from Eq. (26), i.e.,

$$B = [\mathbf{D}_1 \wedge \mathbf{D}_2 \wedge ({}^3\mathbf{S}_1 \wedge^3 \mathbf{S}_3)I_6^{-1}]I_6 = 0, \tag{28}$$

where B is a scalar-valued (grade 0) function of design and input parameters and it is parametrized by the three angles of rotation (θ_1, θ_2 and θ_3).

The singularity surface obtained from B (Eq. (28)) and the workspace of the manipulator are shown in Fig. 5 in terms of the three joint angles θ_1, θ_2 and θ_3.

The singularity surface and workspace are obtained for the following design parameters:
$\mathbf{OA}_1 = (-0.20, 0.52, 0.56)^T$; $\mathbf{OA}_2 = (0.20, 0.52, 0.56)^T$; $\mathbf{OA}_3 = (0, 0.52, 0)^T$; $\mathbf{O}_4\mathbf{B}_1 = (-0.1075, 0.05, 0)^T$; $\mathbf{O}_4\mathbf{B}_2 = (0.1075, 0.05, 0)^T$; $\mathbf{O}_4\mathbf{B}_3 = (0, 0, 0)^T$; $\alpha_1 = 55^{\circ}$; $\alpha_2 = 43^{\circ}$; $d_4 = 0.52$ m. Also, the following constraints on the motion are imposed in the workspace derivation: $L_{min} = 0.30$ m; $L_{max} = 0.58$ m (minimum and maximum lengths of the SPU limbs); minimum angle between each SPU limb and the plane of the base platform = 30°. A section of the singularity surface and workspace are shown in Fig. 6 for the angle $\theta_3 = 0$. The singularity point given in this figure corresponds to the robot configuration from Figs. 3 and 4. A more detailed analysis of the workspace of this robot is presented in [21].

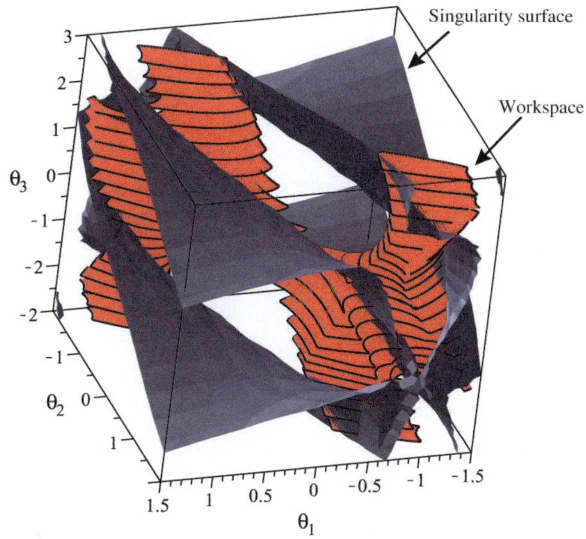

Fig. 5 The singularity surface and workspace boundary of the robot

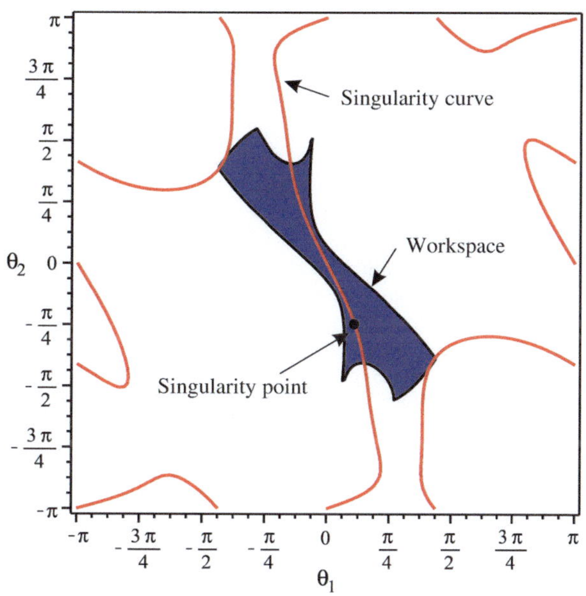

Fig. 6 The singularity curve and workspace boundary of the robot for $\theta_3 = 0$

5 Conclusions

The geometric algebra approach proves its ability of providing a good geometrical insight into the singularities of parallel manipulators with limited mobility as in the case of the proposed novel parallel manipulator for minimally invasive surgery. Using this approach, the geometrical condition for singular configuration of the proposed robot is obtained in a basis-free form. The obtained geometric condition for singularities allows to derive the algebraic formulation and to present the singularity surface in terms of three angles. The results, obtained in this paper, are essential for the robot path planning, where the singular configurations for the proposed novel type of minimally-invasive-surgery parallel robot should be avoided. This is especially important for the medical parallel manipulators from the point of view of the successful surgical outcome and the patient's safety. It could be concluded from the presented graphical results that adding a new degree of freedom (the fifth one), namely a redundant rotation around the surgical instrument (end-effector), will result in a more dexterous hybrid manipulator which will be able to easily avoid the singular configurations. This additional rotation would be a redundant one and could be realized by a modification either of the robot or the surgical instrument.

References

1. Ben-Horin, P., Shoham, M.: Singularity of a class of Gough-Stewart platforms with concurrent joints. In: Lenarčič, J., Roth, B. (eds.) Advances in Robot Kinematics, pp. 265–274. Springer, The Netherlands (2006)
2. Dalvand, M.M., Shirinzadeh, B.: Remote Centre-of-Motion control algorithms of 6-RRCRR parallel robot assisted surgery system (PRAMiSS). In: IEEE International Conference on Robotics and Automation (ICRA), pp. 3401–3406. Saint Paul, Minnesota, USA, 14–18 May 2012
3. Doran, C., Lasenby, A.: Geometric Algebra for Physicists. Cambridge University Press (2007)
4. Dorst, L., Fontijne, D., Mann, S.: Geometric Algebra for Computer Science, An Object Oriented Approach to Geometry. Morgan Kaufmann Publishers (2007)
5. Guthart, G., Salisbury, J.K.: The Intuitive telesurgery system: overview and applications. In: IEEE International Conference on Robotics and Automation, pp. 618–621 (2000)
6. Hao, F., McCarthy, J.: Conditions for line-based singularities in spatial platform manipulators. J. Robot. Syst. **15**(1), 43–55 (1998)
7. Hestenes, D.: New Foundations for Classical Mechanics, 2nd edn. Kluwer Academic Publishers, Dordrecht (1999)
8. Hestenes, D., Li, H., Rockwood, A.: New algebraic tools for classical geometry. In: Sommer, G. (ed.) Geometric Computing with Clifford Algebra. Springer, Berlin (1999)
9. Kanaan, D., Wenger, P., Chablat, D.: Singularity analysis of limited-DOF parallel manipulators using Grassmann-Cayley algebra. In: Lenarčič, J., Wenger, P. (eds.) Advances in Robot Kinematics, Analysis and Design, pp. 59–68. Springer (2008)
10. Khan, M.A., Zoppi, M., Molfino, R.: 4-DOF parallel architecture for laparoscopic surgery. In: Lenarčič, J., Wenger, P. (eds.) Advances in Robot Kinematics: Analysis and Design, pp. 119–126. Springer (2008)
11. Kuo, C-H., Dai, J.S.: Robotics for minimally invasive surgery: a historical review from the perspective of kinematics. In: International Symposium on History of Machines, pp. 337–354. Springer Science+Business Media B.V. (2009)

12. Lipkin, H., Duffy, J.: The elliptic polarity of screws. ASME J. Mech. Transm. Autom. Des. **107**, 377–387 (1985)
13. Li, T., Payandeh, S.: Design of spherical parallel mechanisms for application to laparoscopic surgery. Robotica **20**, 133–138 (2002)
14. Liu, G., Lou, Y., Li, Z.: Singularities of parallel manipulators: a geometric treatment. Trans. Robot. Automat **19**(4), 579–594 (2003)
15. Lum, M.J.H., et al.: Kinematic optimization of a spherical mechanism for a minimally invasive surgical robot. In: Proceedings of IEEE International Conference on Robotics and Automation, New Orleans, La, May 2004
16. Merlet, J.-P.: Singular configurations of parallel manipulators and Grassmann geometry. Int. J. Robot. Res. **8**(5), 45–56 (1989)
17. Pisla, D., et al.: Kinematic modelling of a 5-DOF hybrid parallel robot for laparoscopic surgery. Robotica **30**(07), 1095–1107 (2012)
18. Rosen, J., et al.: The BlueDRAGON—a system for measuring the kinematics and the dynamics of minimally invasive surgical tools in-vivo. In: Proceedings of IEEE International Conference on Robotics and Automation, Washington, USA, pp. 1876–1881 (2002)
19. Sima'an, N., Glozman, D., Shoham, M.: Design considerations of new six degrees-of-freedom parallel robots. In: Proceedings of IEEE International Conference on Robotics and Automation, pp. 327–1333. Leuven, Belgium (1998)
20. Tanev, T.K.: Geometric algebra approach to singularity of parallel manipulators with limited mobility. In: Lenarčič, J., Wenger, P. (eds.) Advances in Robot Kinematics, Analysis and Design. Springer (2008)
21. Tanev, T.K.: Minimally-invasive-surgery parallel robot with non-identical limbs. In: Proceedings of 10th IEEE/ASME International Conference on Mechatronic and Embedded Systems and Applications, (MESA2014), Senigallia, Italy, 10–12 Sept 2014. doi:10.1109/MESA.2014.6935558
22. Tanev, T.K.: Singularity analysis of a 4-dof parallel manipulator using geometric algebra. In: Lenarčič, J., Roth, B. (eds.) Advances in Robot Kinematics, Mechanism and Motion, pp. 275–284. Springer (2006)
23. Taylor, R.H., Stoianovici, D.: Medical robotics in computer-integrated surgery. IEEE Trans. Robot. Autom. **19**(5), 765–781 (2003)
24. Zemiti, N., et al.: Mechatronic design of a new robot for force control in minimally invasive surgery. IEEE/ASME Trans. Mechatron. **12**(2), 143–153 (2007)
25. Zlatanov, D., Bonev, I.A., Cosselin, C.M.: Constraint singularities of parallel mechanisms. In: Proceedings of IEEE International Conference on Robotics and Automation, vol. 1, pp. 496–502. Washington, DC (2002)

ISO 13482:2014 and Its Confusing Categories. Building a Bridge Between Law and Robotics

Eduard Fosch Villaronga

Abstract Because of the fast technological development of the past few years, understandable bridges between the technical and the legal domains are urgently needed. In this respect, this paper pioneers the identification and examination of confusing categories among ISO 13482:2014 'Robots and Robotics Devices—Safety Requirements for Personal Care Robots'. It aims to make roboticists aware of the importance of clearer definitions for legal compliance purposes: although clarity may be missing in the legal domain, robot creators are still legally liable for their creations. The choice of the robot category is also controversial: a robot should be assigned to a category if it does not fully fit in it, as this may even lead to an abuse of the Law. A precise categorization is necessary and based on the robot category specific regulations and laws should be taken into consideration and respected.

Keywords Personal care robot · Legal compliance · Confusing categories · Robotics · Law

1 Introduction

Precise terminology has always been important [1–3], even if 'definition is not a final outcome but a single step in a long process of understanding' [4]. Terminology is still the main reference we have to acknowledge and define concepts, ideas or notions. This is a key element when we try to use the same definitions (in our case 'personal care robots') in different fields (the legal and technological fields) because those definitions will lead us to know the 'exact statement or description of the nature, scope or meaning of *[that]* thing' [5]. Moreover, by only knowing the

E. Fosch Villaronga (✉)
University of Bologna, Bologna, Italy
e-mail: eduard.fosch@unibo.it; tot_nira_be@hotmail.com

E. Fosch Villaronga
IDT-UAB, Universitat Autònoma de Barcelona, Barcelona, Spain

P. Wenger et al. (eds.), *New Trends in Medical and Service Robots*,
Mechanisms and Machine Science 39, DOI 10.1007/978-3-319-30674-2_3

accurate description of that thing we will be able to carefully discern what regulation applies to it.

Of note, personal care robots are only formally regulated by standards, and ISOs are the only instruments dealing with this kind of robots. However, this does not mean that they are exempt from legal or other compliances. In reality, four are the constraints that by default regulate any thing: their architecture, social norms, the market and, in any case, the Law [6].

First, the architecture of personal care robots needs to follow not only this specific technical standards but also other standards related to other sub-fields, like acoustical engineering, automotive engineering, artificial intelligence, computational linguistics, mechatronics engineering, machine learning, safety engineering, software engineering, telecommunications, and so on. Second, depending on their aim and purpose, robots should follow particular social norms. That would mean the creators of the robot will have to come to terms with cognitive science, behavioural science, philosophy, ethics, sociology, physics (dynamics, kinematics), education, empathy, etc. Third, only marketable robots are introduced in nursing homes, medical care facilities or the dwellings of disabled people. Consequently, the robot will have to comply with the laws governing the market. Fourth, personal care robots need to be compliant with the existing legal framework. Indeed, even if a precise definition in the legal domain is lacking, personal care robots need to follow some pre-established rules (and sometimes using the Dworkinian way of reasoning/interpreting [7]).

In the present case, ISO 13482:2014 'Robots and Robotics Devices—Safety Requirements for Personal Care Robots' is the only instrument to provide a definition of personal care robots up to now. According to it, personal care robots are 'service robots that perform actions contributing directly towards improvement in the quality of life of humans, excluding medical applications' [8]. After setting that it 'might include physical contact with the human to perform the task' this ISO also provides some typical examples of personal care robots, including: mobile servant robots, physical assistant robots and person carrier robots.

From a legal perspective, this definition is not really accurate. This is very important because ISOs are considered to be *soft law* instruments, that is, 'normative provisions contained in non-binding texts' [9]. Indeed, *improvement in the quality of life of humans* is rather vague and more precise definitions are needed. This is what we call an 'undefined legal concept': not only the word 'improvement' pictures a blurred reality (it is not clear exactly when we can really talk of improvement, if that improvement is general for everyone, etc.) but also 'quality of life' is quite unclear (it depends on several factors such as cultural, age, or gender differences, and different interpretations of *quality of life* could be given).

Vagueness in technical definitions leads us to misunderstand in legal terms what kind of thing we are dealing with, and under what regulation this thing should fall. This could lead the way to unforeseeable scenarios where one could be compliant with wrong instruments and, for that reason, expose themselves to sanctions and further responsibilities due to lack of diligence.

Thus, roboticists and standard bodies need to be acquainted with the importance of defining the type of robot they are creating concretely and unequivocally. To do this, not only the characteristics of the robot will be important, but also how the end users will use it. For instance, if an exoskeleton was born to be a physical assistant robot, personal care robot ISO will apply; however, if the same exoskeleton is used for rehabilitation purposes, then the applying ISO would be the one regarding medical devices because rehabilitation falls under that specific ISO (and also the European directive 93/42/EEC on medical devices, or Directive 90/385/EEC on active implantable medical devices).

In ISO 13482:2014 some confusing categories can be found and they are worth analyzing. First an overview of the state of the art of the 'personal care' level in personal care robots will be provided; after that, confusion issues regarding the subcategories of personal care robots will be addressed. These categories are: mobile servant robot, physical assistant robot and person carrier robot.

2 A Brief Overview of the Level of 'Personal Care' in Personal Care Robots

The international standard ISO 13482:2014 was born to specify 'requirements and guidelines for the inherently safe design, protective measures, and information for use of personal care robots' [8]. In it, this kind of robots is defined as: 'service robot that performs actions contributing directly towards improvement in the quality of life of humans, excluding medical applications'. Such a definition however is rather vague, as it leaves some uncertainty regarding exactly what robots we are dealing with.

The negative taxonomy given by the ISO could be of help, as this standard clearly states what remains outside of it. For instance, robotic devices will be covered by this ISO if used in personal care applications, while other applications will be excluded. ISO 13482:2014 also establishes that it 'is limited to earthbound robots'. In more details, it precisely establishes that:

This International Standard does not apply to:

- robots travelling faster than 20 km/h;
- robot toys;
- water-borne robots and flying robots;
- industrial robots, which are covered in ISO 10218;
- robots as medical devices;
- military or public force application robots.

Firstly, and very importantly, as already mentioned in the personal care robot definition, this ISO covers robotic devices used in personal care applications. Indeed, those devices used in other applications, e.g. rehabilitation, should fall outside this regulation. Yet, reality will tell us that this is not as simple as it seems (see infra).

Secondly, neither the definition of personal care robot nor the negative taxonomy actually explain what 'personal care' is. Collins dictionary defines it as the 'help given to elderly or infirm people with essential everyday activities such as washing, dressing and meals'. Elderly Accommodation Counsel of the UK (EAC) sustains that it is the 'assistance with dressing, feeding, washing and toileting, as well as advice, encouragement and emotional and psychological support' [10]. EAC adds that 'the Department of Work and Pensions of the UK (DWP) defines this as attention required in connection with bodily functions. Bodily functions can include dressing, washing, bathing or shaving, toileting, getting in or out of bed, eating, drinking, taking medication, [*and*] communicating. Seeing and hearing are also considered to be bodily functions'.

The definition of *personal care* is somehow related with the Instrumental Activities of Daily Living [11], something that seems to have nothing to do with medical activities. Robots described as personal care robots (mobile servant robot, physical assistant robot and person carrier robot), though, do not still comply with all these functions, and this is a major issue. Actually, the state of the art is a bit behind this definition. For instance, mobile servant robot is defined as a robot that handles objects and exchange information, but nothing is said regarding other uses like helping users with dressing or feeding. Another example is Resyone of Panasonic, the first robot that obtained the ISO 13482:2014 certification. This is a robotic bed that transforms into a reclining wheelchair. It is true that it can help patients to get in or out of bed, and that is considered part of personal care, but it still does not perform any of the main actions within the range of 'personal care' activities. For more information on Resyone, see below in Sect. 3.3.

3 Confusion Within the Categories Identified by ISO 13482:2014

In theory, the usage of a robot should not determine the regulation under which it falls. On the contrary, a robot should be compliant by its inner and default capacities, not by its use; otherwise legal compliance could be at risk. Indeed, a robot may have some default capacities (communication capabilities, a data collection system, autonomous behavior, etc.) that could in fact cause different problems in legal terms, independently of how the robot is used and of the ISO certifications it may have obtained. Roboticists should thus be particularly careful: for instance, if a robot is not used as a medical device, that does not consequently mean that its by-default capacities do not need to comply with the current laws.

From a legal perspective, if a robot does not involve any new scenario and the existing laws already address every legal aspect associated with that robot, then there will be no need to create new laws. Indeed, if a personal care robot has some characteristics that are already well described and regulated in the ISO for medical devices and personal care robots, it will not be necessary to require additional or other legal compliances. Actually, it would be easier if some basic regulatory models for the by-default capacities existed; and then some regulatory complements were added depending on the specific situations and the new capacities involved. Unfortunately, such models do not exist yet.

In fact, robot regulatory definitions are missing. In some cases, some regulations are available (for instance regarding data collection), yet they are scattered throughout the legal(s) system(s); and that seriously hinders legal compliance for roboticists. Definitions embracing real cases are needed to give response and fill this gap; this way we could have compliant robots no matter what use we assign to them.

By analyzing the reality and the categories enshrined in ISO 13482:2014, some major other problems can also be identified, as detailed in Table 1.

In the following sub-sections, we will present the characteristics that identify each of the robot categories according to the ISO (namely, their main characterizing features) and then we will highlight some confusions we encountered during our investigations.

These confusions normally tend to be between the in-scope and the out-scope robots of the ISO 13482:2014 (such as the use of some robot toys as person carrier robots); sometimes confusion can arise regarding a concrete sub-category of personal care (physical assistant robots used in warfare environments), other times it is just with the general category of personal care robots (if a surveiling drone in a hospital could be considered a personal care robot); and sometimes there are other existing robots that, given their functionalities, could be included somehow as part of personal care robots (like the seal robot used with Alzheimer patients).

3.1 Person Carrier Robots

Person carrier robots are defined by ISO 13482:2014 as 'personal care robot [*s*] with the purpose of transporting humans to an intended destination'. In other words, these robots are meant to convey persons from one place to another one. The restrictions made by the ISO are: robots traveling faster than 20 km/h and robot toys are expressly excluded in its scope. In the following sub-sections we will show that sometimes reality goes beyond some existing categories (e.g. a robot toy car used as a person carrier robot).

Table 1 ISO 13482:2014 Confusing categories

Robot	*Confusion*
Robot toy car	Person carrier robot
Exoskeleton	Medical device/military robots
Therapeutic robot	Personal care robot
Resyone	Person carrier robot
Drone surveiling	Personal care robot
Segway, –20 km/h	Personal care robot

3.1.1 Robot Car Toys and Person Carrier Robots

There are so many different kinds of robot toys for children: educational robots [12, 13], robot pets [14, 15], etc. Their purposes are many depending on the goal they are designed for. Surely, they are expressly excluded by ISO. It seems they do not meet the personal-care target mentioned in this International Standard. The famous Pleo (a cute four-life-stage dinosaur robot toy that you can feed, play with, teach) is a clear example for this, because, unfortunately, its functions do not include taking care of any user.

Reality shows that there are several robot toys that help children with disabilities, a targeted group within personal care robots. This is the case of electric-powered child-sized toy cars that offer mobility to children with disabilities [16]. As explained by Galloway [17], wheelchairs are reserved for children over 3 years old and new robotic devices to help disabled children's mobility cost tens of thousands of euros (and they are very heavy). To cope with such limitations, he founded the project 'Go Baby Go' in order to take already commercialized car toys and to transform and adapt them for children with cerebral palsy or Down syndrome to move.

These robots are not simply toys; they are robots, whose goal is to improve the reduced mobility capabilities of children. They could be considered part of ISO 13482:2014 under the category of person carrier robots. The question here is: could car toys be understood like person carrier robots as described in the ISO when they are modified to fulfill the needs of a disabled child? Or, on the contrary, the exclusion of robot toys from the ISO scope makes the ISO itself not applicable to them? And consequently, what soft-law could regulate those robots? Could they be not compliant with the law?

3.1.2 The Case of Segways and the Extension of Legal Compliance in Outdoor Spaces

Toth argues that there are two sub-types of person carriers within the person carrier robots category: indoor person carriers and outdoor person carriers [18]. According to him and to ISO 13482:2014 categories [8], inside this sub-types there are other sub-categories:

(a) Indoor Person Carriers:

   a. A carrier-with-passenger-standing-on-the-foothold is a robot that transports people throughout domestic properties at very slow speeds, appropriate to moving about the house; and
   b. A carrier-whose-passenger-sits-on-a-monocycle, is for large indoor public spaces such as airport terminals or large exhibition centers, or shopping malls, which may be used for transporting persons at quite slow speeds.

(b) Outdoor Person Carriers:

   a. A wheeled-passenger-carrier used at speeds, could be up to the equivalent of slow cycling pace; and
   b. A legged-passenger-carrier for transporting persons off-road and in non-urban (rural/semi-rural) locations at a speed of a walker.

It is worthwhile noticing that there are more and more there are segways in the market, which may fall under the first category (indoor person carriers) but they are used in fact in outdoor contexts and by non-disabled people. Should segways be regulated for personal care robots ISO then? Don't they contribute *towards improvement on the quality of life of humans* and shouldn't they be considered as medical applications? If not, what regulation should apply to them?

The extension of legal compliance for outdoor spaces is another fundamental point. Depending on the ownership of the person carrier robot, the responsible should be aware of the possibility of the outdoor use of this type of robot. Therefore, when considering a wheelchair that belongs to a hospital but it is used for patients to go in and outside it, the responsibilities of the patient and of the hospital, respectively should be clearly specified and distinguished. This will be a bit more complicated with brain-controlled wheelchairs [19].

3.2 Physical Assistant Robots

Physical assistant robots are defined in ISO 13482:2014 as: 'personal care robot [*s*] that physically assists a user to perform required tasks by providing supplementation or augmentation of personal capabilities'.

User is understood by ISO as *either the operator of the personal care robot or the beneficiary of the service provided by the personal care robot* [8]. Therefore, these robots do not strictly interact with humans (because they do not talk to them nor, for instance, do they serve them a cup of tea), but they are directly laced to them. In fact, and according to ISO 13482:2014, this entwinement within this sub-type of personal care robot creates two new sub-categories: restraint and restraint-free types of physical assistant robots.

(a) The first one is for physical assistant robots *that* are *fastened to a human during use* (and this would include wearable suits or non-medical physical assistance exoskeletons, that is to say, robots that directly help users by being attached to the humans).
(b) The second one is a physical assistant robot that, on the contrary, *is not fastened to a human during use* (this could include power assisted devices or powered walking aids).

After this categorization, ISO distinguishes between supplementation and augmentation. Supplementation could be understood as the 'assistance that restores a normal level of human capability to persons who may otherwise have difficulty in doing so (due to fatigue, handicap, etc.)'. This supplementation can, at the same time, be divided into two sub-categories: the up-to-50 % and the 50–100 % categories. According to Toth, this can be done 'for the cases the physical assistant is providing the lesser or the greater part of the work or effort involved in a physical task'; and this is very important 'because it determines whether or not the robot is physically more powerful than the human user, and whether or not the human user is capable of overpowering the robot in the case of failure'.

Augmentation is envisaged as the 'physical assistance giving humans the capability to perform physical tasks that exceed what can normally be expected without assistance (e.g. extreme strength, endurance, etc.)'.

Considering the difference between the two categories above, the problems that may be associated with both of them will be totally different. Indeed, having a robot device directly attached to one's body is not the same as a robotic device that one takes or applies only when needed. Accordingly, from an ethical point of view, differences between these devices will also differ substantially.

The following sub-sections will address two issues arisen by these sub-types of personal care robots: first, the case of physical assistant robots used in rehabilitation contexts; and second, physical assistant robots used in warfare environments.

3.2.1 Physical Assistant Robots in Rehab Contexts

In both cases (restraint and restraint-free physical assistant robots) the robotic device tracks the movements of the patient in order to record, control and monitor its use. This information could be used for different purposes: mainly to function itself (the robot needs information about the movements of the patient to react and work normally), but also for physicians or the therapists to know what treatment they need to apply, if there is any improvement in the patient's disease, etc.

ISO 13485:2013 defines medical devices as 'any instrument [...] to be used, alone or in combination, for human beings for one or more of the specific purpose (s) of: diagnosis, prevention, monitoring, treatment or alleviation of disease [...]. For instance, if exoskeletons were meant to be robotic devices just to help users in their daily routines (similarly to robotic prostheses), then Personal Care Robots ISO would apply. However, if their aim is to enhance patients' sanity and they are designed to be used in rehabilitation contexts, the medical devices' regulation would have to apply.

In any case, the recommendation to roboticists is to apply for both ISOs to be sure that there are no extra responsibilities derived from usage not covered by the scope of the chosen instrument. Of course, two ISOs will entail increased costs and longer procedures. However, there will be more benefits for the end-users to buy the medical device, and that could counterbalance the loss of time/money.

3.2.2 Physical Assistant Robots in Warfare Contexts

Similarly to drones, the scope of ISO 13482:2014 consists in addressing safety requirements for personal care robots. These robots have a precise and well-defined goal, that is, to improve the life of the intended users. Indeed, they are referred to as 'service robots' because they perform tasks for the sake of human care. Conversely, military robots are completely out of this scope.

The reality seems anyway to intertwine both kinds of robots. HULC is an exoskeleton intended to be used in warfare environments [20]. This exoskeleton gives supplementation of force and increases ability, strength and endurance. What kind of regulation (even if soft-law) is governing this use of exoskeletons?

In fact, this situation poses lots of yet unanswered ethical questions: is it ethical to use physical assistant robots to increase human force in warfare? Can physical assistant robots be considered part of the human body and be treated as human parts for indemnification reasons in case of harm? How can we address the delegation that human gives to the machine when using an exoskeleton? Is the law prepared to deal with 'super-humans' due to exoskeletons that, in theory, were intended to be just simple personal care robots?

As we argued before, the use of a robot should not determine the regulation that governs it. If HULC does not differ from other exoskeletons, from a legal perspective it should be regulated in the same manner. This has nothing to do with the existence of military codes, which normally govern the conduct of persons in the Armed Forces. A person (the creator of the robot/exoskeleton in this case) cannot choose the policies that govern a robot. If a robot has some given capabilities, consequently it will also have some particular regulations to follow. This is a guarantee for the user. Otherwise robot creators could exonerate themselves from any liability very easily, by claiming that they are not responsible for uses in other, different contexts (see below in the conclusion).

3.3 Mobile Servant Robots (Non Healthcare Facilities)

ISO 13482:2014 defines mobile servant robots as: 'personal care robot [*s*] that is capable of travelling to perform serving tasks in interaction with humans, such as handling objects or exchanging information. The confusion that mobile servant robots pose is basically regarding the main definition of 'personal care' and also the state of the art of these devices.

Regarding the latter, there are already marketable mobile servant robots even if they are not expressly designed for being in Healthcare Institutions. Already existing mobile servant robots are conceived to be able to perform some undefined intended tasks that will vary depending on their buyer/user: in schools as an extra-curricula support, in airports as attendants, or directly in hospitals as helpers/attendants [21].

The state of the art reveals that nowadays these robots are commonly used just for advertisement purposes rather than as real attendants or helpers. In fact, society does not seem to be ready for the implementation of these robots yet [22]. Yet, they have become part of a new trendy marketing strategy which has a high success: robot catches the attention of users and people take pictures with it and post them on Facebook, Twitter, and other social networks. A major worry and concern is the fact that these robots are capable of taking pictures themselves, they can upload it directly to Twitter, they are able to collect and store all the data of the event, such as how many people took a picture with them (and how many times the same person took a picture). Clearly, not only data protection issues are involved in this frame but also the behavior of the interactors of the robot (and that is called behavioral targeting [23]). This basically means that European data protection regulations based on the anonymisation of the person (and his/her personal information) scarcely capable to handle this new phenomenon where the individualization of the person is no longer needed to achieve the industry goals [24].

Furthermore, depending on robots' functions, there can be sub-categories within this sub-type of personal care robot not reflected yet in the ISO. Those could be: cleaning robot, delivery service robot, docent robot or security robot. The involved risks will vary substantially depending on the specific scenario (cleaning, surveillance or servant environment) the functions of the robots. Furthermore, this kind of robots will pose some ethical questions like: is it fair to have robot servants? What treatment/protection should they receive? Are they going to have salary (energy as a method of payment)? Is it legal to hit a mobile servant robot? What happens if the servant cannot understand a hear-impaired person? If serving harm occurs, who is responsible for that? These questions need to be carefully addressed.

The case of Resyone of Panasonic is quite interesting and worth mentioning. This robot is the first to obtain ISO 13482:2014. Resyone, is a robotic device built on an entirely new concept which fuses an electric care bed with an electric reclining wheelchair [25]. Part of the electric care bed detaches off to serve as the electric reclining wheelchair, thus allowing the user to easily transfer from bed to wheelchair without placing burden on the caregiver. With Resyone, only one caregiver is required to support safe and simple transfer between bed and wheelchair, thus lightening the load for care givers and making it easier for care receivers to get out of bed whenever they desire.

Nevertheless, the major concern lies in the fact that Resyone is assessed according to the criteria for mobile servant robots. Mobile servant robots are meant to travel to perform serving tasks in interaction with humans, such as handling objects or exchanging information, as described above. Whereas Resyone seems to be more a restraint-free assistant robot because ISO defines them as those who 'assist elderly/tired person to and from a chair, bed, etc. To assist in basic mobility tasks on flat ground with or without help from partner. To help provide more ease and comfort in daily life for independent living [8]'.

If that definition does not seem to be really in line with the characteristics of Resyone, Resyone should be considered in any case, as a person carrier robot (or a sub-type of person carrier robot) because it transforms into a wheelchair, and wheelchairs are person carrier robots.

This kind of confusions inevitably creates confusions to legal practitioners who find it hard to understand exactly what kind of 'thing' they are talking about. Thus they are uncertain about exactly what regulation needs to be applied. This aspect is very important because when performing the Care Robot Impact Assessment described in [26], risks and solutions will vary substantially between the different types of robots under the category of personal care robot.

3.4 Others: Therapeutic Robotics

Could therapeutic robots be considered part of the ISO 13482:2014? Therapeutic robotics are not a category inside ISO yet, but they in fact *perform actions contributing directly towards improvement in the quality of life of humans*, which is the definition given to personal care robots in the same *corpus*. There are two sub-types of therapeutic robots: physiotherapeutic robots (Fisiobot) and cognitive therapeutic robots (PARO).

Fisiobot is a robot that helps executing physiotherapies previously programmed and established by a physiotherapist [27]. Whereas, PARO is a cognitive therapeutic seal robot used in nursing homes for cognition disorder patients (mainly elderly) to improve brain function, as well as for other benefits [28]. This seal reduces patients' stress, it stimulates interaction between patients and caregivers, and it enhances socialization. These benefits do not have to be related to any specific treatment.

Indeed, not all the rehabilitation contexts are used expressly for rehabilitation. As an exoskeleton, which was created to be a physical assistant robot, could be a medical device if used for treatments, then it could also be the other way round: robots born to be medical devices could be used in other contexts. Indeed, a person could go to visit Fisiobot for a pleasure massage, or use PARO without being under a treatment. The seal is neither monitoring the person's activity nor diagnosing anything (which are typical activities for medical devices).

From a legal perspective, clarity is a must in this regard: are therapeutic robots part of personal care robots regulation? Or are they medical devices? Do they have to have both certifications?

4 A Final Legal Remark

Available robots are countless but marketable robots are fewer. This is because obtaining the certification is very complicated (and sometimes very costly). There are cases where the applicants seek the medical device certification regardless of whether their product really falls under the category of medical devices. For instance, the creators of a robot may be interested in obtaining the certification not because they need to comply with particular regulations, but only to get some benefits. In fact, end users could get discounts for medical devices, consequently this would inevitably increase the number of buyers, and thus the income of the company.

The Law does not permit that. Actually, it is a bit dangerous for the creators of a robot. When deciding what characteristics the robot will have (especially if it is intended to be introduced in the market), and when deciding who will be the end users, they need to think what regulations will apply to them. Of course they also need to be aware that they do not get only rights from regulations but also duties and obligations.

Yet, there is also another case to take into account, namely the same device may be considered in different ways in different countries. This is the case of PARO [29]. In the USA, according to the FDA, the seal robot is considered a medical device, whereas in Europe it only fulfills the Restriction of Hazardous Substances Directive 2011/65/EC. Actually, PARO has the Conformité Européenne mark but it is still not considered as a medical device in Europe. If PARO was considered as that, otherwise all the regulations regarding medical devices should apply to it.

This raises a lot of concerns among jurists, especially regarding the above mentioned 'preciseness' of definitions. How can lawyers expect clarity from the technical side when clarity is first lacking in the legal domain?

5 Conclusions

Great efforts from both legal and technical communities need to be made in order to create understandable bridges within both communities. Lawyers and practitioners normally tend to define too much the reality but engineers tend to define too vaguely some key concepts jurists need to understand. We need something in between.

This article is a first attempt to create these bridges. From one side, it is argued that we need more clarity in personal care robots regulations. At the same time, lawyers need to understand that the progress and the devolvement of certain technology is something inevitable, with related pros and cons. If Internet there would not be many problems, but the great recent advances in would not exist either.

Roboticists need to be acquainted with the importance of clear definitions of their robots. A blurred category could bring about lots of benefits (like receiving financial aids to purchase some products) but could also bring lots of wrong and unlawful constraints, future responsibilities, etc. Although clarity may be missing in legal domain, robot creators still remain responsible for their creations and may be punished. Of note, the consequences could be catastrophic, for instance, in the extreme case of death of someone due to a robotic device. Liability rules will apply anyway if some of the requirements have not been successfully fulfilled and if the creators of the robot have not expressly claimed that they are not responsible for any different use than the one/s for which the robot was made.

Roboticists need to be aware that the theoretical categorization of robots through function leads to confusion in the legal layer. Indeed, a robot poses several legal and ethical challenges overlooked by technical standards. Therefore, apart from the existing technical classification, a categorization in legal terms that could be a guarantee for the users is needed. ISO 13482:2014 classifies personal care robots from a technical perspective. That might be very useful to create new robot applications, but not to give protection to consumers in legal terms. In fact, compliance with some technical safety requirements does not necessarily imply compliance with the entire existing legal framework.

Having only those international standards might lead us to an infra-/over-regulated scenario where users could be in fact not protected. A robot needs to be compliant with the existing legal framework according to its own capacities/capabilities, besides their compliance with technical guidelines.

Above all, it is clear that there is an urgent need to address this new robot phenomenon. Robotic technology will become part of healthcare strategies to deal with current inefficiencies, and will dramatically change how care is delivered. Consequently, lots of questions will arise and lawyers and jurists will be required to give sensible and concrete responses.

Acknowledgments I would like to thank my supervisor Antoni Roig Batalla to be with me in this passionate journey and also Giorgio Schirripa who helped me to edit the wording, the sense and the purpose of this article.

References

1. Scott, N.: Ambiguity versus precision: the changing role of terminology in conference diplomacy. In: Kurbalija, J., Slavik, H.(eds.) Language and Diplomacy, p. 153 (2001)
2. Hoeflich, M.H.: Roman and Civil Law and the Development of Anglo-American Jurisprudence in the Nineteenth Century, pp. 9–30. University of Georgia Press (1997)
3. Chapin, F.S.: Definition of definitions of concepts. Soc. Forces **18**(2), 153–160 (1939)
4. Fetzer, J.H., Schlesinger, G.N., Shatz, D.: Definitions and definability philosophical perspectives. In: Synthese Library Studies in Epistemology, Logic, Methodology, and Philosophy of Science, vol. 216 (1991)
5. Oxford Dictionary. http://www.oxforddictionaries.com/definition/english/definition
6. Lessig, L.: Code Version 2.0, p. 121. Basic Books, NY (2006)
7. Dworkin, R.: Taking Rights Seriously, p. 295. Harvard University Press, Cambridge (1977)
8. ISO 13482:2014. Robots and Robotics Devices—Safety Requirements for Personal Care Robots, 3.13
9. Shelton, D.: Commitment and Compliance: The Role of Non-binding Norms in the International Legal System, p. 292. Oxford University Press, Oxford (2000)
10. Vid. http://www.housingcare.org/jargon-personal-care-ea2e2.aspx
11. Lawton, M.P., Brody, E.M.: Assessment of older people: self-maintaining and instrumental activities of daily living. Gerontologist **9**(3), 179–186 (1969)

12. Mondada, F., et al.: The e-puck, a robot designed for education in engineering. In: Proceedings of the 9th Conference on Autonomous Robot Systems and Competitions, vol. 1, no. LIS-CONF-2009-004, pp. 59–65. IPCB: Instituto Politécnico de Castelo Branco (2009)
13. Schweikardt, E.: Modular robotics studio. In: Proceedings of the Fifth International Conference on Tangible, Embedded, and Embodied Interaction, pp. 353–356 (2011)
14. Bartneck, C., Suzuki, T., Kanda, T., Nomura, T.: The influence of people's culture and prior experiences with Aibo on their attitude towards robots. AI Soc. **21**(1–2), 217 (2007)
15. Tamura, T., Yonemitsu, S., Itoh, A., Oikawa, D., Kawakami, A., Higashi, Y., Nakajima, K.: Is an entertainment robot useful in the care of elderly people with severe dementia? J. Gerontol. A Biol. Sci. Med. Sci. **59**(1), M83–M85 (2004)
16. Kravetz, A.M.: Toys cars offer mobility to children with disabilities. Live Science (2012)
17. Galloway, J.C., Ryu, J., Agrawal, S.K.: Babies driving robots: self-generated mobility in very young infants. Intel. Serv. Robotics **1**, 123–134 (2008)
18. Toth, A.: Domeo project. AAL-2008-1-159, R-BME-1_0-D4.3 D4.3 Risk Assessment/ISO
19. Carlson, T., Millán, J.R.: Brain-Controlled wheelchairs: a robotic architecture. IEEE Robot. Autom. Mag. **20**(1), 65–73 (2013)
20. HULC: An exoskeleton in Berkeley Robotics and human engineering laboratory. bleex.me.berkeley.edu/research/exoskeleton/hulc/
21. Marti, P., et al.: A robotic toy for children with special needs: from requirements to design. In: IEEE 11th International Conference on Rehab Robotics. Kyoto International Conference Center (2009)
22. Special Eurobarometer 382's report Public attitudes towards robots, Wave EB77.1—TNS Opinion and Social (2012)
23. Beales, H.: The value of behavioral targeting. Network Advertising Initiative (2010)
24. Roig Batalla, A.: Privacy and social networks. In: From Data Protection to Pervasive Computing, pp. 146–149. AAAI Publications (2010)
25. Panasonic Global News Exclusive: Care service robot is the first in the world to obtain ISO 13482. http://news.panasonic.net/archives/2014/0319_26411.html
26. Fosch-Villaronga, E.: Creation of a care robot impact assessment. In: XVII International Conference on Social Robotics (2015)
27. angel.co/fisiobot
28. Griffin, R.L.: Changing the Culture for Dementia Care—The Path to a Better Quality of Life for People with Alzheimer's Disease. PESI Healthcare Publishing Group (2012)
29. Tergesen, A., Inada, M.: It is not a stuffed animal, it is a $6000 medical device. paro the robo-seal aims to comfort elderly, but is it ethical? Wall Street J (2010). http://www.wsj.com/articles/SB10001424052748704463504575301051844937276

Variable Stiffness Mechanism in Robotized Interventional Radiology

L. Esteveny, L. Barbé and B. Bayle

Abstract During the last two decades, a large number of robotic assistants have been developed to help surgeons place surgical tools. Until now, research in this field has mostly focused on rigid robotic structures, which make safety issues difficult to deal with. In this paper, we consider a new collaborative manipulation approach based on a variable stiffness mechanism. By controlling the stiffness perceived by the user when he/she manipulates the device, it then becomes possible to guide his/her gesture in a safe way. This strategy is first presented, before detailing the design, optimization and experimental validation of the proposed mechanism based on leaf springs.

Keywords Variable stiffness mechanism · Compliant mechanism · Leaf spring · Interventional radiology · Collaborative manipulation

1 Introduction

The initial motivation for the presented work is to propose an innovative strategy for robotic assistance in interventional radiology [1, 3]. During image-guided percutaneous procedures, needles are used to perform diagnosis or therapy. Robotic assistance has emerged in this field throughout the last 15 years to help develop these very minimally invasive medical techniques [14]. However, existing systems are usually quite rigid and non-backdrivable, which leads to limit undesirable tissue lacerations by:

L. Esteveny (✉)
PMA, Katholieke Universiteit Leuven, Leuven, Belgium
e-mail: laure.esteveny@kuleuven.be

L. Esteveny · L. Barbé · B. Bayle
EAVR, ICube-Strasbourg University, Strasbourg, France
e-mail: laurent.barbe@unistra.fr

B. Bayle
Institute of Image-Guided Surgery, Strasbourg, France
e-mail: bernard.bayle@unistra.fr

P. Wenger et al. (eds.), *New Trends in Medical and Service Robots*,
Mechanisms and Machine Science 39, DOI 10.1007/978-3-319-30674-2_4

- compensating for the patient physiological motions [10], when robots are attached to the operating table [12];
- releasing the tool from time to time, even when robots are directly mounted on the patient [9].

To cope with these drawbacks, a statically balanced 3-DOF system has been introduced in [4] so as to position tools with a limited amount of energy. Built with light links and a mechanical gravity compensation system, this backdrivable device is designed in order to perform collaborative manipulation tasks, and could offer solutions for the guidance of medical gestures. Nevertheless, it was designed to be as passive as possible, and so it cannot apply enough controllable forces to guide the surgeon gesture. Usually, such a guidance requires to implement virtual fixtures [11], which consist in software constraints imposed by powerful actuators. In this type of guidance, safety is a major issue since the necessary torques, directly produced by the robotic device joints, are not limited. An alternative strategy to fulfill the guidance is proposed hereafter. It consists in using a variable stiffness mechanism (VSM), able to impose controllable resistive forces to the surgeon, when this latter moves away from his/her target. With this strategy, the robotic device does not produce more energy than it has received, making interactions safer.

To better understand the purpose of a VSM, let us first comment on variable stiffness actuators (VSA), whose development in the field of robotics has been growing for the last 10 years. VSA allow to control a joint in both position and stiffness (around its position) by typically adding controllable elasticity, via mechanical flexible transmissions such as springs [17, 18]. Various solutions have been proposed to design VSA but one particularly interesting family of device is the 'series configuration', where one actuator is dedicated to vary the position while the other one adjusts the stiffness. This second actuator coupled with the flexible transmission is what we call a VSM. The stiffness modulation can be obtained by prestressing a flexible element as in [16] or [20]. However, the actuation energy remains high. An alternative consists in varying the fixation point of the flexible element as performed in [8, 15]. In this configuration, the force required to modulate the stiffness is lower since it is perpendicular to the one developed by the flexible transmission. The flexible transmissions are often made out of linear springs, low-cost and widespread but still unidirectional and cumbersome. Compliant mechanisms seem thus more relevant since they are able to deform themselves under a load according to a specific characteristic [6, 7]. As such mechanisms already have an intrinsic stiffness, they are especially well adapted to obtain small displacements under high loads, as exploited in leaf springs [2, 19]. However, VSM based on leaf springs still remain non-totally optimized in term of stiffness adjustment strategy. Indeed, sliders are usually moved along the leaf springs to modify their effective lengths. Ideally, only the leaf spring part situated after the support, known as the effective length, deforms itself. However, in practice, the leaf spring is also deformed before the support. Such non-desired deformation then leads to reduced stiffness range and increased energy consumption.

The paper is organized as follows. The general principle of the proposed guidance strategy is described in Sect. 2. The final envisioned mechanism is composed of a clutch, not implemented here, and a VSM that would be added to each joint to obtain a resistive effect. Then, the main features of the developed VSM are presented. Its structure is based on an existing compliant mechanism, whose intrinsic stiffness can be adjusted by changing the effective length of its leaf springs thanks to sliders. The originality of the proposed VSM lies in the slider design, which is described and analyzed in Sect. 3. We show that the VSM performances for both the stiffness range and the device energy consumption can be greatly enhanced by increasing the number of supports on each slider. In Sect. 4, the VSM implementation and its experimental characterization are presented. Finally, Sect. 5 concludes the paper and provides the perspectives of this work.

2 Guidance Strategy for Collaborative Manipulation

2.1 General Principle

During collaborative manipulation, the robot and the physician work together to perform tasks such as positioning a tool. In order to ensure safety, the user should be the only one to bring energy, the robot producing only resistive forces to guide his/her gesture. To achieve such a strategy, first consider a statically balanced mechanism, as the one proposed in [4]. Now assume that there exists a clutch, at each joint, able to connect/disconnect the VSM proposed hereafter, in order to change the joint stiffness around the system position. The clutch and the VSM are passive systems [13], leading to the safe working principle:

1. When the user goes toward the target, the clutches decouple the VSM from the robotic balanced structure. This latter can be freely moved by the user, almost without effort.
2. When the user moves away from the target, the clutches connect the VSM to the robotic structure and the stiffness of the VSM is automatically adjusted depending on the distance to the target. The user then feels a resistive torque, guiding him/her back to the correct trajectory.

The guidance strategy is illustrated in Fig. 1. The robot is defined as a statically balanced structure, to which a clutch and a VSM are added at each joint. The user acts on the robotic structure by applying joint torques denoted as τ_u. The guidance algorithm computes the clutches state $\mathbf{state}^*$ and VSM stiffness $\mathbf{k}^*$ required to follow the desired trajectory, according to the robot configuration $\mathbf{q}$. Depending on these values, the clutches can be closed or opened, so that the VSM may or may not produce resistive torques τ_r. Though the clutches design will deserve some interest, the rest of the paper is concerned with the design of the VSM.

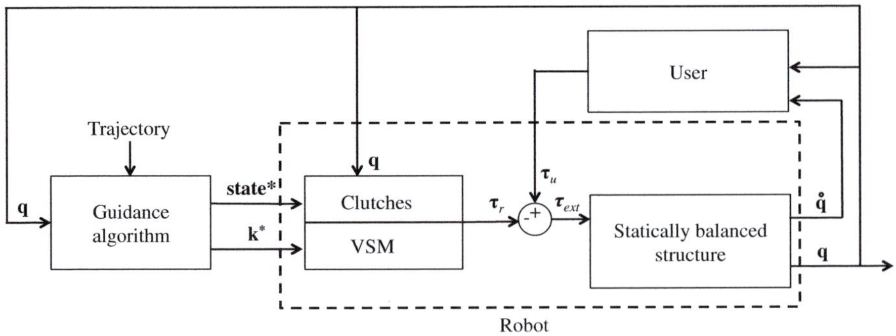

Fig. 1 Guidance strategy

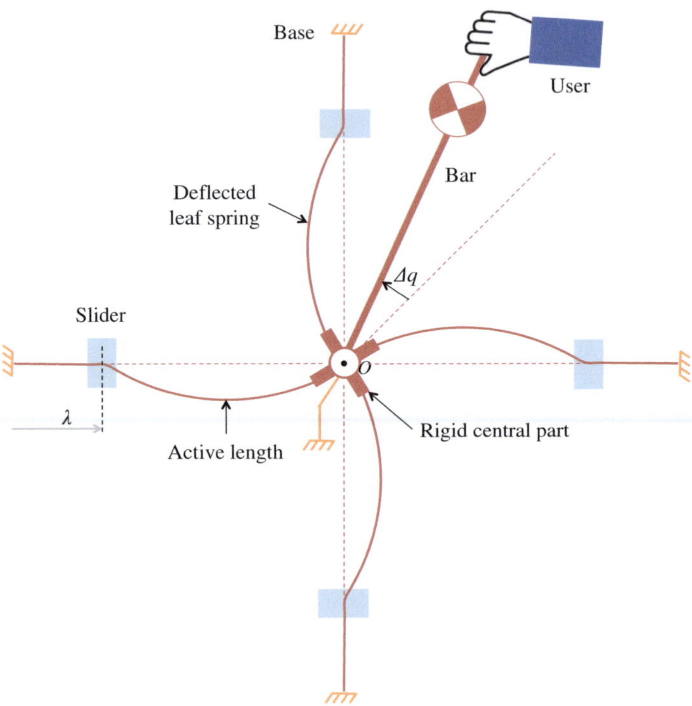

Fig. 2 Principle of the VSM

2.2 *Variable Stiffness Mechanism*

The example of a bar in rotation, represented in Fig. 2 (rotary joint at point O), is used to highlight the major challenges of the VSM.

The VSM is composed of 4 thin beams similar to leaf springs connected to a rigid central part, where dotted lines represent the VSM equilibrium position. Such architecture results from the arrangement of two compliant mechanisms known as Remote Center Compliance (RCC) [6], originally composed of only two perpendicular leaf springs. The external part is attached to the base, leading to the leaf spring deflection when a torque is applied on the central rigid part. Such mechanism has been selected due to its stiffness expression, which draws an hyperbolic curve from the infinite to 0 when the effective length of the leaf springs increases. Furthermore, its simplicity and integration possibilities due to its cleared centrum are non negligible. We have considered two RCC to obtain a stiffer mechanism, statically balanced whatever the gravity direction is. As a consequence, the joint stiffness is independent from the load.

The leaf springs deflect when a Δq displacement is imposed by the user to the bar, providing a resistive torque to the bar. We then propose to modulate this resistive torque by translating four sliders of a distance λ along each leaf spring. As a consequence, the deflections of the leaf springs are modified, leading to a joint stiffness change. The stiffness is ideally minimal when $\lambda = 0$ and tends towards the infinite when the sliders are close to the rigid central part. As the sliders move along the leaf springs with respect to the base, they do not add embedded inertia to the bar. Note that the slider displacements should be synchronized to ensure that O remains the pivot point, removing the possible transversal forces at point O.

2.3 Structure Based on Leaf Springs

To our knowledge, the sliders proposed in the literature to change the effective length of leaf springs are based on a single localized support [2, 19], such as the one illustrated in Fig. 3, which is applied on a quarter of the previous VSM (as the other parts are identical) under a loading torque applied at point O. In the ideal case to achieve, only the part of the leaf spring between the slider and the rigid central part is deformed. As a consequence, the stiffness can be high and the line tangent to the leaf spring at the support is null, as visible in Fig. 3. If the support meets the leaf spring in a point as it happens with rollers, the leaf spring deflects itself before and

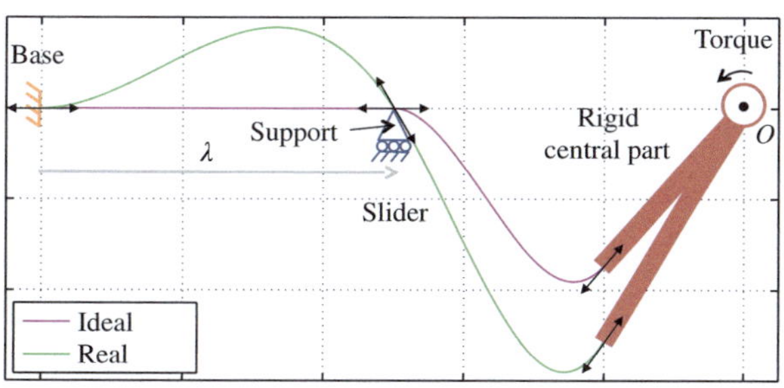

Fig. 3 Deflection of the leaf spring in the ideal and the real cases

after the support. As a result, the stiffness is less important than in the previous case, leading to a lower range of stiffness. Furthermore, the tangent line at the support is non-null, as clearly visible in Fig. 3. This leads to more energy consumption to maintain and move the slider since the slider direction of motion is not anymore perpendicular to the spring force direction.

3 Stiffness Enhancement Methodology

3.1 Parameters Influences

This part describes a new design method for the sliders. Each proposed slider is composed of two supports, referred as points B and C in Fig. 4. The distance between the two supports is δ, such as $\lambda > \delta > 0$, where λ gives the position of the slider. The letters p and r respectively stand for the length of the leaf spring and the length of the rigid part. Then, let k be the VSM stiffness and E and I be the Young's modulus of the leaf spring and its moment of inertia with respect to **z** axis.

The structural analysis theory [5] applied on such a structure leads to the following VSM stiffness:

$$k = \frac{c_1}{c_4} \tag{1}$$

where c_1 and c_4 are reported in the appendix. To illustrate this part in a more general formulation, all the figures included in this section are plotted considering $r = 0.2(r+p)$, $p = 0.8(r+p)$, $\lambda \in [0.1(r+p); 0.65(r+p)]$, which are consistent with a realistic design. The external torque applied on the VSM is known as τ.

The stiffness-slider displacement characteristics for the ideal, 1 support and 2 supports cases are reported in Fig. 5. As anticipated, the stiffness increases with λ, following an hyperbola behavior. By comparing the ideal and 1 support cases, this figure clearly shows that a large part of stiffness is lost when λ increases, with a ratio of 2 when $\lambda = 0.65(r+p)$. The same characteristics are plotted for the 2 supports case according to Eq. (1), for different values of δ. A decrease of δ results in a behavior tending towards the ideal behavior, so with a larger range of stiffness. On the contrary, when δ tends to λ, point B gets closer to the base, leading to the

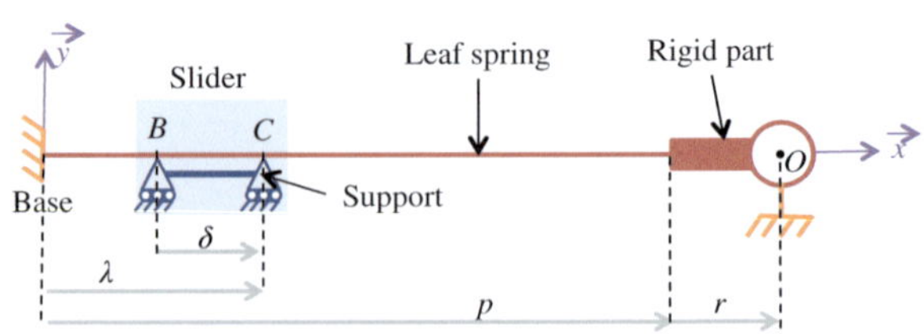

Fig. 4 Parameters used for defining a quarter of the VSM

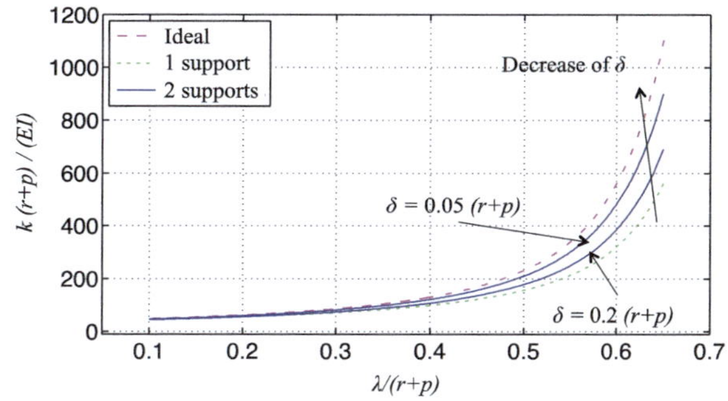

Fig. 5 VSM stiffness behavior according to the slider positions

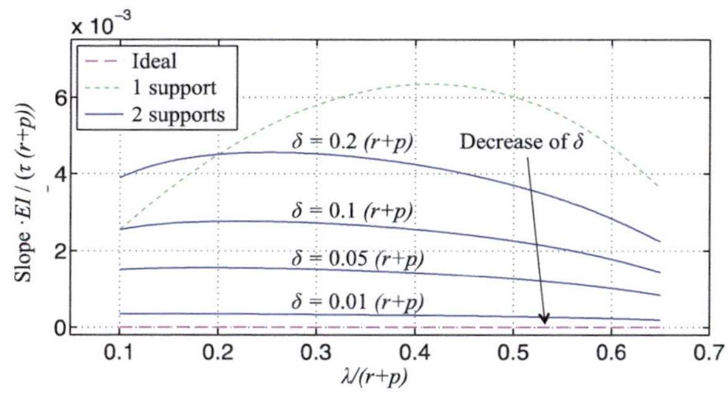

Fig. 6 Slope behavior of the tangent to the deflected curve at λ, according to the slider positions

case of a single support. These observations mean that a same stiffness range can be obtained with a more compact VSM if it is based on sliders with two supports close to each other.

It is also interesting to look at the slope of the tangent to the deflected curve of the leaf spring at λ reported in Fig. 6. This slope remains null in the ideal case scenario, meaning that the only forces applied to the sliders are perpendicular to them. As a consequence, no energy is required to maintain the position of the sliders while the only energy required to move the sliders is used to counteract frictions. However, as visible in Fig. 6, they are not ensured anymore in the case of sliders with a single support. Sliders with 2 supports can almost solve this issue. Indeed, the slope of the tangent tends towards 0 when δ decreases.

3.2 Material and Dimensioning

The leaf spring material is crucial. Ideally, creep and stress relaxation have to be minimal so as to ensure repeatability and to limit non-linear effects. Polymers are then excluded while metal alloys are preferred. In [7], one criteria consists in keeping the metal with the highest ratio of yield strength to Young's modulus.

Concerning the dimensioning, the parameters r, p and δ are chosen to ensure the conception specifications and the desired dimensions of the whole joint. In order to compact the device and increase the stiffness range, r and δ should be chosen as low as possible. The main criteria to dimension the leaf springs are then: (1) keeping the spring stresses σ inferior to the admissible stress σ_{ad} so as to stay in the material linear range of deformation; (2) obtaining a stiffness range included in $[k_{min}; k_{max}]$.

The leaf spring stress is maximal when the spring deflection is maximal, i.e. when the stiffness is minimal. Considering $\lambda = \delta = 0$, such stress is equivalent to the one of the RCC [6] and is given by:

$$\sigma_{ad} > \sigma = \frac{\Delta q E h (2p + 3r)}{p^2} \tag{2}$$

where h the leaf thickness. The desired minimal stiffness leads to the maximal angle Δq_{max}. Then, we can deduce h such as:

$$h < h_{max} = \frac{\sigma_{ad}\, p^2}{Eh(2p + 3r)} \tag{3}$$

Equation (1) is then used to calculate the spring width b when λ is minimal and $k = k_{min}$. The maximal value of λ is then deduced from the same equation where $k = k_{max}$.

4 Prototype and Experimental Results

4.1 Prototype

The VSM prototype is represented in Fig. 7 (only mechanical part, without any actuation).

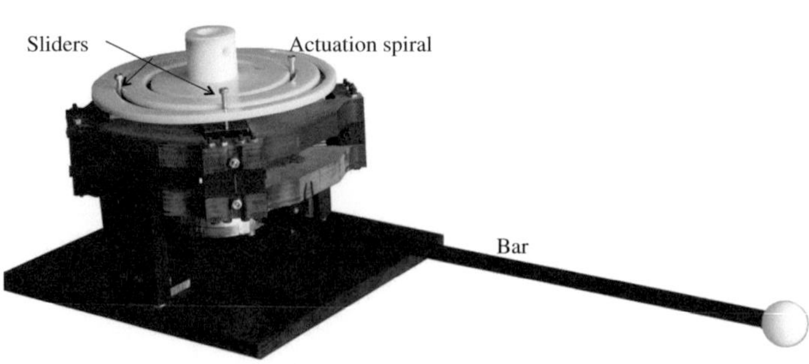

Fig. 7 Overall view of the realized prototype

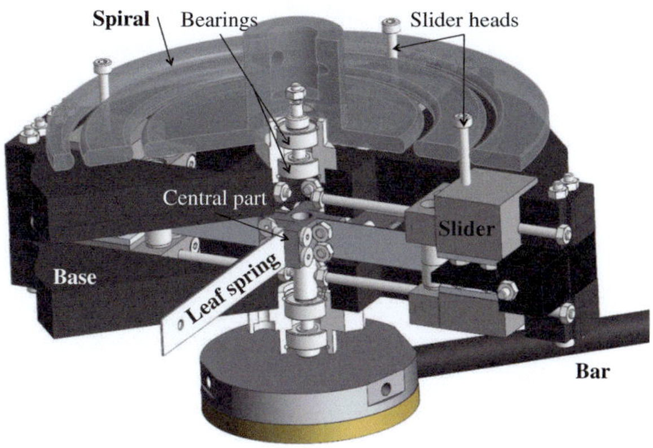

Fig. 8 VSM assembly CAD view

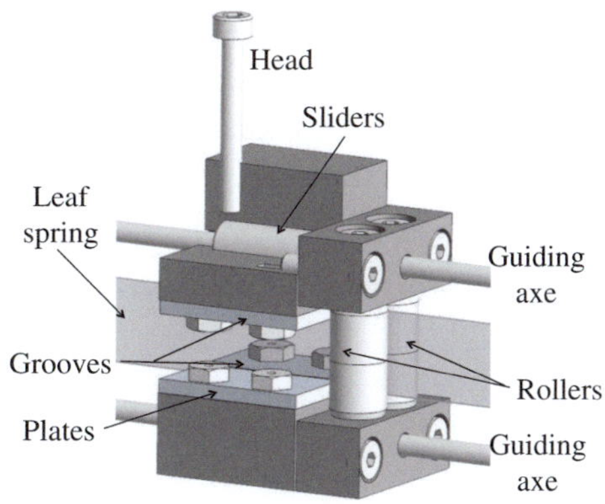

Fig. 9 Slider CAD view

According to the previous part, we have selected a 304-H metal with a thermally augmented yield strength while the other parts are mainly composed of stainless steel and polyamide 6 to lighten the prototype. The leaf springs are fixed to a metallic rigid central part linked to the bar, as illustrated in Fig. 8. The two contact points are implemented so as to have good sliding properties, limited backlashes, using two rollers pressed against the leaf springs in C and two grooves in B to have δ as low as possible (see Fig. 9). Finally, an Archimedean spiral is used to move simultaneously all the sliders. Once the spiral is kept at a position, neither slider is able to move.

We first chose: $r = 8.5$ mm and $p = 44$ mm, so that k varies in the range [0.057; 0.25] N·m/deg. Assuming that $E = 200$ GPa, these values enable us to get the following angular displacements of the bar under a 1 N·m torque: a 4.4 deg displacement when the stiffness is minimal, and a 1 deg displacement when the stiffness is maximal. According to the dimensional criteria proposed in part Sect. 3.2, the maximal value of h is 0.7 mm. We select a standard leaf spring of experimentally checked thickness $h = 0.46$ mm. Then, b is calculated based on the minimal stiffness, obtained when $\lambda = \delta = 5.3$ mm and is equal to 11.4 mm. The desired stiffness

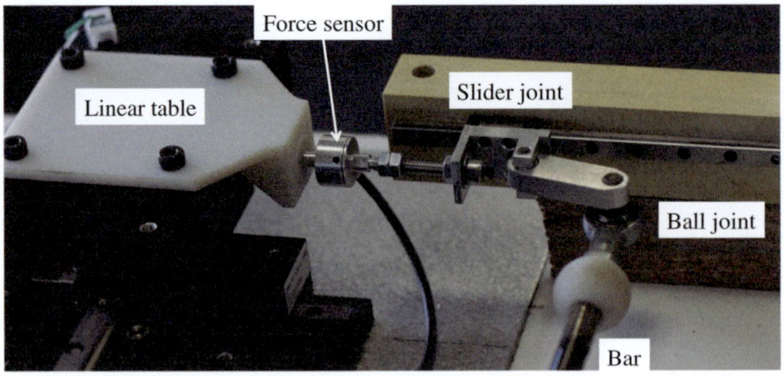

Fig. 10 Test-bed used to characterize the variable stiffness mechanism

range is then totally accessible when λ varies from 5.65 mm to 28.8 mm. The maximal forces applied to the rollers are then limited to 40 N while those applied to the grooves remain inferior to 250 N, in the worst case scenario where λ is minimal.

4.2 Setup and Protocol

This section aims at characterizing the mechanical behavior of the developed prototype to compare it with the theoretical dimensioning. Quasi-static experiments have been considered for different positions of the sliders. We have first evaluated the angular displacement of the bar subject to a specific torque. To that purpose, different positions have been imposed at the tip of the arm while the resistive force has been measured, thanks to the test-bed illustrated in Fig. 10. The latter is based on a linear table (FB075 series actuated by HR4-Nanomotion motors), whose position is known with a 10^{-3} mm-accuracy. An unidirectional force sensor (Scaime K1107) is attached to the table and makes the force estimation possible with a 0.8 N accuracy. To suppress transversal forces, the latter translates along the frame. The motion of the bar is then transmitted to the force sensor thanks to a connecting rod, connected to the bar via a ball-joint and connected to the sensor via a pivot joint.

The linear table has been controlled to have specified positions of the bar for a given position of the sliders (1 mm steps at 0.5 mm/s), and the force has been measured simultaneously. These steps have then been repeated back and forth for all the admissible displacements of the bar.

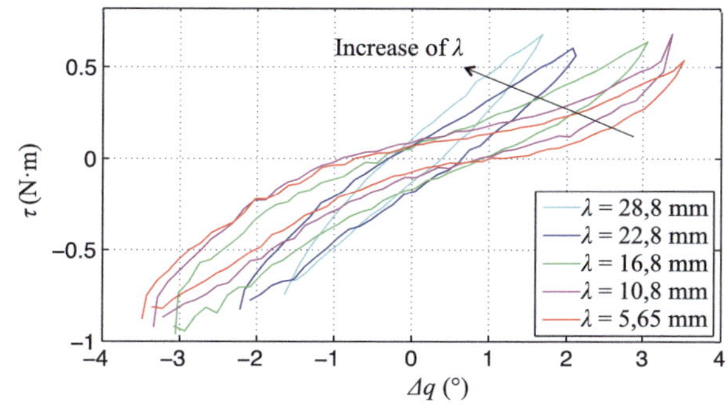

Fig. 11 Torque-displacement of the bar characteristics for several positions λ of the sliders

4.3 Results

4.3.1 Torque-Displacement Characteristics of the Bar

Figure 11 reports the characteristics of τ depending on Δq for several values of λ, where the leaf springs stay in their linear range of deformation. An hysteresis cycle is visible. It can easily be explained by the backlashes that exist between leaf springs and rollers/grooves. Indeed, for a given solicitation, the leaf springs are pushed against some rollers while under the opposite solicitation, they are pushed against the opposite rollers. This same behavior is also observed with the grooves. The stiffness of the VSM is then obtained by calculating $\tau/\Delta q$ for a given λ and for a given direction when following the torque-displacement characteristic. According to Fig. 11, the mean stiffness obtained for each position Δq is the slope value of the torque-displacement characteristics at a given λ. According to Eq. (1), these values should be linear. However, experimental results show non-linear areas, starting when the torque increases and the stiffness decreases, i.e. when the sliders are away from the center (λ small). In these cases, forces due to the leaf spring deformations and applied on the VSM base are extremely high. This results in low deformations of the base, which slightly change the attached point of the leaf springs, leading to stiffness variations.

4.3.2 Stiffness-Slider Position Characteristics

The previous data, where only the linear parts around the central position are considered, are hereafter used to express the mean stiffness of each curve. Figure 12 reports thus the experimental stiffnesses for different positions λ of the sliders. These values differ from the dimensioning because of some spring parameter inaccuracies such as on E and I. However, according to the experimental stiffnesses, we are able to evaluate a mean value for EI (cf. Eq. (1)) and then to plot the theoretical stiffness. As visible in Fig. 12, the experimental values fit the theoretical ones. With such 2

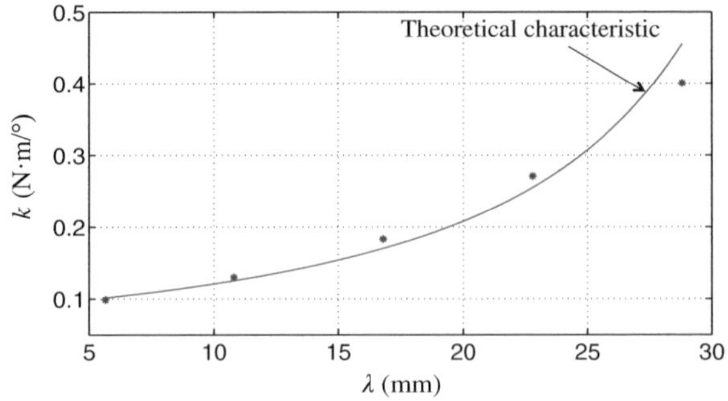

Fig. 12 Stiffness variation depending on λ

contact sliders, we achieve, in the worst case scenario where λ is maximal, more than 93.5 % of the stiffness obtained in the ideal case. With only one support, this achievable stiffness would have been dropped to 66 %.

5 Conclusions and Perspectives

In this paper, we have first introduced a new strategy based on flexibility addition at the joint level to impose resistive torques to a user to help him/her perform tasks safely. Such a strategy meets safety requirements since it is entirely based on passive components. We have then focused on the design of a VSM based on leaf springs. After detailing its principle, we have proposed to improve both the stiffness range and the energy consumption of such a device by the use of two support sliders. Their analysis has made possible the design of a prototype, and the proof of enhancement of the VSM properties. We have shown that the experimental characterization fits correctly the model even if several nonlinearities remain. Such behaviors can be explained by the fact that the leaf springs are assembled.

In the future, manufacturing the springs, the central part and the frame in a monolithic part will suppress a large number of backlashes, ensure the leaf spring perpendicularity and properly set the attachment points of the leaf springs. Furthermore, choosing material with a really high ratio of yield strength to Young's modulus such as titanium or Copper-Beryllium will improve the device compactness. Note that such choices were not selected here to have a quick and non-expensive prototype to test. Other future works will focus on the actuation and control of the VSM. The spiral will be associated with an actuator to enable a controllable change of stiffness and the clutch will be designed and implemented. The whole proposed guidance strategy will be evaluated on a 1 DOF setup before being used on a multiple DOF robotic device.

Acknowledgments The authors acknowledge the support of the Region Alsace, the Institute of image-guided surgery (IHU Strasbourg) and the Foundation ARC. This work has been sponsored by the French government research program Investissements dAvenir through the Robotex Equipment of Excellence and Labex CAMI (ANR- 10-EQPX-44 and ANR-11-LABX-0004).

Appendix: c_i Expressions

$$c_1 = 8EI(\delta - \lambda)\delta[(2\delta + 6\lambda)p^3 + (9r\lambda + 9\lambda r - 18\lambda^2 + 3\delta r + 3\delta r)p^2 + (18\lambda r^2 - 18\lambda^2 r - 18r\lambda^2 + 18\lambda^3 + 6\delta r^2 - 6\lambda^2\delta)p + (-6\lambda^4 - 3r\lambda^2\delta - 3\delta\lambda^2 r + 9\lambda^3 r - 18r^2\lambda^2 + 4\lambda^3\delta + 9\lambda^3 r)]$$

$$c_4 = -\delta(\lambda - p)^3(\delta - \lambda)(3\delta\lambda + \delta p - 3\lambda^2 + 3\lambda p)$$

References

1. Bayle, B., Piccin, O., Barbé, L., Renaud, P., Mathelin, M.: Image-guided interventions and robotics. In: Garbey, M., Bass, B.L., Collet, C., Mathelin, M., Tran-Son-Tay, R. (eds.) Computational Surgery and Dual Training, pp. 191–205. Springer, US (2010)
2. Choi, J., Hong, S., Lee, W., Kang, S., Kim, M.: A robot joint with variable stiffness using leaf springs. IEEE Trans. Robot. **27**(2), 229–238 (2011)
3. Cleary, K., Melzer, A., Watson, V., Kronreif, G., Stoianovici, D.: Interventional robotic systems: applications and technology state-of-the-art. Minim. Invasive Ther. **15**(2), 101–113 (2006)
4. Esteveny, L., Barbé, L., Bayle, B.: A novel actuation technology for safe physical human-robot interactions. In: IEEE International Conference on Robotics and Automation, pp. 450–457. Hong Kong, China (2014)
5. Gere, J.: Mechanics of Materials. Thomson, Brools/Cole (2004)
6. Henein, S.: Conception des structures articulées à guidages flexibles de haute précision. Ph.D. thesis, École polytechnique fédérale de Lausanne (2000)
7. Howell, L.: Compliant Mechanisms. Wiley (2001)
8. Jafari, A., Tsagarakis, N., Caldwell, D.: Awas-ii: a new actuator with adjustable stiffness based on the novel principle of adaptable pivot point and variable lever ratio. In: IEEE International Conference on Robotics and Automation, pp. 4638–4643. Shanghai, China (2011)
9. Maurin, B., Bayle, B., Piccin, O., Gangloff, J., de Mathelin, M., Doignon, C., Zanne, P., Gangi, A.: A patient-mounted robotic platform for ct-scan guided procedures. IEEE Trans. Biomed. Eng. **55**(10), 2417–2425 (2008). doi:10.1109/TBME.2008.919882
10. Riviere, C., Gangloff, J., de Mathelin, M.: Robotic compensation of biological motion to enhance surgical accuracy. Proc. IEEE **94**(9), 1705–1716 (2006)
11. Rosenberg, L.: Virtual fixtures: Perceptual tools for telerobotic manipulation. In: IEEE Virtual Reality Annual International Symposium, pp. 76–82 (1993). doi:10.1109/VRAIS.1993.380795
12. Stoianovici, D.: Urobotics—urology robotics at Johns Hopkins. Comput. Aided Surg. **6**(6), 360–369 (2001)
13. Swanson, D., Book, W.: Path-following control for dissipative passive haptic displays. In: 11th Symposium on Haptic Interfaces for Virtual Environment and Teleoperator Systems, pp. 101–108. Los Angeles, CA, USA (2003). doi:10.1109/HAPTIC.2003.1191245
14. Troccaz, J. (ed.): Medical Robotics. Wiley (2012)
15. Tsagarakis, N., Sardellitti, I., Caldwell, D.: A new variable stiffness actuator (compact-vsa): Design and modelling. In: IEEE/RSJ International Conference on Intelligent Robots and Systems, pp. 378–383. San Francisco, USA (2011)
16. Van Ham, R.: Compliant actuation for biologically inspired bipedal walking robots. Ph.D. thesis, Vrije Universiteit Brussel (2006)

17. Van Ham, R., Sugar, T., Vanderborght, B., Hollander, K., Lefeber, D.: Compliant actuator designs. Review of actuators with passive adjustable compliance/controllable stiffness for robotic applications. IEEE Robot. Autom. Mag. **16**(3), 81–94 (2009)
18. Vanderborght, B., Albu-Schaeffer, A., Bicchi, A., Burdet, E., Caldwell, D., Carloni, R., Catalano, M., Eiberger, O., Friedl, W., Ganesh, G., Garabini, M., Grebenstein, M., Grioli, G., Haddadin, S., Hoppner, H., Jafari, A., Laffranchi, M., Lefeber, D., Petit, F., Stramigioli, S., Tsagarakis, N., Van Damme, M., Van Ham, R., Visser, L., Wolf, S.: Variable impedance actuators: a review. Robot. Auton. Syst. **61**(12), 1601–1614 (2013)
19. Wang, R.J., Huang, H.P.: Mechanically stiffness-adjustable actuator using a leaf spring for safe physical human-robot interaction. Mechanika **18**(1), 77–83 (2012)
20. Wolf, S., Hirzinger, G.: A new variable stiffness design: Matching requirements of the next robot generation. In: IEEE International Conference on Robotics and Automation, pp. 1741–1746. Pasadena, CA, USA (2008)

Application of Nonlinear Dynamics to Human Knee Movement on Plane and Inclined Treadmill

D. Tarnita, M. Georgescu and D.N. Tarnita

Abstract The objective of this study is to quantify and investigate nonlinear motion of the human knee joint for a sample of 7 healthy subjects on plane treadmill and inclined treadmill with an angle of 10° and for both knees of a sample of 3 patients who suffer of osteoarthritis, only on the plane treadmill, using nonlinear dynamics stability analysis. The largest Lyapunov exponent (LLE) and correlation dimensions are calculated as chaotic measures from the experimental time series of the flexion-extension angle of human knee joint. Larger values of LLEs obtained for patients group suffering by osteoarthritis are associated with more divergence and increase of knee variability, while smaller values obtained for healthy subjects reflect increase of local stability, less divergence and variability, less sensitivity to perturbations and higher resistance to stride-to-stride variability. The use of nonlinear tools may provide additional insight on the nature of the step-to-step fluctuations present in human and robotic locomotion.

Keywords Human knee · Osteoarthritic knee · Treadmill · Nonlinear dynamics · Lyapunov exponents

D. Tarnita (✉) · M. Georgescu
University of Craiova, Craiova, Romania
e-mail: tarnita.daniela@gmail.com

M. Georgescu
e-mail: georgescumarius@livel.com

D.N. Tarnita
University of Medicine and Pharmacy, Craiova, Romania
e-mail: dan_tarnita@yahoo.com

P. Wenger et al. (eds.), *New Trends in Medical and Service Robots*,
Mechanisms and Machine Science 39, DOI 10.1007/978-3-319-30674-2_5

1 Introduction

Variability of gait can be defined as the variance of the gait parameter around the mean, and a broad range of variability measures has been reported in literature [1–3]. The measure of gait variability assumes that each stride is unrelated to strides in the past, and that inter-stride variations are random [2]. Temporal-distance measures of gait have been used to evaluate gait function and dysfunctions in the elderly and fall prediction [4, 5]. The kinematics of artificial structures used in medical field as prosthetic devices, humanoid robots and robotic structures used in minimal invasive surgery is studied in [6–8]. Many studies that investigated the relationship of gait speed and variability were conducted using different walking speeds that were measured from overground walking [9–11]. In healthy adults, the kinematics of walking is more variable as people walk slower or faster than their preferred speed [12–14]. Motorized treadmills are widely used in research in biomechanical studies of human locomotion or in clinical therapy. The purpose of [15] was to characterize the differences between overground and treadmill walking in terms of stride-to-stride variability. Biomechanics research in gait has focused largely on walking on the horizontal [16–18], with less attention for inclined surfaces [19–21].

During the last decades, a lot of new mathematical tools have been used to better characterize the stability and the nonlinear features of gait variability. Local dynamic stability refers to the behavior of a system in response to very small perturbations [22]. It is quantified by the maximum Lyapunov exponent which is a measure of the ability of the walking subject to maintain continuous motion and to attenuate the effects of the local perturbations [2, 18, 23]. Yang and Wu [24] showed the potential of the largest Lyapunov exponents used to measure the balance control of human standing, an important aspect in the development of bipedal walking machines.

The hand trajectories for adults were compared with the trajectories of robotic systems using nonlinear dynamic tools in [7, 25]. Experiments on the application of chaos theory to describe a robot's behavior quantitatively, using the Lyapunov exponent of robot trajectories are presented in [26–29].

The objective of this study is to quantify and investigate nonlinear motion of the human knee joint on plane and inclined treadmill, using nonlinear dynamics stability analysis. The largest Lyapunov exponent (LLE) and correlation dimension will be calculated as chaotic measures from the experimental time series of the flexion-extension angle of human knee joint.

2 Nonlinear Dynamics

2.1 State Space Reconstruction

One method to reconstruct the state space S is to generate the so-called delay coordinates vectors [30]. The space constructed using the vector

$$x_n = \{s(t_0 + nT_s);\ s(t_0 + nT_s + T);\ \ldots;\ s(t_0 + nT_s + (d_E - 1)T\}; \qquad (1)$$

is called the reconstructed space, where the integer d_E is the embedding dimension. In relation (1) s(.) is a measured scalar function and T_s is the sampling time, n = 1, 2,…, d_E, $T = kT_s$ an appropriately chosen time delay.

It is assumed that the geometry and the dynamics of the trajectory obtained using the vectors x_n are the same as the geometry and the dynamics of the trajectory in the actual phase space of the system. This assumption is verified with a proper choice of time delay and embedding dimension. The embedding dimension d_E must be large enough so that the reconstructed orbit does not overlap with itself. The dynamics in the reconstructed state space is equivalent to the original dynamics, so an attractor in the reconstructed state space has the same invariants, such as Lyapunov exponents and correlation dimension [31].

2.2 Correlation Dimension

An attractor's dimension is a measure of its geometric structure. The correlation dimension, d_F, is one of the most used measures of the fractal dimension, and one of the chaotic characteristics which allows to define the dimension of an attractor and shows the existence of the self-similarity [23]. The correlation dimension, $C_2(l)$, represents the probability that the distance between two arbitrary points x_i and x_j of the reconstructed space will be l.

$$C_2(l) \cong l^{d_F}. \qquad (2)$$

The correlation dimension is given by the saturation value of the slopes of the curves for an increasing embedding dimension. If there is no saturation of the slopes, and they keep increasing with the increasing of the embedding dimension, then the system is stochastic.

2.3 Embedding Dimension

The embedding is a mapping from one dimensional space to a m-dimensional space and is based on the principle that all the variables of a dynamical system influence one another. In conformity with the theorem of Takens, a map exists between the original state space and a reconstructed state space and the dynamical properties of the system in the true state space are preserved under the embedding transformation, [32]. One of the most used method for measuring the minimal embedding dimension is introduced by Kennel et al. [33] and it is called the false nearest neighbor (FNN) method. The main idea of the method is to unfold the observed orbits from self overlap arising from the projection of an attractor of a dynamical system on a lower dimensional space [34]. To properly reconstruct the chaotic flow, a minimum dimensionality is needed and this is marked by a vanishing fraction of FNN [35]. If two nearest neighbors are nearest neighbors in the d_i dimension, but they are not in the d_{i+1} dimension they are called false nearest neighbors [2, 23, 35]. The value where the percentage of false nearest neighbors approaches zero is chosen as d_E value [23, 26, 35]. The local dimension of the dynamics determinated by the local FNN method shows how many dimensions can be used to model the dynamics of the studied system.

2.4 Lyapunov Exponents

Lyapunov exponents are used to distinguish the chaotic and non-chaotic behavior because they exhibit the rate of divergence or convergence of the nearby trajectories from each other in state space [26], providing a measure of the system sensitivity to its initial conditions. For a 3-dimensional state space there will be an exponent for each dimension: all negative exponents will indicate the presence of a fixed point; one zero and the other negative indicate a limit cycle; one positive indicate a chaotic attractor [23]. If the system has more than one positive Lyapunov exponent, the magnitude of the LLE indicates the maximum amount of instability in any direction in the attractor. Therefore, in order to characterize the behavior of a dynamical system, the sign of LE must be determined. The value of the LLE is expressed in bits of information/second and it is the main exponent that quantifies the exponential divergence of the neighboring trajectories in the reconstructed state space and reflects the degree of chaos in the system. The obtained information is necessary to identify the stability of the time series.

3 Experimental Study

The experimental method which allows obtaining the kinematic parameters diagrams for the human knee joint uses a data acquisition system based on electrogoniometers [7]. The electrogoniometer is made of one potentiometer and two rods; one of them is fixed on the longitudinal axis of femur bone, while the other is fixed on the longitudinal axis of the tibia. The rods are fixed with elastic straps, type Velcro. The acquisition data and control board Arduino Mega 2560 has the role of acquisition data from the potentiometer and it stocks up this data in files data which will be processed. In the command board it is upload the code written in C/C++ which returns the angular values function of time [7]. The board and the computer are interconnected by serial interface and the acquisition data series are displayed on the monitor. The block schema of the acquisition data system based on a electrogoniometer is presented in Fig. 1.

In Fig. 2 the data acquisition system mounted on the subject is shown. Measurements were performed on a sample of 7 healthy subjects and on a sample of 3 patients who suffer of knee osteoarthritis. The experimental data for healthy subjects were acquired for walking cycles of the right knee on plane treadmill (TM 0) and on inclined treadmill at 10° (TM 10). They were pain-free and had no evidence or known history of motor and skeletal disorders or record of surgery to the lower limbs. For healthy persons the experimental tests were approved by the University of Craiova human ethics research committee and they were performed in the biomechanics laboratory at the Faculty of Mechanics, University of Craiova.

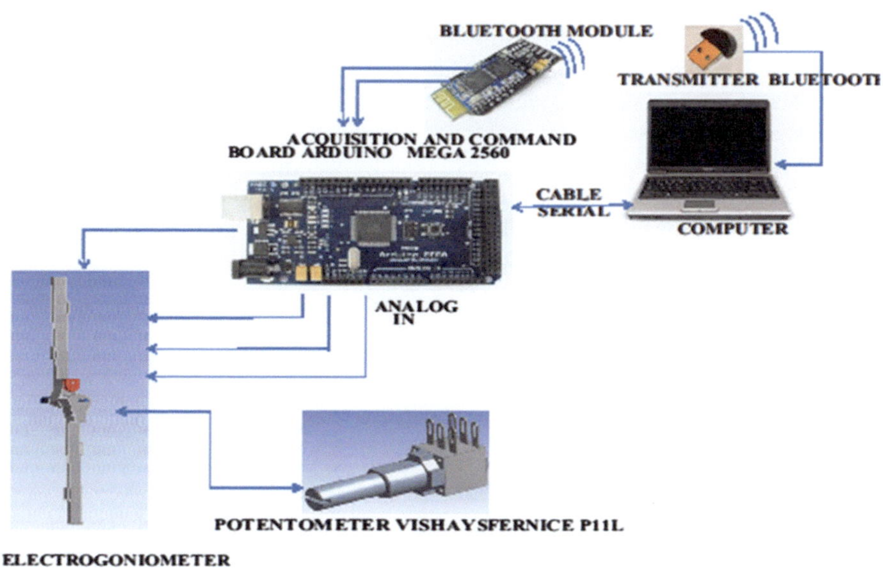

Fig. 1 Block schema of the acquisition data system based on electrogoniometer

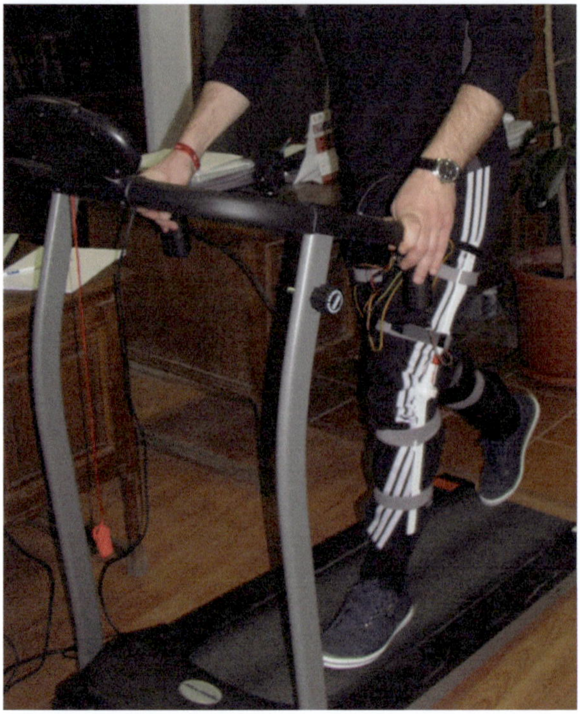

Fig. 2 Subject with data acquisition system

The patient group was evaluated in second stage knee osteoarthritis. Before starting the experiments there were collected anthropometric data both from healthy subjects and from subjects with osteoarthritis.

In Table 1 and Table 2 the mean values and standard deviations for anthropometric data of healthy subjects and, respectively of patients are presented.

The healthy subjects execute two tests for which the experimental data were acquired for continuous walking cycles: Test 1—walking on the plane TM 0 for 3 min at a normal speed of 3.6 km/h; Test 2—walking on the inclined TM 10 for 3 min at a normal speed of 3.6 km/h. The suffering subjects performed only Test 1 in one recovery room of the Emergency Dolj Hospital.

Table 1 Healthy subjects—mean values and standard deviations of anthropometric data

Subject	Age (years)	Weight (kg)	Height (cm)	Leg length (cm)	Hip–knee length (cm)	Knee–ankle length (cm)
Average	31.57	77	174.71	85.286	45.28	40
St. dev.	4.27	6.63	4.27	6.5	4.75	1.91

Table 2 Patients group—mean values and standard deviations of anthropometric data

Patient	Age (years)	Weight (kg)	Height (cm)	Leg length (cm)	Hip–knee length (cm)	Knee–ankle length (cm)
Average	55.7	81	172.27	82.35	43.15	39.2
St. dev.	3.86	8.16	8.14	3.72	2.85	1.21

4 Results

The angular amplitudes of human knee flexion-extension during the gait on the treadmill were obtained for each test as data files. In the data analysis the beginning region and the end region of the time series were cut off in order to remove the transient data. In Fig. 3 the diagram of the knee flexion-extension angles Φ_1 for Test 1 and Φ_2 for Test 2, [degrees] in respect with time [s] for subject 1. The knee flexion-extension movements occur entirely within the normal range of motion according to normative data. The maximum amplitudes of the healthy subjects knees ranged from 57.38° to 69.01°. For patients, the maximum amplitudes ranged from 45.53° to 51.73° for the OA knees and from 50.86° to 64.23° for the healthy knees. The flexion angle during the gait cycle revealed differences between patients and healthy subjects. There were not big differences in the shape of the flexion angle. The patients had less range of motion during the gait cycle than the healthy subjects, their knees were on average less flexed throughout the gait cycle than the healthy subjects but, also, the healthy knees of the patients were on average less flexed than the knees of healthy subjects. This is explained by the influence of the

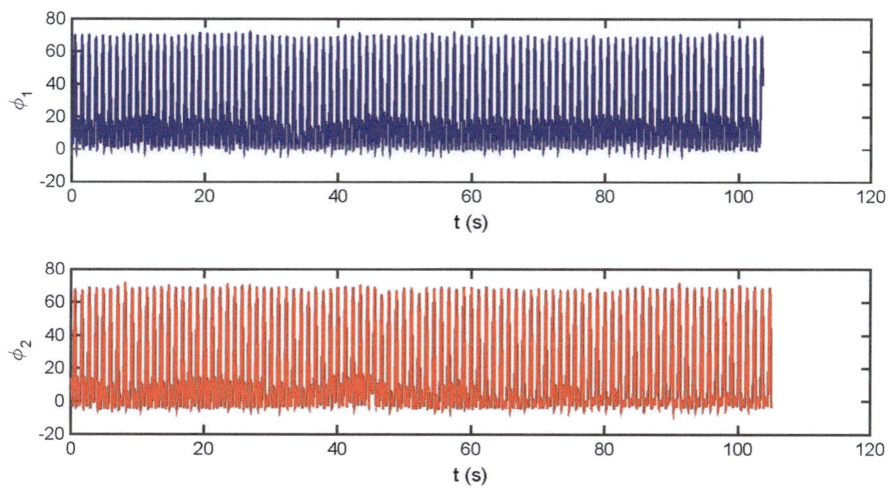

Fig. 3 Diagram of the knee flexion-extension angles Φ_1 [deg] for test 1 and Φ_2 [deg] for test 2 in respect with time [s] for subject 1

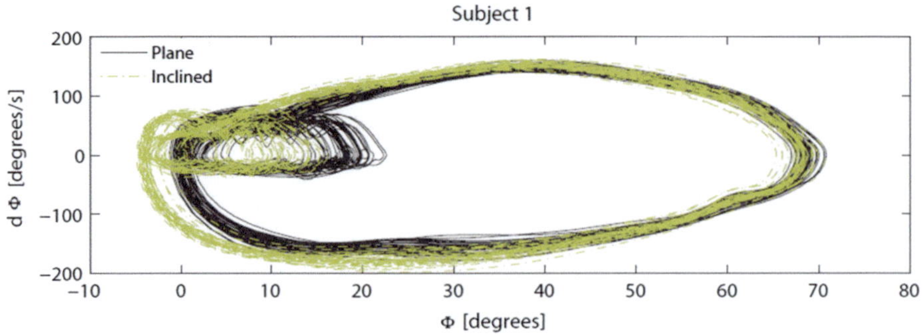

Fig. 4 Phase plane plots for both plane TM and for inclined TM for subject 1

OA knees pain and by body tendency of maintaining the stability when reaching the knee flexion amplitude.

In this study the human lower limb was considered as a nonlinear system that can achieve dynamic equilibrium. Standard plots in which the knee joint displacements are plotted against time do not provide sufficient information about the dynamics of the system. Phase plane portraits will be used to characterize the kinematics of the system when it attained this equilibrium. Using phase plane portraits one can correlate the joint rotations with the respective joint velocities.

The phase plane plot is a two-dimensional plot in which the time derivative $\phi^{\cdot}$ is plotted versus ϕ at each data point. The phase plane plots, shown in Fig. 4, contain information as the graph of data for both tests for subject 1. For all other subjects, the phase plane plots are similar. The plots traced for plane treadmill show less divergence in their trajectories, while the trajectories obtained for inclined treadmill at 10° are confined within a tighter space. The phase plane curves are more compact for walking on TM 0 than for walking on TM 10.

Phase plane portraits can be utilized to compare the joint kinematics of clinical patients with normal subjects or to compare the joint kinematics for plane walking versus inclined walking, and, also to differentiate the variations among the groups. In Fig. 5 the phase plane portraits for both knees of patient 1 are shown. For all patients, the right knee is the pathological one and the left knee is the normal one.

A comparison of phase plane portraits of Patient 1 versus Subject 1 (Fig. 6) show us evident differences between the angular amplitudes and between the gradients values. Comparing the four phase-plane graphics, it can be seen that for healthy subject the cycles curves of both tests are more compact and their spread is decreasing, while the plots traced for patient show more divergence in their trajectories. So at normal speed the amplitude of consecutive steps tend to be constant, while in the case of patient's kneees the amplitude varies. It can be seen that the phase planes are almost concentric curves, inside is the curve corresponding to the osteoarthritic knee, and outside are the curves corresponding to the healthy subject.

Similar comparatives curves of phase plane portraits are obtained for all seven subjects and for all three patients. Traditional measures of variability, which only

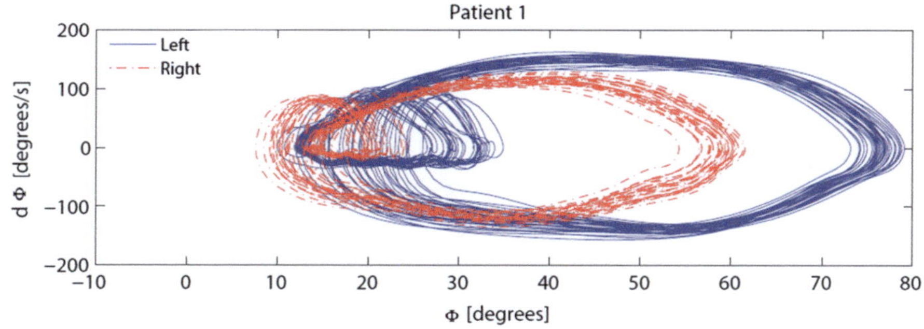

Fig. 5 Phase plane plots for both knees of patient 1

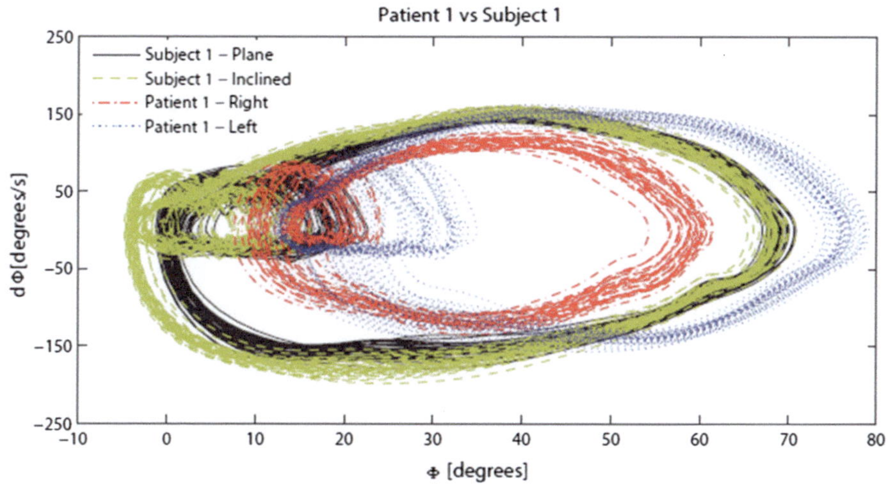

Fig. 6 Phase plane plots for patient 1 versus subject 1

provide estimates of the average magnitude of variations across strides, are therefore insufficient to characterize the local dynamic stability properties of locomotor behavior.

To characterize the underlying complexity during movement, the experimental data are analyzed using the LE and correlation dimensions of angular amplitude in the human knee joint as a measure of the stability of a dynamical system.

The time delays were calculated for each of the 20 data set (2 tests for 7 subjects and 2 knee, same test for 3 patients) from the first minimum of the Average Mutual Information (AMI) function [23, 26]. The adopted value for time delay is equal to 8.

A suitable embedding dimension was chosen by using the false nearest neighbour (FNN) method [23, 26]. Embedding dimension is the minimum value that trajectories of the reconstructed state vector may not cross over each other in state space. Total percentage of false neighbours for the human knee joint was computed

Fig. 7 Embedding dimension chosen by using the false nearest neighbor (FNN) method

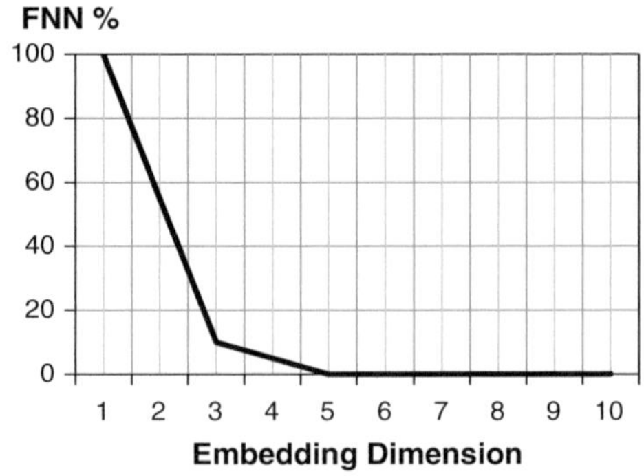

by FNN method and the number of dimensions was chosen where this percentage approaches zero. The results were similar for all time series collected for both tests and for all subjects and patients and indicated an appropriate embedding dimension of $d_E = 5$ (Fig. 7).

Using Chaos Data Analyzer (CDA) software, we calculated Mean Correlation Dimension for each time series obtained in the both experimental tests. This values are presented in Table 3 and, respectively, in Table 4. As we can see, the correlation dimensions were increasing, the higher the dimension D becomes and, also, they increase in the case of inclined treadmill comparing with plane treadmill walking. The values of correlation dimension were the similar with results obtained by other researchers in their nonlinear dynamics studies applied at human joints movements [2, 12].

For test 1, graphics of correlation dimension values in respect with embedding dimension D (Fig. 8a) for each subject and, respectively, in respect with all subjects for each embedding dimension D (Fig. 8b) are presented.

We calculated the LLE values for all time series using special software to analyze nonlinear time series data, Chaos Data Analyzer, based on the method by Wolf et al. [27]. The value of the LLE is the main exponent that quantifies and reflects the degree of chaos in the system. If the system is known to be deterministic, a positive Lyapunov number can be taken as proof of a chaotic system. The LLE calculated for all time series were positive, so we can conclude that the

Table 3 Mean correlation dimension test 1—walking on plane treadmill

	D = 3	D = 4	D = 5	D = 6	D = 7	D = 8	D = 9	D = 10
Sub.1	2.043	2.178	2.219	2.43	2.515	2.560	2.596	2.765
Sub.2	1.968	1.983	2.056	2.069	2.175	2.156	2.232	2.305
Sub.3	1.957	1.973	2.023	2.056	2.240	2.352	2.398	2.461
Sub.4	2.048	2.218	2.299	2.454	2.590	2.657	2.645	2.752
Sub.5	1.966	2.009	2.043	2.162	2.152	2.245	2.262	2.283
Sub.6	1.995	2.138	2.319	2.457	2.546	2.619	2.646	2.848
Sub.7	1.961	2.102	2.278	2.405	2.500	2.572	2.618	2.837

Table 4 Mean correlation dimension test 1—walking on inclined treadmill

	D = 3	D = 4	D = 5	D = 6	D = 7	D = 8	D = 9	D = 10
Sub.1	2.134	2.297	2.338	2.459	2.547	2.593	2.619	2.788
Sub.2	2.055	2.277	2.405	2.601	2.646	2.918	3.023	3.024
Sub.3	1.981	2.105	2.159	2.394	2.353	2.408	2.602	2.625
Sub.4	2.186	2.402	2.503	2.805	2.782	2.819	2.903	3.093
Sub.5	1.986	2.123	2.323	2.398	2.417	2.378	2.396	2.542
Sub.6	2.111	2.29	2.397	2.479	2.572	2.765	2.783	2.909
Sub.7	1.996	2.138	2.284	2.434	2.529	2.589	2.658	2.737

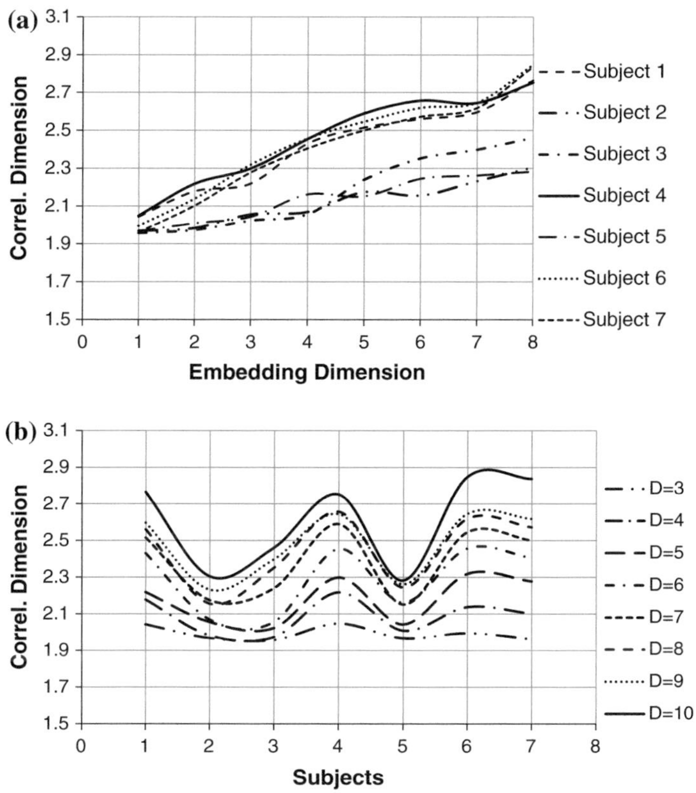

Fig. 8 **a** Graphics of correlation dimension values in respect with embedding dimension D for each subject; **b** Graphics of correlation dimension in respect with all subjects for each D (test1)

time series of amplitude of the human knee joint movement were chaos and the human lower limb is a deterministic chaotic system. In Table 5 and Table 6 the LLE values of both tests of healthy subjects and, respectively, of both knees of patients group, are presented. The values are given in units of bits per data sample. The

Table 5 Largest Lyapunov exponent values for healthy subjects

	Sub1	Sub2	Sub3	Sub4	Sub5	Sub6	Sub7
TM 0	0.047	0.078	0.049	0.057	0.042	0.058	0.055
TM 10	0.048	0.082	0.056	0.06	0.047	0.058	0.06

Table 6 Largest Lyapunov exponent values for patients

	Sub1	Sub2	Sub3
Left	0.132	0.098	0.108
Right	0.163	0.131	0.157

existence of the positive Lyapunov exponent indicates that the time series of the movement amplitude has instability. The results are similar with those obtained by other researchers in their nonlinear dynamics studies applied at human joints movements [2, 18].

In Fig. 9 we can see that the LLE values are smaller on the plane treadmill (the range values is 0.047–0.078) than on the inclined treadmill for healthy subjects (the range values is 0.047–0.082). One of the explanations could be that the effects of the inclined plane on the variability are more pronounced than in the situation of plane walking. The LLE values are bigger for the normal knees of the patients and much bigger for osteoarthritic knees. The LLE values are comprised between 0.098 and 0.132 for normal knees and, respectively, between 0.131 and 0.163 for osteoarthritic knees (Fig. 9) . Larger values of LLEs obtained for normal knees of patients are explained by the influence of the osteoarthritic knees pain and instability.

Larger values of LLEs obtained for patient's knees are associated with more divergence, a decrease of local stability and increase of knee flexion variability, more sensitivity to perturbations, while smaller values obtained for plane treadmill of healthy subjects reflect a local stability, less divergence and variability, less sensitivity to perturbations and higher resistance to stride-to-stride variability.

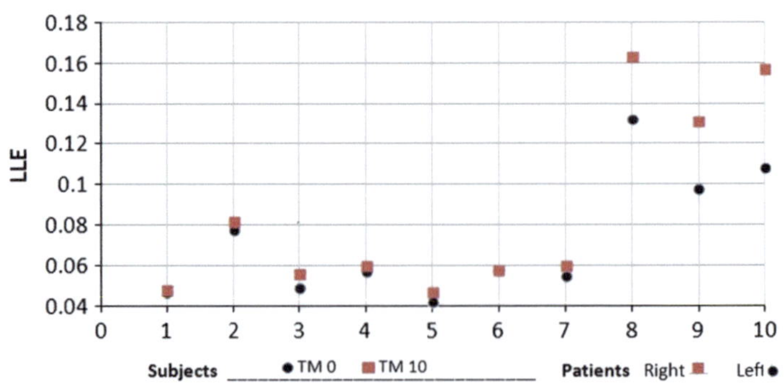

Fig. 9 LLE values of healthy subjects and of patients

5 Conclusions

A study based on the tools of nonlinear dynamics to visualize the steady state kinematics of human knee movement is presented. The kinematic data of the flexion extension angles for two tests of human knee joint motion were analyzed. The purpose of this study was to investigate the spatio-temporal characteristics, the biomechanics of chaotic characteristics of movements of the knee joint. We applied the chaotic analysis to the rhythmic flexion-extension movements of human knee joint and showed that there existed the chaotic feature of angle positions using the chaotic measure such as the largest Lyapunov exponent and the correlation dimension. The LLE obtained for each test of human knee joint were positive values which suggest that human knee motions show chaotic characteristics. In this paper, the LLEs represent measures of the exponential divergence from trajectories in the state space domain reconstructed from knee motions in the time domain. The mean LLE values for healthy human knee joints ranged from 0.042 to 0.082, while for the osteoarthritic knees of patients LLE values ranged from 0.131 to 0.163. Larger values of LLEs obtained for patients are associated with more divergence and increase of knee flexion variability, while smaller values obtained by healthy group for plane treadmill walking and inclined treadmill walking reflect a local stability, less divergence and variability, less sensitivity to perturbations and higher resistance to stride-to-stride variability.

The flexion-extension movement of the human knee during the locomotion presents interest for the kinematic and dynamic study of the bipedal locomotion applied to humanoid robots. The results obtained can be used as a reference for the normal knee joint movement for further studies of abnormal movement. The results can show the potential of the Lyapunov exponents used to measure the balance control of human walking, an important aspect in the development of bipedal walking machines.

It is difficult to make conclusions about the underlying source of the positive LLEs, but an important purpose in the research of human joint kinematics is to investigate the nature and origin of differences in variability characteristics and to understand the underlying process that controls their variability [15]. The use of nonlinear tools may provide additional insight on the nature of the step-to-step fluctuations present in human and robotic locomotion. The results of this study can be used in the medical field to develop new artificial devices that could reproduce the motion of the lower limb, in robotics for humanoid robots which movements are inspired by human movement or as educational robot in order to study the complex process of locomotion.

References

1. Hausdorff, J.M., Rios, D.A., Edelberg, H.K.: Gait variability and fall risk in community-living older adults: a 1-year prospective study. Arch. Phys. Med. Rehabil. **82**(8), 1050–1056 (2001)
2. Dingwell, J.B., Cusumano, J.P., Cavanagh, P.R., Sternad, D.: Local dynamic stability versus kinematic variability of continuous overground and treadmill walking. J. Biomech. Eng. **123** (1), 27–32 (2001)
3. Hausdorff, J.M.: Gait dynamics, fractals and falls: finding meaning in the stride to-stride fluctuations of human walking. Hum. Mov. Sci. **26**(4), 555–589 (2007)
4. Menz, H.B., Lord, S.R., et al.: Age-related differences in walking stability. Age Ageing **32**(2), 137–142 (2003)
5. Owings, T.M., Grabiner, M.D.: Variability of step kinematics in young and older adults. Gait Posture **20**(1), 26–29 (2004)
6. Plitea, N., Pisla, D., et.al: On the kinematics of a new parallel robot for brachytherapy. Proc. Rom. Acad. Ser. A: Math. Phys. Tech. Sci. Inf. Sci. **15**(4), 354–361 (2014)
7. Tarnita, D., Marghitu, D.: Analysis of a hand arm system. Robot. Comput.-Integr. Manuf. **29** (6), 493–501 (2013)
8. Pisla, D., Szilaghyi, A., Vaida, C., Plitea, N.: Kinematics and workspace modeling of a new hybrid robot used in minimally invasive surgery. Robot. Comput.-Integr. Manuf. **29**(2), 463–474 (2013)
9. Ottaviano, E., et al.: An experimental evaluation of human walking. In: International Congress Design and Modelling of Mechanical Systems, Hammamet, 16–18 Mar 2009
10. Winter, D.A.: Biomechanical motor patterns in normal walking. J. Mot. Behav. **15**(4), 302–330 (1983)
11. Moe-Nilssen, R., Helbostad, J.L.: Interstride trunk acceleration variability but not step width variability can differentiate between fit and frail older adults. Gait Posture **21**(2), 164–170 (2005)
12. Dingwell, J.B., Marin, L.C.: Kinematic variability and local dynamic stability of upper body motions when walking at different speeds. J. Biomech. **39**(3), 444–452 (2006)
13. Jordan, K., Challis, J.H., et al.: Walking speed influences on gait cycle variability. Gait Posture (2006). doi:10.1016/j.gaitpost.2006.08.010
14. Oberg, T., Karsznia, A., et al.: Joint angle parameters in gait: reference data for normal subjects, 10–79 years of age. J. Rehab. Res. Develop. **31**(3), 199–213 (1994)
15. Terrier, Ph, Dériaz, O.: Kinematic variability, fractal dynamics and local dynamic stability of treadmill walking. J. NeuroEngineering Rehabil. **8**, 1–13 (2011)
16. Winter, D.A.: The Biomechanics and Motor Control of Human Gait: Normal, Elderly and Pathological, 2nd edn. Waterloo, Canada (1991)
17. Davis, R., Ounpuu, S., Tyburski, D., Gage, J.: A gait analysis data collection and reduction technique. Hum. Mov. Sci. **10**, 575–587 (1991)
18. Tarnita, D., Catana, M., Tarnita, D.N.: Nonlinear analysis of normal human gait for different activities with application to bipedal locomotion. Ro. J. Tech. Sci. Appl. Mech. **58**(1–2), 177–192 (2013)
19. Kawamura, K., Tokuhiro, A., Takechi, H.: Gait analysis of slope walking: a study of step length, stride width, time factors and deviation in the centre of pressure. Acta Med. Okayama **45**(3), 179–184 (1991)
20. Leroux, A., Fung, J., Barbeau, H.: Postural adaptation to walking on inclined surfaces: I. Normal strategies. Gait Posture **15**(1), 64–74 (2002)
21. Sun, J., Walters, M., Svensson, N., Lloyd, D.: The influence of surface slope on human gait characteristics: a study of urban pedestrians walking on an inclined surface. Ergonomics **39**(4), 677–692 (1996)
22. Kang, H.G.: Kinematic and motor variability and stability during gait: effects of age, walking speed and segment height, Doctoral Thesis, The University of Texas, Dec 2007

23. Dingwell, J.B., Cusumano, J.P.: Nonlinear time series analysis of normal and pathological human walking. Chaos **10**, 848–863 (2000)
24. Yang, C., Wu, Q.: On Stabilization of bipedal robots during disturbed standing using the concept of Lyapunov exponents. Robotica **24**(5), 621–624 (2006)
25. Han, J., Moussavi, Z.: Application of nonlinear dynamics to human postural control system. Eng. Med. Biol. Soc. Conf. Shanghai, 1–4 Sept 2005
26. Abarbanel, H.D.: Analysis of Observed Chaotic Data. Springer, New York, Inc. (1996)
27. Wolf, A., Swift, J., Swinney, H., Vastano, J.: Determining Lyapunov exponents from a time series. Physica **16D** (1995)
28. Nehmzow, U., Walker, K.: Quantitative description of robot-environment interaction using chaos theory. In: Proceedings of ECMR 03, Warsaw (2003)
29. Small, M., Tse, C.: Applying the method of surrogate data to cyclic time series. Physica D **164**, 187–201 (2002)
30. Packard, N.H., Crutchfield, J.P., et al.: Geometry from a time series. Phys. Rev. Lett. **45**, 712–716 (1980)
31. Nayfeh, A.H.: Introduction to Perturbation Techniques. Wiley-Interscience, NY (1981)
32. Takens, F.: Detecting strange attractors in turbulence. In: Rand, D.A., Young, L.S. (eds.) Lecture Notes in Mathematics, vol. 898, pp. 366–381 (1981)
33. Kennel, M.B., Brown, R., Abarbanel, H.D.I.: Determining embedding dimension for phase space reconstruction using a geometrical construction. Phys. Rev. A **45**, 3403–3411 (1992)
34. Perc, M.: The dynamics of human gait. Eur. J. Phys. **26**, 525–530 (2005)
35. Boccaletti, S., Valladares, et al.: Reconstructing embedding spaces of coupled dynamical systems from multivariate data. Phys. Rev. E **65**(035204(R)), 1–4 (2002)

Training of Robot to Assigned Geometric and Force Trajectories

A. Leskov, V. Golovin, M. Arkhipov and L. Kocherevskaya

Abstract The features of training by demonstration in robotics for restorative medicine are considered in the article. They are caused by the fact that during training the robot interacts with patient's soft tissue. The regime of training by demonstration is more natural for physician than training of force points using the manual by physician. Also the training by demonstration is more precise method of input of assigned geometric and force trajectories.

Keywords Force trained points · Training by demonstration · Force sensors · Soft tissue deforming · Geometric and force trajectories

1 Introduction

Position/force control is necessary for some procedures of restorative medicine robotics. They are various massage movements of extremities in joints [1, 6] and ultrasonic diagnostics. Kernel of these science works is robot mechanical noninvasive interaction with living, biological, viscous elastic, nonlinear soft tissue [4]. The soft tissue elasticity and thickness of every patient can not be determined beforehand.

It is necessary to solve the following tasks of control:

A. Leskov (✉)
Bauman Moscow State Technical University, Moscow, Russia
e-mail: medicalrobot973@gmail.com

V. Golovin · M. Arkhipov
Moscow State Industrial University, Moscow, Russia
e-mail: medicalrobot@mail.ru

L. Kocherevskaya
National University of Science and Technology MISIS, Moscow, Russia

P. Wenger et al. (eds.), *New Trends in Medical and Service Robots*,
Mechanisms and Machine Science 39, DOI 10.1007/978-3-319-30674-2_6

- to generate and to remember set of points characterizing form and state of soft tissues,
- to perform the manipulations on soft tissues using training points,
- to change manipulations kind to achieve necessary patient's psychological state.

The noninvasive mechanical influences at position/force control are used to solve the first problems.

The position/force aim is the following [1, 4, 11, 12]:

$$\mathrm{X}(t) \rightarrow X_0(t) \text{ and } F(t) \rightarrow F_0(t), \tag{1}$$

where $\boldsymbol{X}_0(t)$ and $\boldsymbol{F}_0(t)$ are assigned geometric and force trajectories, $\boldsymbol{X}(t)$ and $\boldsymbol{F}(t)$ are real geometric and force trajectories. At the same time the following equation is performed on a given trajectory:

$$\mathbf{F}_0(t) = f(\mathbf{X}_0(t)). \tag{2}$$

Further the various input methods in robot $\boldsymbol{X}_0$ (t) and $\boldsymbol{F}_0$(t), namely, training methods will be considered.

In the second section the special case of robot training by showing along tool axis for force point getting is considered, in the third and fourth sections the general spatial case of training is given.

2 Training with the Help of Force Points

The values of $X_0(t)$ and $F_0(t)$ can be introduced by separate points and then the interpolation will be performed. They can be force trained points A_i which contain geometric and force information about the interaction of robot tool and soft tissue.

$$A_i = (x, y, z, o, a, t, F_z), \tag{3}$$

where x, y, z are geometric coordinates of robot tool position; o, a, t are geometric coordinates of robot tool orientation; F_z is component of force of the interaction of robot tool and soft tissue [3].

The set of points A_i can be determined experimentally using movement of robot tool by manual or joystick. The block diagram of system of force points training is given on Fig. 1. The system contains drive with inner position feedback. The F'_{z0} is force assigned along robot tool axis in direction normal to the body surface.

The following notations are introduced in Fig. 1: $q(t)$ is n-dimensional vector of generalized robot coordinates; $F_r(t)$ is n-dimensional vector of forces (moments) generated by the robot drives; $F(t)$ is m-dimensional vector of generalized forces acting on end-effector from environment; $J(q)$ is m × n Jacobian matrix; $f(q)$ and

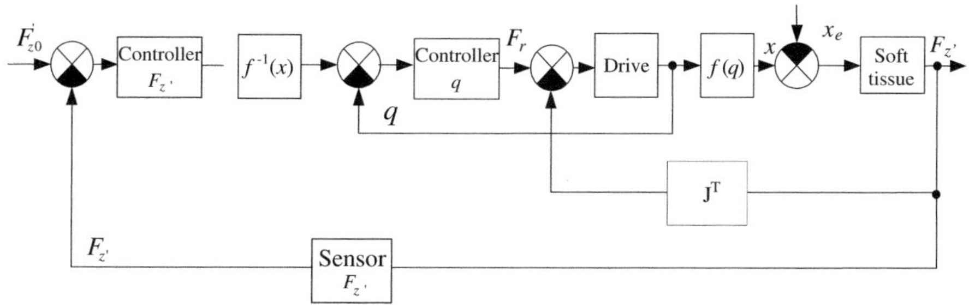

Fig. 1 Block diagram of system of force points training

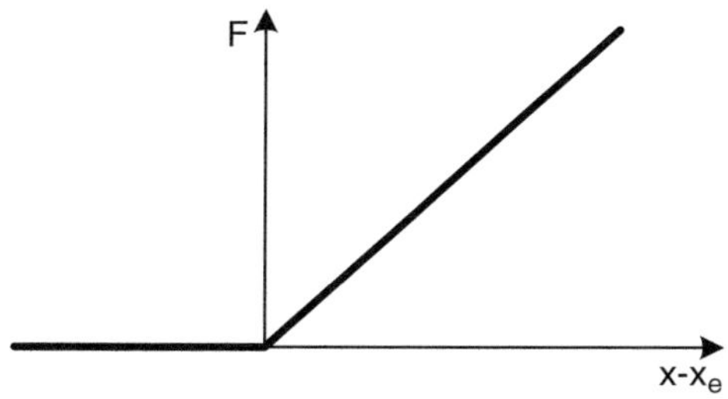

Fig. 2 The static characteristic of soft tissue and robot tool interaction

$f^{-1}(x)$ are the coordinate transformations in direct and inverse kinematic task; $x(t)$ is vector of aim coordinates and $x_e(t)$ is vector of soft tissue relief.

If robot tool does not touch the soft tissue and robot moves in free space then force $F = 0$ (Fig. 2).

The conditions of approaching to assigned forces are shown below.

$$\begin{gathered}\text{if } F_{Z'} \le F_{Z'0} - \Delta F \text{ then } \Delta z'_{i+1} = \Delta, \\ \text{if } F_{z'0} - \Delta F < F_{z'} < F_{z'0} + \Delta F \text{ then } \Delta z'_{i+1} = 0, \\ \text{if } F_Z \ge F_{Z0} + \Delta F \text{ then } \Delta z'_{i+1} = -\Delta,\end{gathered} \tag{4}$$

where ΔF is deviation from assigned force; Δ is step of moving in tool axis direction.

As in this scheme the moving in tool axis direction is step by step then big steps for rapid motion cause significant force errors. In the Fig. 3 the force caused by discreteness of moving along patient's spine long muscles are shown. The assigned force is equal to 15 N.

Similar experiments were performed on patient's spine long muscles at two back-forward movements. The force curve $F(t)$ for the points trained with step of 0.5 mm and the curve of displacement deviations $\xi(t)$ are resulted on Fig. 4.

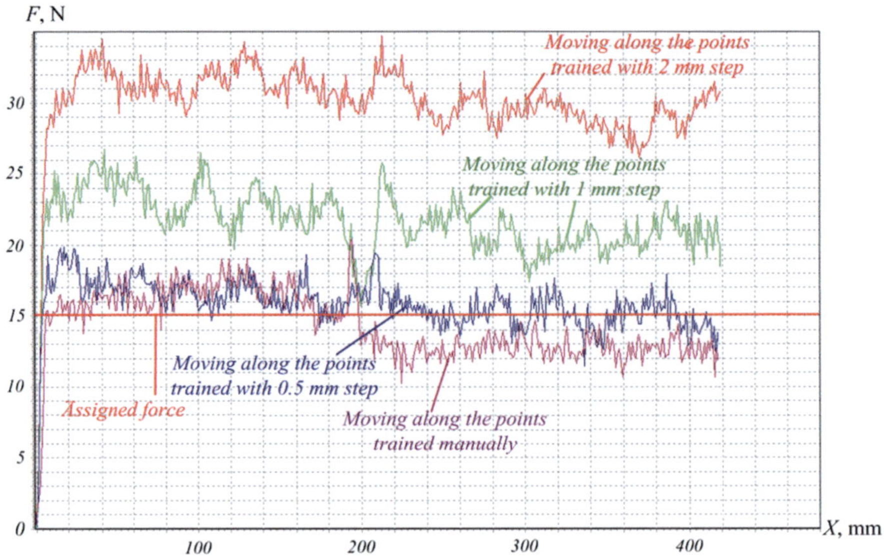

Fig. 3 Curves $F(t)$ arising at passage of points trained with various steps

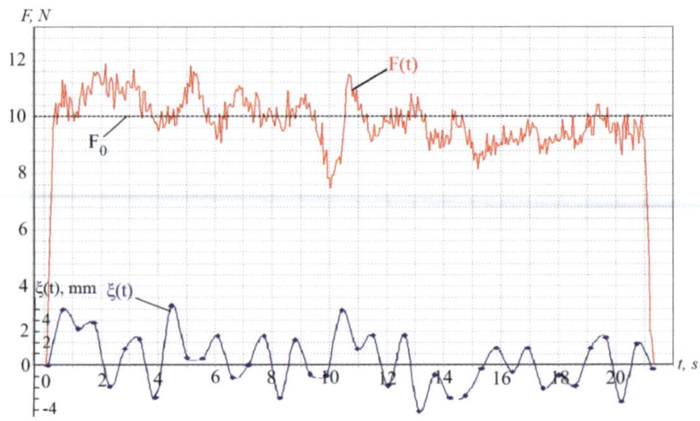

Fig. 4 Curves of $F(t)$ and $\xi(t)$ obtained at passage along patient's long muscles

3 Training by Demonstration

There is another method of obtaining of set of points A_i by demonstration in view of soft tissue deforming [5]. If it is training of geometric points without forces then it is known as training by showing when operator holding robot tool by his hand moves robot in free space [7]. Firstly this is training of paint robots. The experienced house painter moves airbrush by his hand. The special springs help to be unloaded from links weight. The trajectory of hand moving is written and then it is repeated.

Now there are unloading by program methods with using force information. But in contrast to geometric training the robot interacts with environment causing soft tissue force reaction.

The differential equation of robot interacting with soft tissue and masseur's hand has the following form:

$$H(\mathbf{q})\,\ddot{\mathbf{q}} + \mathbf{h}(\mathbf{q},\dot{\mathbf{q}}) + \mathbf{C}(\mathbf{q}) = \mathbf{F}_r + J^T(\mathbf{q})\mathbf{F}_e, \tag{5}$$

where $H(\mathbf{q}) \in R^{n\times n}$ is matrix of manipulation inertia, $\mathbf{h}(\mathbf{q},\dot{\mathbf{q}}) \in R^n$ is nonlinear function of centrifugal and Coriolis' forces (moments), $\mathbf{C}(\mathbf{q}) \in R^n$ is nonlinear function of gravitational forces (moments), $\mathbf{F}_e \in R^m$ is vector of generalized forces (moments) acting on end-effector from environment.

The mode of slow and smooth massage movements can be approximated to the static one. Then we have:

$$H(\mathbf{q})\,\ddot{\mathbf{q}} = \mathbf{h}(\mathbf{q},\dot{\mathbf{q}}) = 0, \tag{6}$$

$$\mathbf{C}(\mathbf{q}) = \mathbf{F}_r + J^T(\mathbf{q})\mathbf{F}_e, \tag{7}$$

$$\mathbf{F}_e = \mathbf{F}_0 - \mathbf{F}, \tag{8}$$

where F_0 is vector of forces (moments) from operator's hand.

Finally we have:

$$\mathbf{C}(\mathbf{q}) - J^T(\mathbf{q})(\mathbf{F}_0 - \mathbf{F}) = \mathbf{F}_r, \tag{9}$$

where F_r is vector of force (moment) made by robot drives. The forces (moments) acting on robot end-effector are shown on Fig. 5 and scheme of training by demonstration in view of soft tissue deforming is given on Fig. 6.

On Fig. 5 T_1 is vector of forces (moments) measured by upper force sensor, T_2 is vector of forces (moments) measured by lower force sensor.

This system is similar to system of training of force points, but in system of training of force points the force is given by program and in system of training by demonstration the force is given by operator's handle.

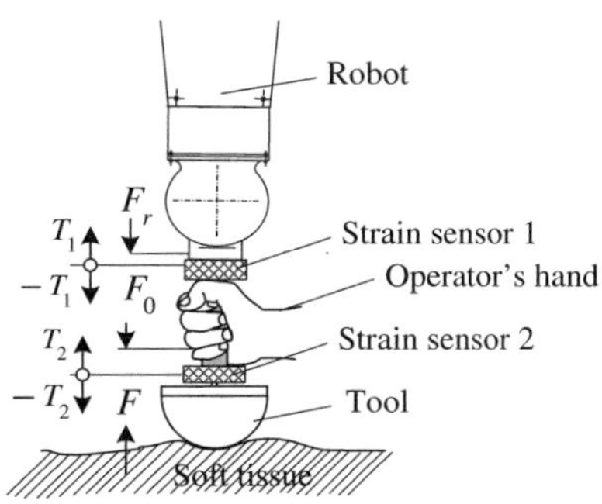

Fig. 5 The forces (moments) acting on robot end-effector

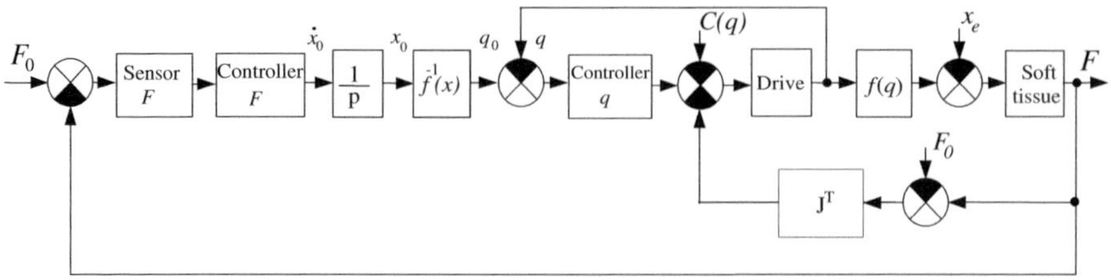

Fig. 6 Scheme of training by demonstration in view of soft tissue deforming

If the mass of robot end-effector is concentrated in tool, then the sensors placed above and below the operator's hands will measure various forces.

$$T_1 = F_r = F - F_0 - C(q), \tag{10}$$

$$T_2 = -F + C(q) = -F_0 - F_r \tag{11}$$

The upper sensor measuring force $T_1 \approx F - F_0$ is *sensor F* in system on Fig. 6. The lower sensor measuring force $T_2 \approx F - F_0$ can be used for visual observation of the force reaction of soft tissue.

During training the movements in robot joints are recorded from coders as separate training points or as continuous trajectory.

For realization of training by showing the force information from strain sensor located on robot hand isn't single. The force information can be obtained from joint force sensors and converted by Jacobian matrix how it's done in LWR Kuka robot. Also the force information can be obtained from joint drive currents.

4 The System of Training by Demonstration Using Measured Drives Currents for Calculation Soft Tissue Resistance Forces

The currents of robot drives include some information about load moments. On Fig. 7 the system of training by demonstration using measured drive currents for calculation soft tissue resistance forces is given. The block $(J^T)^{-1}(q)$ is necessary for

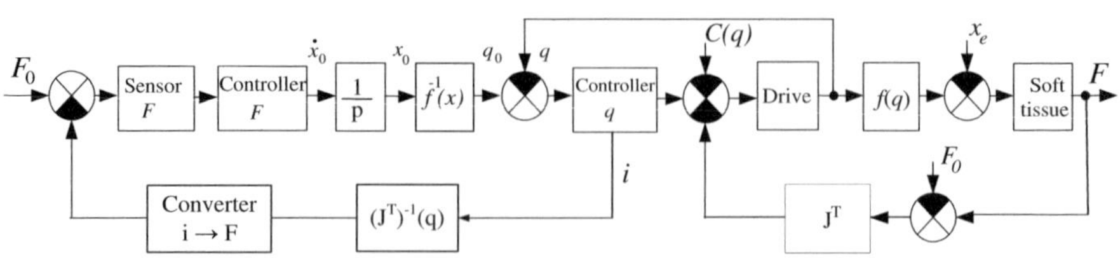

Fig. 7 Scheme of training by demonstration in view of soft tissue deforming using measured drive currents for calculation soft tissue resistance forces

transformation of measured drive currents in currents of aim coordinates system. Then these currents are transformed by converter in forces (moments).

The idea of using of measured drive currents for calculation soft tissue resistance forces is realized in UR5 and UR10 robots.

5 The Features of Training by Demonstration in View of Soft Tissues Deforming

The ideal massage is when masseur deforms patient's soft tissues by his sensitive hand. As to unload the robot action on masseur's hand completely is impossible then the training of masseur to perform massage techniques by robot tool with interfering robot is a must.

The training by demonstration is example of interaction of robot and human-operator in total working area when robot can work without enclosure. In robotics for restorative medicine the patient and robot interact in total working area also. In contrast to usual ergonomic scheme where robot performs manipulations with technical environment, in this case third component is human also [2]. The scheme of interaction between components of physician-operator, robot, patient is presented in Fig. 8. New connections appear in this three-component system.

The possible connections between components and modes are the following: 1—command control signals from a physician for change of modes and procedure parameters, including training mode; 2—use by the physician of the data, received in the previous sessions and knowledge base replenishment (system Medsoft); 3—psychological influence of the physician on the patient; 4—manual execution of procedure by the physician (solo or with a robot); 5—signals of subjective patient's state transmitted to the physician including verbal feedback; 6—assigned values of forces, movements, velocities for position/force control and nominal date for biotechnical control; 7—signals of real state of soft tissues for position/force control; 8—signals of real state of soft tissues for biotechnical control; 9—signals of individual robot control from patient, 10—robot action on patient.

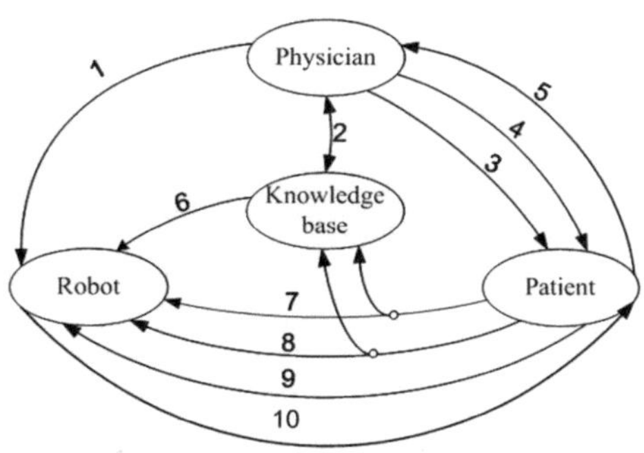

Fig. 8 Scheme of interaction between components of physician-operator system, robot, patient

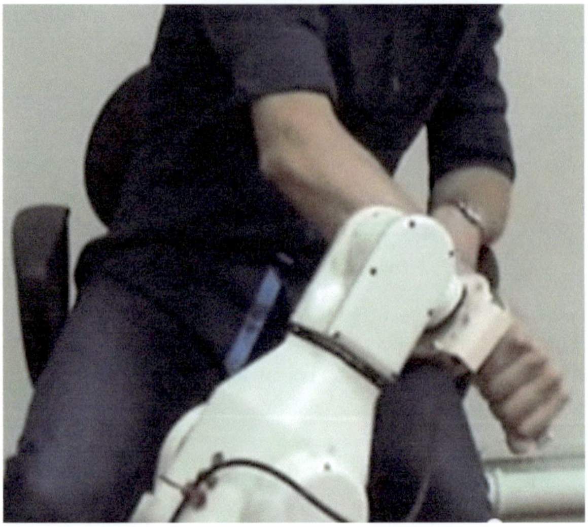

Fig. 9 The training of Kawasaki FS-003 N robot by demonstration with using six-component train sensor

The influences, signals and modes given on the scheme form several control counters: automatic position/force control (6 + 7 + 10), automatic biotechnical control (6 + 8 + 10), command control (1 + 2 + 10), manual performing of procedure (4 + 5), mutual performance of procedure by physician and robot (1 + 2 + 3 + 4 + 5 + 6 + 7 + 8 + 9 + 10), individual robot control from patient (9 + 10).

The last mode of individual robot control from patient is similar robot training by operator [10].

The training of Kawasaki FS-003 N robot by demonstration with using six-component strain sensor is shown in Fig. 9. The general form of six-component strain sensor Schunk FTD-Delta SI-330-30 using for training by demonstration and controller is given in Fig. 10.

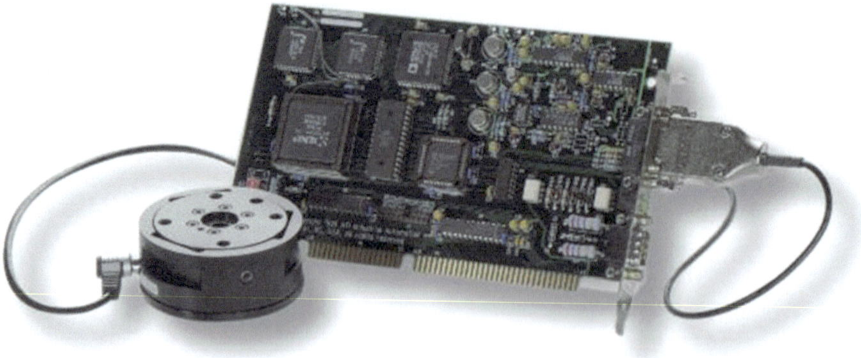

Fig. 10 Six-component strain sensor Schunk FTD-Delta SI-330-30 and controller

New relations between the robot and the person arise not only in a medical robotics. In non-structured environments and extreme situations, the robot should be not "stupid" but the intellectual assistant to the person. There are problems of equality in rights of interaction of the robot and the assembly worker on the conveyor, when in unscheduled situations, the assembly worker not only controls the robot but also he adapts to its work, providing both the friendly interface and his own safety. Mutual work of robot and operator is necessary in cosmos condition when the robot repeats the movements shown by operator or the operator controls robot perceiving the force interaction of robot with equipment [8, 9].

6 Conclusions

The training of separate force points has the benefit no requiring expensive six component strain sensor for force measurement. However it is slow training requiring large number of points.

The method of training by demonstration of moving in free space is known in industrial robotics for example for spray painting and arc welding. The method of training by demonstration with deformation of environment can be used for massage. It is more natural and quick method than the training of separate force points.

Both methods have significant drawback requiring immobility of the object on which manipulations are performed. This drawback can be excluded by using dynamic position/force control to correct object movements.

Acknowledgments The scientific work described in this paper was supported by Russian presidential grant № MK-2511.2014.

References

1. Golovin, V., Samorukov, A.: Massage method and device for its implementation, Russian Patent, № 2145833 (1998)
2. Golovin, V., Arhipov, M., Zhuravlev, V.: Ergatic and biotechnical control in medical robotics. J. Mechatron. Autom. Control **18**, 54–56 (2011)
3. Golovin, V., Arkhipov, M. Zhuravlev, V.: Force training for position/force control of massage robots. In: Mechanisms and Machine Science. New Trends in Medical and Service Robots. Springer International Publishing, Switzerland, pp. 95–109 (2014)
4. Golovin, V., Grib, A.: Mechatronic system for manual therapy and massage. In: Proceeding of 8th Mehatronics Forum International Conference, University of Twente, Netherlands (2002)
5. Golovin, V., Zhuravlev, V., Arkhipov, M.: Robotics in restorative medicine. In: Robots for mechanotherapy p. 280. LAP LAMBERT Academic Publishing, GmbH & Co. KG (2012)
6. Golovin, V.: Robot for massage. In: Proceedings of JARP, 2nd Workshop on Medical Robotics. Heidelberg, Germany (1997)
7. Grollman, D., Jenkins, O.: Can we learn finite state machine robot controllers from interactive demonstration? Studies in Computational Intelligence, vol. 264, pp. 407–430 (2010)

8. Kryuchkov, B., Kulakov, F., Karpov, A., Nechaev, A., Usov,V., Chernakova, S.: A way of integration of a robot-assistant in joint activities with cosmonauts by "Teaching by showing" method. Robot. Tech. Cybern. **2**(3) (2014)
9. Leskov, A., Illarionov, V., Zimin, A., Moroshkin, S., Kalevatykh, I.:Distance robotics learning using hybrid simulating testbed//REV2014. In: 11th International Conference on Remote Engineering and Virtual Instrumentation. Porto, pp. 225–226 (2014)
10. Medvedev, V., Leskov, A., Yushenko, A.: Control Systems of Manipulation Robots, p. 416. Science Publishing (1978)
11. Vukobratovic, M., Surdilovic, D., Ecalo Y. and Katic, D.: Dynamics and robust control of robot—environment interaction. In: Monograph series in the World scientific publishing under the title "New Frontiers in Robotics", p. 660. World Scientific Publishing Company (2009)
12. Vukobratovic, M.: Unified approach to control laws synthesis for robotic manipulators in contact with dynamic environment. In: IEEE International Conference on Robotics and Automation, p. 213–229, Atlanta, USA (1993)

Kinematic Analysis of an Innovative Medical Parallel Robot Using Study Parameters

Calin Vaida, Doina Pisla, Josef Schadlbauer, Manfred Husty and Nicolae Plitea

Abstract The paper investigates the kinematic analysis of an innovative 5-DOF parallel medical robot used for brachytherapy. Robotic assisted brachytherapy involves the targeted treatment of cancerous cells delivering high dosages of radiation inside the tumor, using as guiding tool a highly accurate robotic arm. The kinematic modeling of this mechanism is addressed using algebraic constraint varieties and the Study parametrization of the Euclidean displacement group. Algebraic methods in connection with classical multi-dimensional geometry have proven to be very efficient in the computation of direct and inverse kinematics of mechanisms as well as the explanation of strange, pathological behavior. The obtained results are simulated and compared with the results obtained by the evaluation of the determinants of the A and B Jacobi matrices. This complete kinematic analysis of the robot will largely increase its safety during the medical procedure.

Keywords Parallel robot · Kinematics · Study parameters · Singularities analysis · Brachytherapy

C. Vaida · D. Pisla (✉) · N. Plitea
CESTER, Technical University of Cluj-Napoca, Cluj-Napoca, Romania
e-mail: doina.pisla@mep.utcluj.ro

C. Vaida
e-mail: calin.vaida@mep.utcluj.ro

N. Plitea
e-mail: nicolae.plitea@mep.utcluj.ro

J. Schadlbauer · M. Husty
Unit for Geometry and CAD, University of Innsbruck, Innsbruck, Austria
e-mail: josef.schadlbauer@uibk.ac.at

M. Husty
e-mail: manfred.husty@uibk.ac.at

P. Wenger et al. (eds.), *New Trends in Medical and Service Robots*,
Mechanisms and Machine Science 39, DOI 10.1007/978-3-319-30674-2_7

1 Introduction

Cancer represents one of the main causes of death nowadays, due to a complex set of uncontrollable natural and artificial factors. Huge efforts have been made by the entire scientific community to provide better solutions and new techniques for the curative and palliative treatment of malignant tumors. In the recent years, studies have led to the development of the local, targeted treatment of cancer tumors, using a technique called brachytherapy (BT). This procedure involves the placement of tiny radioactive miniaturized sources very precisely in the tumor area, delivering high dosages of radiation in the cancerous cells. Its effectiveness is clearly demonstrated, its side effects are reduced to a minimum, but it involves an important condition: the catheters delivering the radioactive sources must be placed precisely as the radiation dose decreases abruptly from the base and incorrect positioning causes the necrosis of healthy tissue without affecting the tumor. Brachytherapy is commonly used as an effective treatment for cervical, prostate, breast, and skin cancer and can also be used to treat tumors in many other body sites [12]. Robot-assisted brachytherapy proves to be a necessity in order to: improve accuracy of the needle placement and seed delivery; improve the consistency of the seed implant; avoid critical healthy areas; reduce radiation exposure [8, 12]. All these aspects, along with the latest achievements in robotic brachytherapy are summarized in [8]. This study represents a report of the AAPM (American Association of Physicists in Medicine) which analyzes most robotic systems for brachytherapy and their development stage. The report points out that almost all systems target only the prostate (with one robot reported for lung brachytherapy) with only one being FDA approved. The same report [8] points out the importance and advantages of using robotic systems in brachytherapy along with the need of further development of this field to extent the application of this focused therapy to all areas of the body. H. Bassan et al. built a 5-DOF hybrid robotic system to perform 3D ultrasound guided percutaneous needle insertion surgery [1]. The macro stage is responsible for the orientation of the needle with a parallel mechanism and the micro stage for needle insertion and rotation. Yu et al. developed a 16 DOF robotic system, with 9 DOF for the positioning module and 7 for the surgery module, for prostate BT [14]. In [9] the same team developed another robotic system, entitled MIRAB designed for the simultaneous insertion of multiple needles. G. S. Fischer et al. introduced a 4-DOF hybrid robot for real-time control transperineal prostate needle orientation under MRI guidance [2]. Pisla et al. performed an overview study regarding the main innovative achievements regarding robotics systems for brachytherapy [4]. A team coordinated by prof. Plitea develops an innovative robotic structure for brachytherapy, entitled PARA-BRACHYROB, capable of targeting tumors located in any area of the thoraco-abdominal area of the body working with the real-time CT monitoring of the needle position [5, 6].

In this paper the authors will focus on the investigation of singularities of the PARA-BRACHYROB. The motivation for this research is given by the high level of safety the robot has to achieve, due to the intimate interaction with the human body. During the needle insertion procedure, the patient and the robot are located in the CT room without any assistant in their vicinity (due to radiation). The robot is teleoperated from a neighboring room, but any erroneous robot motion (e.g. caused by a singular configuration) must be avoided to ensure the patient safety.

It is possible to give a complete global description of the manipulators kinematic characteristics using an algebraic approach. This is due to the fact that Study's parametrization of the 3-dimensional Euclidean motion group is free of parametrization singularities. The complete kinematic description is inherent in the constraint equations, derived by using the linear implicitization algorithm (LIA), introduced by Walter and Husty [13], as well as the geometric description of the manipulator.

The paper uses Study's parametrization of the Euclidean motion group, the ideals belonging to mechanism constraints and methods to solve polynomial equations the are the mathematical equivalents of the mechanism constraints.

The structure of this paper is as follows: In Sect. 2 a complete description of the medical parallel robot is given. Using the implicit functions the determinants of the Jacobi matrices are computed to evaluate the singular configurations of the robot. Section 3 presets the kinematic modeling and singularities analysis using Study parameters. Next, the experimental model of the robot is presented, followed by the assessment of the results of the mathematical models presented before.

2 The Medical Parallel Robot

The kinematic structure of the PARA-BRACHYROB innovative parallel robot for brachytherapy is presented in Fig. 1. The robot has been developed starting from an initial solution presented in [7], by adding to it an additional mechanism with 1-DOF, representing the active joint, dedicated for the needle insertion.

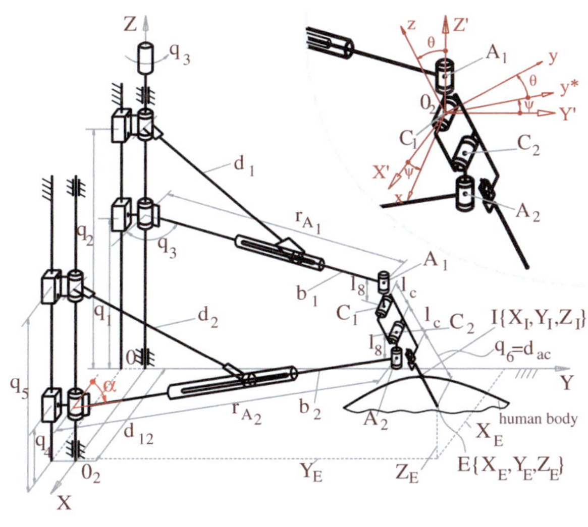

Fig. 1 The kinematic structure of PARA-BRACHYROB

Based on the kinematic scheme, the PARA-BRACHYROB cylindrical parallel robot consists of two modules, the first one having 3-DOF and 3 active joints (q_1, q_2,q_3) and a second module with 3-DOF and 2 active joints (q_4, q_5). The first two joints of each cylindrical module are translational joints, while the third motion is a rotational one around the axis of the first joints, whereas the first module has an active joint while the second one a passive joint. The modules end points are denoted with A_1 and A_2. For each module two rod lengths (b_1, d_1 and b_2, d_2) are introduced as geometrical parameters. At this point a fixed coordinate system is introduced, OXYZ, with the Z axis along the active rotational axis of the first module. The second module has its origin in the point O_2, which is positioned on the OX axis at a distance d_{12} from the origin of the OXYZ coordinates system. The two modules are interconnected with two passive Cardan joints having the first rotation axis around the Z axis (A_1 and A_2) and the second one perpendicular to it (C_1 and C_2). A geometrical parameter (l_8) describes the distance between the axis of the Cardan joints. The second rotational axes of each of the two Cardan joints are connected and they guide the needle holder. The distance between the points C_1 and C_2 respectively C_2 and the retracted position of the needle is denoted with (l_C). The needle holder integrates a translational actuator (q_6), which has a redundant motion (with respect to the robotic structure) enabling the needle insertion to the target point with all the other actuators fixed (blocked). Besides the two passive Cardan joints, the robot has also six passive rotational joints and two passive translational joints.

The robot task can be defined based on the robotics assisted brachytherapy protocol [4]: the robot should introduce, based on radiologic data, needles with diameters varying from 0.6 mm up to 2 mm and lengths from 100 mm up to 250 mm, on distances up to 200 mm, following a linear trajectory. For this task the robotic system receives a set of two points: point I (X_I, Y_I, Z_I)—the insertion point and point T (X_T, Y_T, Z_T)—the target point. In addition, a third point is introduced in the algorithm, the current robot position, point C (X_C, Y_C, Z_C, ψ_C, θ_C). Based on this data, the final needle orientation is computed:

$$\begin{cases} \psi_{IT} = atan2\left(Y_T - Y_I, X_T - X_I\right) \\ \theta_{IT} = atan2\left(\sqrt{(Y_T - Y_I)^2 + (X_T - X_I)^2}, Z_I - Z_T\right) \end{cases} \tag{1}$$

This task will be achieved through a motion decomposed in two parts:

- the approach stage (from point C to I), when the first five actuators are used, to reach the point of entry inside the patient, with the final orientation, having the pose (X_I, Y_I, Z_I, ψ_{IT}, θ_{IT});
- the needle insertion stage (from point I to T), when the sixth actuator is used to push the needle, on a straight line, to reach the target point having the pose (X_T, Y_T, Z_T, ψ_{IT}, θ_{IT}).

2.1 Singularities Analysis using the Jacobi Matrices

The kinematic model of the PARA-BRACHYROB structure was presented in [6]. As the needle insertion module does not introduce a DOF (its motion is redundant) the system of implicit functions, which results using the geometrical relations between the coordinates of the active joints, the needle tip and the geometrical parameters of the structure, is:

$$\begin{cases} f_1 : Z_E + l_1 + (q_6 + 2 \cdot l_c) \cdot cos(\theta) - q_1 \\ f_2 : X_E - (q_6 + 2 \cdot l_c) sin(\theta) cos(\psi) - \left[b_1 + \sqrt{{d_1}^2 - (q_2 - q_1)^2} \right] \cdot cos(q_3) \\ f_3 : Y_E - (q_6 + 2 \cdot l_c) sin(\theta) sin(\psi) - \left[b_1 + \sqrt{{d_1}^2 - (q_2 - q_1)^2} \right] \cdot sin(q_3) \\ f_4 : Z_E - l_2 + (q_6 + l_c) \cdot cos(\theta) - q_4 \\ f_5 : {X_{O2}}^2 + {X_E}^2 + {Y_E}^2 + (q_6 + l_c)^2 \cdot sin^2(\theta) - 2 \cdot (q_6 + l_c) \cdot sin(\theta) \cdot \\ \quad \cdot \left[(X_E - X_{O2}) \cdot cos(\psi) + Y_E \cdot sin(\psi) \right] - 2 \cdot X_{O2} \cdot X_E - {b_2}^2 - {d_2}^2 - \\ \quad -(q_5 - q_4)^2 - 2 \cdot b_2 \cdot \sqrt{{d_2}^2 - (q_5 - q_4)^2} \end{cases} \tag{2}$$

Using Eq. 2 the Jacobi matrices can be computed. They represent the partial derivative of the implicit functions with respect to the needle tip coordinates (matrix A) and the active joints (matrix B) with a size of 5 × 5. Their determinants are:

$$det(A) = -2 \cdot {l_c}^2 \cdot sin^2(\theta) \cdot \left[(X_{O2} - X_E) \cdot sin(\psi) + Y_E \cdot cos(\psi) \right] \tag{3}$$

$$det(B) = \frac{(q_2 - q_1) \cdot (q_5 - q_4) \cdot \left[b_1 + \sqrt{{d_1}^2 - (q_2 - q_1)^2} \right] \cdot \left[b_2 + \sqrt{{d_2}^2 - (q_5 - q_4)^2} \right]}{\sqrt{{d_1}^2 - (q_2 - q_1)^2} \cdot \sqrt{{d_2}^2 - (q_5 - q_4)^2}} \tag{4}$$

The singular configurations of PARA-BRACHYROB are determined when the two determinants vanish (A—parallel type singularities and B—serial type singularities). Using Eq. 3 the following cases arise:

- $l_c = 0$—this situation corresponds to the case when the distance between the two cardan joints is zero, meaning that the points C_1 and C_2 superpose; This situation cannot materialize in practice and can be discarded;
- $sin^2(\theta) = 0$—this equation characterizes the vertical position of the needle module, when the two cardan joints are positioned on a vertical axis (parallel with the OZ axis). In this configuration the robot gains one degree of freedom, allowing the rotation of the needle positioning module around the axis defined by the points C_1 and C_2. In the robot control algorithm this situation will be avoided by imposing that $\theta_{IT} \neq \frac{\pi}{2}$;

- $(X_{O2} - X_E) \cdot sin(\psi) + Y_E \cdot cos(\psi) = 0$ which is equivalent with $tan(\psi) = -\frac{Y_E}{X_{O2}-X_E}$. Considering the fact that the needle tip coordinates (point E) will be always located between the two robot arms, the ratio $\frac{Y_E}{X_{O2}-X_E}$ will be always positive, meaning that the angle ψ will take values in the domain $\psi \in \left[\frac{\pi}{2}, \pi\right] \cup \left[\frac{3\pi}{2}, 2 \cdot \pi\right]$. The configuration corresponds to the case when the coordinates of q_4, q_5, C_1, C_2 and E are located in the same plane. In the control algorithm this situation will be tested when a trajectory is generated, and in case a singular configuration an alternate trajectory will be computed.

Using Eq. 4 the following cases arise:

- $q_1 = q_2$, respectively $q_4 = q_5$—these configurations define the case when one of the two pairs of translational active joints of the PARA-BRACHYROB modules superpose. In a real scenario this case cannot appear, the experimental model of the robot having limit switches which avoid this situation;
- $d_1 = q_2 - q_1$, respectively $d_2 = q_5 - q_4$—this configuration defines the maximum distance between the two pairs of translational active joints which corresponds to the case when the rod $d_i, i = 1..2$ will be positioned vertically. This second case defines an extreme configuration which is avoided in the robot control system.

Analyzing the singularities defined using the Jacobi matrices results a series of simple equations, which implemented physically (using sensors) or analytically (using equations) in the control system of the robot, will ensure the proper functioning of the structure.

3 The Kinematics Using Study Parameters

The first step in the analysis of this manipulator is the derivation of the constraint equations. For this purpose this parallel manipulator is decomposed into two serial chains. As shown in Figs. 2 and 3 the serial structures are two identical PRPRR chains, $\mathbf{L}_1$ resp. $\mathbf{L}_2$. The direct kinematics of the chain $\mathbf{L}_i$ is computed via the matrix product

$$\mathbf{L}_i = \mathbf{M}_{i1} \cdot \mathbf{T}_1 \cdot \mathbf{T}_2 \cdot \mathbf{T}_3 \cdot \mathbf{T}_4 \cdot \mathbf{M}_{i2} \cdot \mathbf{T}_5 \cdot \mathbf{M}_{i3}, \tag{5}$$

where the matrices represent transformations according to Table 1. The transformation matrix $\mathbf{L}_1$ resp. $\mathbf{L}_2$ is representing a Euclidean displacement for all sets of parameters. Following Walter and Husty [13] this Euclidean displacements are mapped to the kinematic image space $\mathbb{P}^7$ using the kinematic mapping κ introduced by Study [11]. The parametrization of the image is displayed in Eqs. (6) and (7).

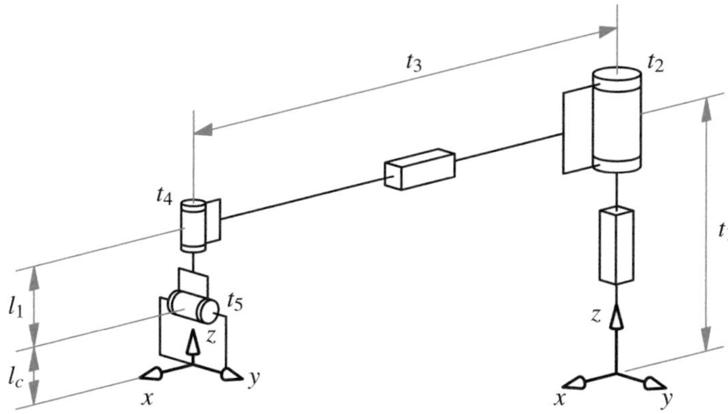

Fig. 2 Basic structure of the first PRPRR chain

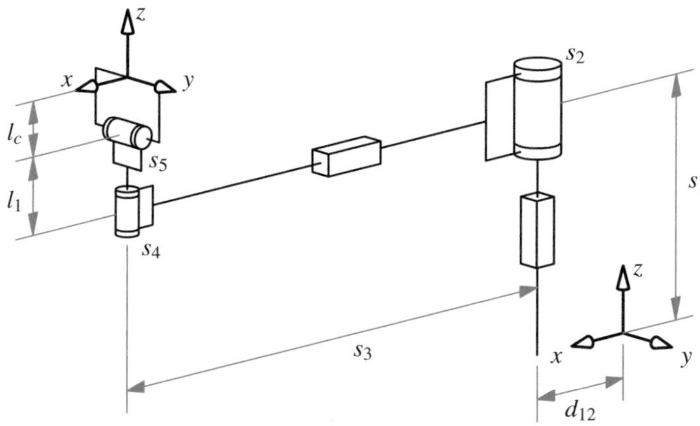

Fig. 3 Basic structure of the second PRPRR chain

$$\kappa\left(\mathbf{L}_1\right)=\begin{pmatrix} 2t_2t_4-2 \\ -2t_5(t_2+t_4) \\ -(2t_2t_4-2)t_5 \\ -2t_2-2t_4 \\ t_2t_3t_5-t_3t_4t_5+l_1t_2+l_1t_4+l_ct_2+l_ct_4-t_1t_2-t_1t_4 \\ l_1t_2t_4t_5-l_ct_2t_4t_5-t_1t_2t_4t_5+t_2t_3t_4-l_1t_5+l_ct_5+t_1t_5+t_3 \\ -l_1t_2t_5-l_1t_4t_5+l_ct_2t_5+l_ct_4t_5+t_1t_2t_5+t_1t_4t_5+t_2t_3-t_3t_4 \\ -t_2t_3t_4t_5+l_1t_2t_4+l_ct_2t_4-t_1t_2t_4-t_3t_5-l_1-l_c+t_1 \end{pmatrix} \quad (6)$$

Table 1 The geometric representation of the transformation matrices for $\mathbf{L}_1$ resp. $\mathbf{L}_2$

Matrix	Representation	Parameter	Type
$\mathbf{M}_{11}$	Basistransformation for leg 1 (identity matrix)	–	–
$\mathbf{M}_{21}$	Basistransformation for leg 2, translation along the x-axis	d_{12}	–
$\mathbf{T}_1$	Translation along z-axis	t_1 resp. s_1	active
$\mathbf{T}_2$	Rotation around z-axis	t_2 resp. s_2	active resp. passive
$\mathbf{T}_3$	Translation along x-axis	t_3 resp. s_3	active
$\mathbf{T}_4$	Rotation around z-axis	t_4 resp. s_4	passive
$\mathbf{M}_{12}$	Translation along z-axis (distance between A_1 C_1)	l_1	–
$\mathbf{M}_{22}$	Translation along z-axis (distance between A_2 C_2)	l_1	–
$\mathbf{T}_5$	Rotation around y-axis	t_5 resp. s_5	passive
$\mathbf{M}_{13}$	Final translation along z-axis	l_c	–
$\mathbf{M}_{23}$	Final translation along z-axis	l_c	–

$$\kappa\left(\mathbf{L}_2\right) = \begin{pmatrix} 2s_2s_4 - 2 \\ -2s_5(s_2 + s_4) \\ -(2s_2s_4 - 2)s_5 \\ -2s_2 - 2s_4 \\ p_1 \\ p_2 \\ p_3 \\ p_4 \end{pmatrix} \tag{7}$$

$$\begin{aligned}
p_1 =& - d_{12}s_2s_5 - d_{12}s_4s_5 + s_2s_3s_5 - s_3s_4s_5 - l_1s_2 - l_1s_4 - l_cs_2 - l_cs_4 - s_1s_2 - s_1s_4 \\
p_2 =& - l_1s_2s_4s_5 + l_cs_2s_4s_5 - s_1s_2s_4s_5 - d_{12}s_2s_4 + s_2s_3s_4 + l_1s_5 - l_cs_5 + s_1s_5 + d_{12} + s_3 \\
p_3 =& l_1s_2s_5 + l_1s_4s_5 - l_cs_2s_5 - l_cs_4s_5 + s_1s_2s_5 + s_1s_4s_5 - d_{12}s_2 - d_{12}s_4 + s_2s_3 - s_3s_4 \\
p_4 =& d_{12}s_2s_4s_5 - s_2s_3s_4s_5 - l_1s_2s_4 - l_cs_2s_4 - s_1s_2s_4 - d_{12}s_5 - s_3s_5 + l_1 + l_c + s_1
\end{aligned}$$

The parametrizations $\kappa\left(\mathbf{L}_i\right)$ are representing 5-dimensional subvarieties of the Study quadric. An implicit representation of this varieties is computed by using the LIA (= Linear Implizitization Algorithm, see Walter and Husty [13]). It has to be noted that the passive joint parameters mentioned in Table 1 are eliminated during this process. The degree of the Ansatz polynomials in the Study parameters $x_0, x_1, x_2, x_3, y_0, y_1, y_2, y_3$ has to be fixed. The LIA shows that there are 4 linear and one quadratic polynomial representing $\kappa\left(\mathbf{L}_1\right)$. Because of the length of the polynomials only the first constraint polynomial is displayed at this point:

$$\begin{aligned}
&(l_1^2t_2^2 - 2l_1t_1t_2^2 - l_c^2t_2^2 + t_1^2t_2^2 + t_2^2t_3^2 + l_1^2 - 2l_1t_1 - l_c^2 + t_1^2 + t_3^2)x_3 \\
&+ (2l_1t_2^2 - 2l_ct_2^2 - 2t_1t_2^2 + 2l_1 - 2l_c - 2t_1)y_0 + 4t_2t_3y_1 + (2t_2^2t_3 - 2t_3)y_2 = 0
\end{aligned} \tag{8}$$

The ideal generated by the 5 polynomials of the first chain is denoted by $\mathscr{I}_1$. The variables in $\mathscr{I}_1$ are the Study parameters. The input parameters of the first chain are t_1, t_2, t_3 and l_1, l_c determine the design of the manipulator.

For $\kappa\left(\mathbf{L}_2\right)$ the LIA is returning no linear polynomial. But it comes up with 10 quadratic polynomials, 56 polynomials of degree 3 and 205 polynomials of degree 4. Further inspection shows that all polynomials of degree 3 and 4 are included in the ideal generated by the quadratic polynomials. The ideal generated by these 10 quadratic polynomials is denoted by $\mathscr{I}_2$. Because of the length only one of these polynomials is explicitly shown here

$$\begin{aligned}&(-l_1 - l_c - s_1)x_0y_2 + (-l_1 + l_c - s_1)x_1y_3 + (l_1 - l_c + s_1)x_2y_0\\&+ (l_1 + l_c + s_1)x_3y_1 - 2y_0y_1 - 2y_2y_3 = 0\end{aligned} \tag{9}$$

One of the quadratic polynomials is the Study quadric itself

$$x_0x_0 + x_1y_1 + x_2y_2 + x_3y_3 = 0. \tag{10}$$

This polynomial is already included in the ideal $\mathscr{I}_1$.

For the solution of the direct kinematic problem the zero set of the union $\mathscr{I} = \mathscr{I}_1 \cup \mathscr{I}_2$ has to be computed for every set of input parameters. The vanishing set of an ideal are all common roots of the polynomial which generate the ideal.

The ideal $\mathscr{I}_1$ is generated by 4 linear polynomials and one quadratic polynomial. Solving for all y_i linearly results in

$$\begin{aligned}y_0 &= -\frac{l_1t_2^2x_3 + l_ct_2^2x_3 - t_1t_2^2x_3 + t_2^2t_3x_1 - 2t_2t_3x_2 + l_1x_3 + l_cx_3 - t_1x_3 - t_3x_1}{2(t_2^2+1)},\\
y_1 &= -\frac{l_1t_2^2x_2 - l_ct_2^2x_2 - t_1t_2^2x_2 - t_2^2t_3x_0 + 2t_2t_3x_3 + l_1x_2 - l_cx_2 - t_1x_2 + t_3x_0}{2(t_2^2+1)},\\
y_2 &= \frac{l_1t_2^2x_1 - l_ct_2^2x_1 - t_1t_2^2x_1 - t_2^2t_3x_3 - 2t_2t_3x_0 + l_1x_1 - l_cx_1 - t_1x_1 + t_3x_3}{2(t_2^2+1)},\\
y_3 &= \frac{l_1t_2^2x_0 + l_ct_2^2x_0 - t_1t_2^2x_0 + t_2^2t_3x_2 + 2t_2t_3x_1 + l_1x_0 + l_cx_0 - t_1x_0 - t_3x_2}{2(t_2^2+1)}.\end{aligned} \tag{11}$$

Substituting these solutions for y_i into the quadratic equation in $\mathscr{I}_1$ results in $x_0x_1 + x_2x_3 = 0$. This equation is also contained in the ideal $\mathscr{I}_2$, so this equation will be considered in the discussion of $\mathscr{I}_2$.

The solutions obtained in Eq. (11) are then substituted into the polynomials of the ideal $\mathscr{I}_2$. This results in the new ideal $\mathscr{I}_2'$ containing the unknowns x_0, x_1, x_2, x_3. The ideal $\mathscr{I}_2'$ is generated by 10 polynomials. It was not possible to compute a general Gröbner Basis for this ideal, but after adding the normalizing condition $x_0^2 + x_1^2 + x_2^2 + x_3^2 - 1 = 0$ Maple was able to compute a basis together with 5 other generating polynomials. As the ordering was chosen to be lexicographic, the basis contains a univariate polynomial which is of degree 8. It has to be noted that up to now all the computations could be done without specifying the design and input parameters.

As an example this basis is computed for the following set of parameters $d_{12} = 500, l_c = 100, l_1 = 65, t_1 = 300, s_1 = 100, t_2 = \frac{1}{2}, t_3 = 700, s_3 = 600$. The ideal $\mathscr{I}_2'$ for this example is

$$\begin{aligned}&\langle 226827960320000001x_3^8 - 306217746432000000x_3^6\\&+ 104408484969185280x_3^4 - 715496995160064x_3^2 + 1115133370245,\\&443023360000000x_3^7 - 598081536000000x_3^5 + 202940527645440x_3^3\\&+ 21867860385x_2 - 734406240672x_3, -443023360000000x_3^7\\&+ 448561152000000x_3^5 - 101960332381440x_3^3 + 157191796503x_1\\&+ 348999698736x_3, 340241940480000000x_3^7 - 461655021568000000x_3^5\\&+158970234397777920x_3^3 + 72736553244285x_0 - 1598728406827896x_3\rangle.\end{aligned} \tag{12}$$

The complete solution of the direct kinematics for this example is shown in Table 2. Table 2 reveals that the solutions 1 and 2 correspond to the same end effector pose. This is due to the fact that there is a quadratic normalizing condition and the Study parameters are homogeneous coordinates. The same is true for the solutions 3–4 as well as the solutions 5–6 and 7–8. This means that there are 4 different solutions for the direct kinematics of this manipulator.

Figure 4 shows all 4 solutions. Figure 5 is a top view of the solutions. The z-axes of the end effector frame of solutions 1 and 3 coincide. The solutions only differ in an 180° rotation about the z-axis. The same holds for the solutions 5 and 7.

Table 2 Solutions of the direct kinematics for $d_{12} = 500, l_c = 100, l_1 = 65, t_1 = 300, s_1 = 100, t_2 =, t_3 = 700, s_3 = 600$

#	x_0	x_1	x_2	x_3	y_0	y_1	y_2	y_3
1	0.996	−0.0410	0.690	0.0594	189	−110	−260	−224
2	−0.996	0.0410	−0.690	−0.0594	−189	110	260	224
3	0.917	0.0527	−0.630	0.0757	−161	−320	−250	84.8
4	−0.917	−0.0527	0.630	−0.0757	161	320	250.	−84.8
5	0.0486	−0.571	0.0394	−0.820	−164	226	−89.9	−170
6	−0.0486	0.571	−0.0394	0.820	164	−226	89.9	170
7	0.0728	0.554	0.157	−0.819	105	240	−285	117
8	−0.0728	−0.554	−0.157	0.819	−105	−240	285	−117

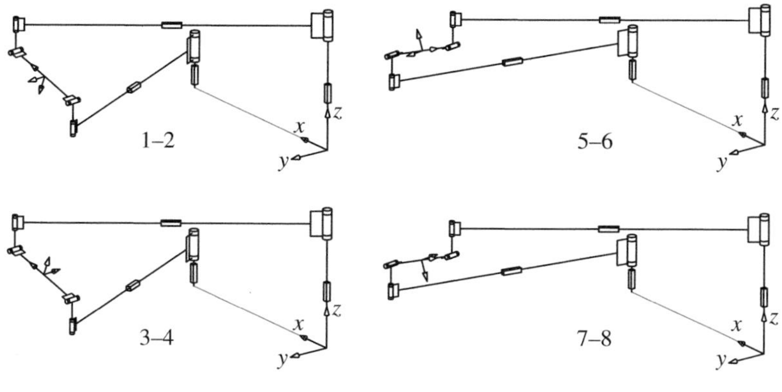

Fig. 4 Solutions of the direct kinematics

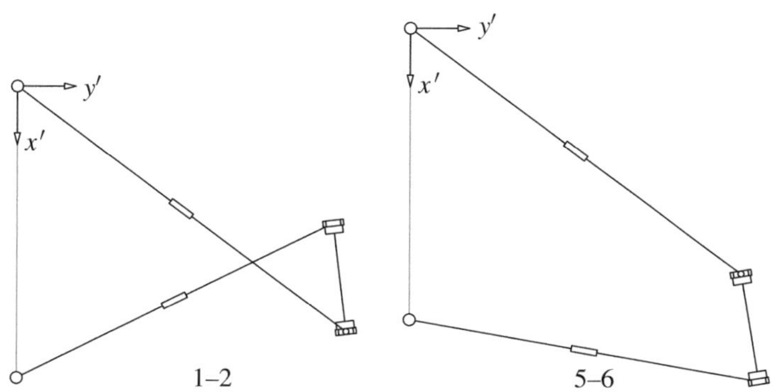

Fig. 5 Solutions of the direct kinematics—*top* views

3.1 Singular Poses of the Manipulator

In this section the singular poses of the manipulator will be discussed. In the kinematic image space singular poses are characterized by taking the Jacobian of the ideal $\mathscr{I} = \langle g_1, \ldots, g_8 \rangle$

$$\mathbf{J} = \left(\frac{g_i}{x_j}, \frac{g_i}{y_j} \right) \tag{13}$$

and computing its determinant $S : \det(\mathbf{J}) = 0$. It is possible to compute the determinant without specifying any design or input parameters. The polynomial S is a polynomial in the variable x_3 and has degree 7. It is a product of 14 factors $f_1, \ldots, f_{14}$. The polynomial S vanishes if $f_i = 0$ for any $i \in \{1, \ldots, 14\}$.

Because of the length of the polynomials f_i only some small examples are mentioned at this place. The general form of these polynomials is

$$f_1 \quad : \quad 2l_1 + 2l_c + s_1 - t_1$$
$$f_2 \quad : \quad 8l_c x_3^2 + 2l_1 - 2l_c + s_1 - t_1.$$

For the following example the design values $d_{12} = 500, l_c = 100, l_1 = 65$ are substituted into f_1 and f_2

$$f_1 \quad : \quad 330 + s_1 - t_1 \tag{14}$$
$$f_2 \quad : \quad 800x3^2 + s_1 - t_1 - 70. \tag{15}$$

The singularity condition S is vanishing for example if $f_1 = 0$ and this is the case if the difference $t_1 - s_1 = 330$. This means that the height of the first two prismatic joints is exactly the distance between A_1 and A_2, for example $t_1 = 430, s_1 = 100$. To compute the solution for this singular pose the input parameters are $t_2 = \frac{1}{2}, t_3 = 700$. Substituting these values into the basis of $\mathscr{I}$ results in

$$\begin{aligned}\mathscr{I} = \big\langle & 390625(s_3^2 - 320000)^4, -109375000(s_3^2 - 320000)^3 x_2, \\ & -31250000(s_3^2 - 320000)^3 x_1, \\ & -19531250(s_3^2 - 320000)^4(7x_0 + 24x_3)\big\rangle\,. \end{aligned} \tag{16}$$

Note that the first polynomial in Eq. (16) is independent of x_3. This means that the value of x_3 can be chosen arbitrarily, so this is a one parametric motion, but value of s_3 has to be $s_3 = 400\sqrt{2}$ to make the first polynomial vanish. In this case the end effector can move without changing the input parameters, a so called self-motion. This motion is a pure rotation about the z-axis of the moving frame, shown in Fig. 6.

The polynomial f_2 vanishes for $d_{12} = 500, l_1 = 65, l_c = 100, \ s_1 = 100, \ s_3 = 10\sqrt{3551 + 336\sqrt{39}}, t_1 = 300, \ t_2 = \frac{1}{2}, t_3 = 700$ and $x_3 = \frac{3}{20}\sqrt{15}$. The numerical values for the remaining Study parameters are

$$\begin{array}{llll} x_0 = -0.578 & x_1 = -0.403 & x_2 = -0.402 & x_3 = 0.580 \\ y_0 = -158 & y_1 = -108 & y_2 = 352 & y_3 = 11 \end{array}$$

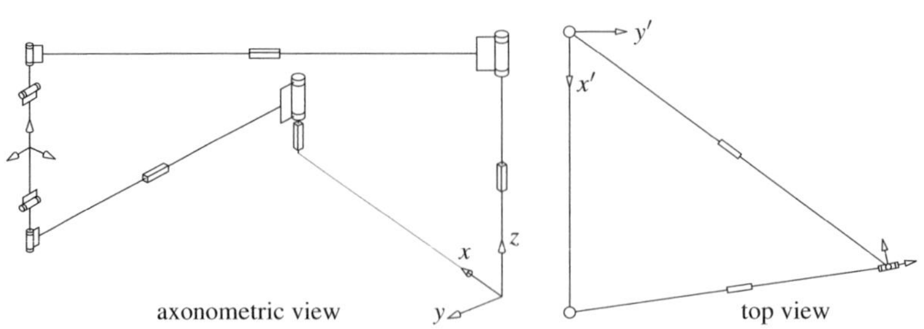

Fig. 6 Self motion of the manipulator

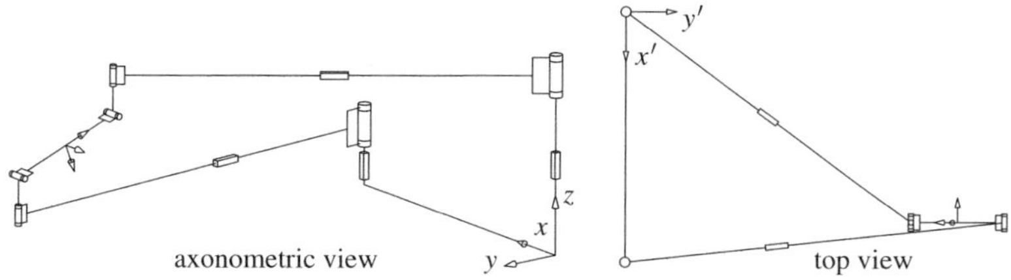

Fig. 7 Singular pose of the manipulator

This solution is shown in Fig. 7. A geometric interpretation of this singular pose is missing up to now and will be subject to future research.

4 The Experimental Model

Starting from a set of working parameters defined together with a team of oncologists from the "Iuliu Hatieganu" University of Medicine in Cluj-Napoca, Romania and the kinematic scheme defined in Fig. 1, the experimental model of the PARA-BRACHYROB parallel robot has been achieved. As the therapeutic protocol in [4] points out, an important step of the procedure is the correct calibration

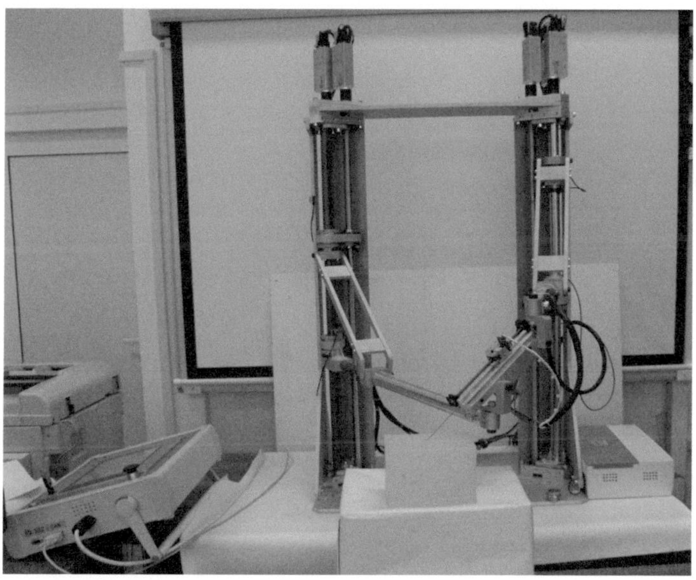

Fig. 8 The experimental model of PARA-BRACHYROB

between the three elements involved: CT-Scan—patient—robot. Figure 8 illustrates the experimental model of PARA-BRACHYROB, designed in accordance with all the requirements defined by the doctors. Based on the conclusions presented in [10] regarding the needle deflection, a force sensor is integrated in the needle insertion mechanism to monitor the force variation during the needle insertion though the body. The different types of tissue (layers of skin, fat, muscles, internal organs parenchyma) have different resistances and whether the force exceeds certain limits, causing the needle deflection from the trajectory, the sensor will trigger a total retraction and the repeating of the procedure. The module has a mechanical release mechanism which enables total control of the needle length inserted inside the patient and also its safe retraction in case of an emergency.

5 Results Interpretation and Implementation

The two approaches used for the singularities analysis of PARA-BRACHYROB enable the implementation of a safe control system for the robot. The simple geometrical interpretation of the singular poses described using the Jacobi matrices enabled the definition of a workspace of the robot limited with position sensors. The complete description of the singular poses of the robot achieved using the Study parameters defined a polynomial (S) of 14 factors which are dependant only on the geometrical parameters of the structure. The presence of the 14 factors in the polynomial (S) suggests that there are singular configurations which have not been described by the analysis of the Jacobi matrices. Thus, in order to ensure the safe behavior of the robot the expression of the polynomial (S) will be used in the singularities avoidance algorithm. During the pre-planning phase, when the trajectory is tested for safe behavior, the first step refers to the determination of the robot position with respect to the tumor location to ensure that it remains inside the robot workspace without being close to its boundaries; secondly, the value of (S) will be assessed in each point, with respect to a boundary value (eps) testing not only the point itself for singularities but also the possible approach towards a singular configuration. Such a situation, illustrated by both approaches, refers to the self motion of the insertion module which arises when the needle axis is parallel with the vertical Z axis. The trajectory generation algorithm will not allow at any moment a value $\theta < 5°$. In case of weak results, the robot position will be adjusted and the trajectory assessment performed again. In this way any possible singular robot configuration during the medical procedure will be avoided. Once the entire trajectory is validated the control system will allow the user to actually actuate the needle.

6 Conclusions

An innovative robotic system for brachytherapy, capable of targeting any tumor in the thoracoabdominal areas of the body with real-time CT monitoring has been presented. The kinematics of the robot have been achieved in two different ways using the Jacobi matrices and the Study parameters. The singularities were studied using the two approaches leading to a complete description of the singular robot configurations. An important aspect is that both approaches characterized the singularities using analytical expressions for the determinants which enabled the implementation of these equations in the control system of the robot which can thus generate safe, singularity free trajectories for the needle.

Acknowledgments This paper was supported by the Project no. 173/2012, code PN-II-PCCA-2011-3.2-0414, entitled "Robotic assisted brachytherapy, an innovative approach of inoperable cancers - CHANCE" and the Bilateral Austria—Romania Project 745/2014, entitled "Developing methods to evaluate the accuracy of potential parallel robots for medical applications" both financed by UEFISCDI.

References

1. Bassan, et al.: A novel manipulator for 3D ultrasound guided percutaneous needle insertion. In: IEEE International Conference on Robotics and Automation, pp. 617–622 (2007)
2. Fischer, G.S., et al.: Design of a robot for transperineal prostate needle placement in MRI scanner. In: IEEE International Conference on Mechatronics, pp. 592–597 (2006)
3. Husty, M.L., Pfurner, M., Schröcker, H.-P., Brunnthaler, K.: Algebraic methods in mechanism analysis and synthesis. Robotica **25**(6), 661–675 (2007)
4. Pisla, D., et al.: Innovative Approaches Regarding Robots for Brachytherapy. New Trends in Medical and Service Robots. MMS, vol. 20, pp. 63–78 (2014)
5. Pisla, D., Cocorean, D., Vaida, C., Gherman, B., Pisla, A., Plitea, N: Application oriented design and simulation of an innovative parallel robot for brachytherapy. In: Proceedings of the ASME 2014 International Conference—IDETC/CIE 2014, Buffalo, New York, USA (2014)
6. Plitea, N., et al.: On the kinematics of a new parallel robot for brachytherapy. Proc. Rom. Acad. Ser. A **15**(4), 354–361 (2014)
7. Plitea, N., et al.: Parallel robot for brachytherapy with two linkages for guiding a platform of CYL-U type, Patent pending: RO129698-A2 (2014)
8. Podder, T., et al.: AAPM and GEC-ESTRO guidelines for image-guided robotic brachytherapy: Report of Task Group 192. Med. Phys. **41**(10), 1–27 (2014)
9. Podder, T., Buzurovic, I., Huang, K., Yu, Y.: MIRAB: an image-guided multichannel robot for prostate brachytherapy, Bodine J. **3**(1) (2010)
10. Strassman, G., et al.: Advantage of robotic needle placement on a prostate model in HDR brachytherapy. Strahlenther Onkol. **187**(6), 367–272 (2011)
11. Study, E.: Geometrie der Dynamen. Teubner (1903)
12. Venselaar, J., Meigooni, A.S., Baltas, D., Hoskin, P.J. (eds): Comprehensive Brachytherapy: Physical and Clinical Aspects (Imaging in Medical Diagnosis and Therapy) (2012)
13. Walter, D.R., Husty, M.L.: On implicitization of kinematic constraint equations. Mach. Des. Res. **26**, 132–151 (2010)
14. Yu, Y., et al.: Robot-assisted prostate brachytherapy. Med. Image Comput. Comput. Assist. Interv. **9**(1), 41–49 (2006)

Visuo-vestibular Contributions to Vertical Self-motion Perception in Healthy Adults

I. Giannopulu, P. Leboucher, G. Rautureau, I. Israël and R. Jouvent

Abstract The intensity of the visuo-vestibular interaction, i.e., visuo-vestibular conflict, would influence upward self-motion and downward self-motion latencies and cardiovascular activity. In order to test this hypothesis, thirty five healthy adults aged 22 years in average have been immersed to a central visual motion via a HMD. During upward and downward self-motion perception, the engagement of vestibular saccular organs seems to contribute differently to latencies and cardiovascular activation depending on the direction of gravitational acceleration. Downward self-motion latencies (same direction acceleration) are shorter than upward self-motion latencies (opposite direction acceleration). In the same vein, cardiovascular autonomic activation, reflecting by heart rate, is lower for downward self-motion than for upward self-motion. Our results provide evidence that visuo-vestibular interaction would contribute to influence both latencies and cardiovascular variation in vertical self-motion perception.

Keywords Visuo-vestibular interaction · Vertical self-motion · Cardiovascular activity · Adults · HMD

1 Introduction

Vertical self-motion perception, i.e., elevator movement, is an embodied sensation of movement in space. It can occur in naturalistic situation when, for example, we take a glass walled elevator to move upward or downward. Though a rapid waterfall is seeable (frequently present in international airports, centers and buildings), we can have the impression that our elevator is moving at the opposite direction (downward or upward). This visually induced self-motion perception is a complex

I. Giannopulu (✉) · P. Leboucher · G. Rautureau · I. Israël · R. Jouvent
Virtual Reality Prism Platform, IHU-a-Brain and Spine Institute (ICM), UPMC, CNRS U7225, Groupe Hospitalier Pitié-Salpêtrière, Paris, France
e-mail: igiannopulu@psycho-prat.fr

P. Wenger et al. (eds.), *New Trends in Medical and Service Robots*, Mechanisms and Machine Science 39, DOI 10.1007/978-3-319-30674-2_8

phenomenon which necessitates bimodal visuo-vestibular interaction at least [1, 2]. It is considered as an archetypal form of virtual reality [3]. The purpose of the present study is to analyse visuo-vestibular interaction of vertical self-motion by investigating the latencies for reporting upward and downward self-motion as well as the variation of autonomic heart rate in human adults using a head mounted display. In that context, visuo-vestibular interaction could be considered as a minimalistic model for efficient spatial navigation in humanoid robots.

The visually induced self-motion perception (whether circular or linear) is characterized by three main perceptual phases. At the begging of the visual motion (peripheral or central), an observer perceives her/himself as stationary and the visual environment as mobile. In a second phase and after some seconds, the observer begins to perceive the mobile visual environment as moving more slowly and her/himself as gradually moving in the opposite direction (latency for reporting self-motion). Finally, in a third phase, the participant receives self-motion only and the visual environment looks stationary (self-motion saturation) [1, 4–6].

Converging neuroanatomical studies carried out that various cortical areas are specialized in visuo-vestibular afferents in humans associating frontal, temporal, parietal and prefrontal cortex [7–9]. Some others have shown that the temporo-parietal cortex would selectively be involved in the treatment of visual and vestibular interactions. Vestibular projection area is rather associated with the neural activity of the occipito-temporo-parietal cortex [10–13], and is involved in the complex representations of egocentric perception of the body in space in both static and dynamic conditions [14, 15].

Self-motion perception results from visual-vestibular interaction and more particular from visual-vestibular conflict. In healthy adults and under normal terrestrial conditions, studies have demonstrated that any reduction of the vestibular information would reduce the visual-vestibular conflict and would have a facilitating effect on self-motion as reflecting to the observed latencies [5, 6]. Similarly, patients with bilateral-labyrinthine damage have shorter latencies for reporting self-motion than healthy observers [16]. Patients with right Menière's disease exhibit shorter latency to reach yaw self-motion to the right than to the left, which is much shorter than of healthy observer to the right [17]. In the same vein, healthy participants have also shorter latencies of self-motion in weightlessness [18] or in microgravity than in gravity conditions [19]. In other words, these studies suggest that the modification of the intensity of the visuo-vestibular conflict influences self-motion latencies.

Suggesting a differential sensitivity between utricular maculae (transduces horizontal accelerations) and saccular maculae (transduces vertical accelerations) in the otolithic system of healthy observers [5, 20], anatomical and functional data are consistent with the aforementioned studies. Moreover, when saccular maculae is maximally aligned with gravitational force, electrophysiological and psychophysical findings have reported a differential sensitivity to opposite accelerations within the vertical axis [4]. Since downward movement is more easily induced than upward movement specially because of the same direction with gravitational acceleration [21, 22], our first hypothesis is associated with the existence of a differentiation on latencies for reporting downward and upward self-motion. More particular, we expect that the latency for reporting self-motion would be shorter for downward self-motion than for upward self-motion. In addition to these measures of self-motion, we will analyze the heart rate of all participants.

Even if little is known about the heart rate variation in self-motion perception, physiological data allow us to formulate various hypotheses. It has been shown that in healthy subjects with erect head aligned in the vertical axis, the otolithic saccular acceleration regulates the heart rate thanks to the activation of the autonomic nervous system [23]. Precisely, otolithic stimulation leads to lower cardiovascular responses (i.e., low heart rate) in patients with bilateral labyrinthine disease than in healthy persons [24]. These results suggest that the cardiovascular responses would be "vestibuloform" by the fact that they are produced only during activation of otolith receptors (saccular and utricular maculaes). In that context, the intensity of the visual-vestibular interaction that modifies self-motion perception would also modify the functioning of the autonomic cardiovascular responses: the lesser the vestibular sensitivity, the lower the cardiovascular reaction. To test this second hypothesis, we will analyze the variation of heart rate in healthy people when vertical self-motion perception is induced. Due to the fact that the otolithic saccular sensitivity for upward motion is higher than for downward motion [21, 22], we expect that the cardiovascular reaction (measured by the heart rate) would be lower for downward than for upward self-motion perception.

Visuo-vestibular interaction can contribute to the navigation of humanoid robots. It is well known that during navigation robots generally deviate from their trajectory due to uncertainty in both equilibrium and position. From neuro-anatomical view point, visuo-vestibular afferences are directly connected with the cerebellum which in turn is interconnected with both sub-cortical and cortical areas [6, 14]. This vestibulo-cerebellum-cortex pathway is critically involved in adaptive changes in gravitational environment. Changes in position can provide noticeable challenges to the conservation of balance and cardiovascular activity as the vestibular system is partly responsible for the regulation of blood pressure [24]. The vestibulo-sympathetic responses integrate various sensory signals reflecting body position in space, somatosensory, viscera and visual information. Even if the integration of the aforementioned signals along the three body axis is crucial for self-position and balance, visuo-vestibular and sympathetic responses along the Z axis (upward and downward self-motion perception) alone could be considered in order to make potential adjustments to robot autonomous navigation.

With this study, we investigate the latencies for reporting upward and downward self-motion, as well as the variation of autonomic heart rate in human adults. The participants were exposed to a pseudorandom dot pattern mixed with a lamellar visual environment via a head mounted display (HMD) when seated in an armchair. If latency for reporting self-motion and cardiovascular responses are modulated by the intensity of the visuo-vestibular conflict, such measures would be shorter for downward self-motion than for upward self-motion since the bimodal sensory would be weaker in the former than in the latter case.

2 Method

2.1 Participants

A total number of thirty five healthy volunteer students (17 men and 18 women) were exposed to a visual stimulation inducing vertical upward and downward self-motion via a Head Mounted Display (HMD). Their average age was 22 years (sd 1 year and 2 months). All participants had normal or corrected-to-normal vision and no history of vestibular, cardiac or neurological disorders of spatial perception and orientation. An additional five participants (three women and two men) participated but were excluded because of numerous dropouts (three persons) or nonsensitive to self-motion (two persons). The study was approved by the national CNRS ethic committee, by the local ethic committee and is conform to Helsinki convention.

2.2 Experimental Apparatus

A head-mounted display (HMD, SONY HMZ-T1) was used to display the visual environment (Fig. 1a). The field of view is 51.6° diagonal at full overplay (45°H × 25.3°V). The HMD optics allow for the full range of depth focus from 25 cm to infinity. The visual environment was a 3D black-white lamellar

(a)

(b)

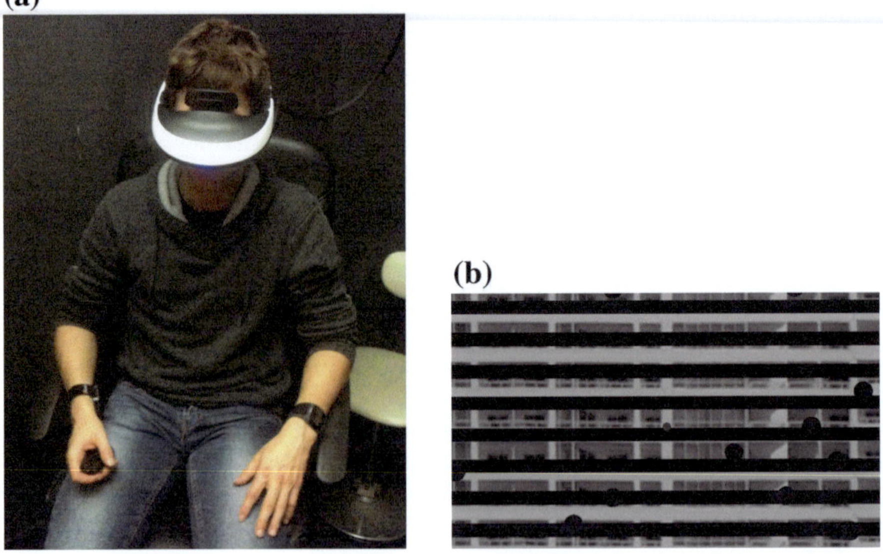

Fig. 1 Head mounted display (**a**) and visual environment (**b**)

stimulation mixed with a pseudorandom dot pattern. It formed an elevator of a 3 m deep, 4 m wide and 3 m high. Its spatial frequency is 0.08 cycle deg^{-1}. It moves upward or downward with a vertical oscillation of 0.6 Hz [25]. The visual environment was controlled by a computer. Two response devices were used: a key response to record latency for reporting self-motion and a cardiofrequencemeter Mio Alpha watch to record heart rate. Mio Alpha measures heart rate on on-line, using two green LED and a photo-electric cell. The LEDs are integrated in the back plate of the watch. They project light on the skin, which allows the photo-electric cell to detect the volume of blood flow. The optical sensor displays an accuracy of -0.1 ± 0.3 bpm.

2.3 *Procedure*

First, the heart rate of each participant was measured during 1 min in silence. After, each participant entered into the "experimental room". With the help of the experimenter, the participant wear the HMD. Only the computer's desktop background was projected on the HMD's scene. A typical trial proceeded as follows. The subject was comfortably seated in an armchair, the vertical axis was aligned with gravitational force. The subject's back and shoulders were in contact with the seat back. The subject was asked to orient the head straight ahead. As soon as the head was correct and after the subject declared that s/he was ready, the visual environment was presented on the HMD's screen. The HMD has built-in stereo headphones thought which rose noise was delivered. The presentation of the visual environment was the beginning of the experiment. The subject correctly installed on the chair was looking at the middle of the visual environment. A small point placed straight ahead at the participant's eye level was used as a fixation stimulus. The experimenter asked the participant "to fixate the point". The cardiofrequencemeter Mio Alpha watch was placed on the participant's left hand; the key response was placed on the participant's right hand (Fig. 1b). The participant was asked to use the same hand for the key response during the experiment. Each subject performed two phases: a selection phase and an experimental phase. The *selection phase* was designed both to test the participants' susceptibility to self-motion perception and to familiarize them with the procedure. It was explained to the subject that the stationary environment will move and during pattern motion they will be able (or not) to identify their self-motion perception. All participants were instructed to press the key as soon as they are able to identify their own motion (and to not press the key in the opposite situation) and to maintain the key pressed during the whole duration of self-motion. Each participant had two directional conditions (upward and downward) the order of which was randomized across the subjects. Each trial lasted 1 min. The inter-trial interval was around 5 s. Within each directional condition, a trial began as soon as the participant reported that s/he was ready. The *selection phase* was considered as completed if the participants provided two consecutive correct trials. A trial is considered as being correct if the participant provided a key press during the allowed duration and give a canonical description of the self-motion. Only the subjects who provided two consecutive correct trials were retained for the experimental phase. During the *experimental phase*, each participant had two direction conditions again. Each participant was given six valid trials for each directional condition the order of which was again randomly. The participant was verbally reminded to orient the head and gaze straight ahead at each directional condition. The inter-trial interval was about 5 s. Once again each participant was asked to instructed to press the key as soon as they are able to identify their own motion (and to not press the key in the opposite situation) and to maintain the key pressed during the whole duration of self-motion. The instructions with respect to the time constrains relative to the trial direction were the same as in the selection phase. At the end of the immersion, the participants were asked to verbalize their sensations and impressions. With this procedure, the thirty five participants reported self-motion perception within the time limit of each trial (1 min) and for all twelve trials (six trials × two directional conditions).

2.4 Dependent Variables and Analysis

The dependent variables were (a) the latency for reporting self-motion; (b) heart rate. All statistical analysis was performed with SPSS Statistics 17.0.

3 Results

The results will be presented into two parts. First we will give the data from the "selection phase", after the data from the "experimental phase".

3.1 Selection Phase

The selection phase was designed with the aim to test the participants' susceptibility to self-motion perception and to familiarize them with the procedure. During the participant's selection and following our criterion, each directional condition was completed when each participant produces two consecutive correct trials. Indeed, the number of trials necessary to reach this criterion theoretically ranges from 4 to 6. The number of trials necessary to reach our criterion was 4.3 ± 1.02, 4.4 ± 1.04 (mean and standard deviation) for the upward and downward self-motion respectively. The given means did not differ between the two directional conditions (student's test, $p > 0.05$).

3.2 Experimental Phase

Under the hypothesis that self-motion perception would be more easily to induce in the downward direction than in the upward direction, latency reporting self-motion is expected to be shorter in the first than in the second direction. Within each of the defined direction, the observed individual distributions of each of the dependent variables approximates a non parametric shaped. The same non parametric distribution is preserved when data are pooled within each of the self-motion directions. With such distribution shapes, the median has been chosen as a central index of each condition. The statistical comparisons have been conducted with the Wilcoxon matched-pairs signed-ranks test. These comparisons have shown that the median latency for reporting self-motion was shorter for downward self-motion than for upward self-motion (two-tailed test $p < 0.01$, T = 66, n = 35) (Fig. 2). The groups' median time was 0.8 and 1.3 s in the former than in the latter condition respectively ($\chi^2 = 3.99$, $p < 0.05$).

Due to the intensity of the visual-vestibular interaction along the vertical axis, we have hypothesized that the cardiovascular reaction (measured by the heart rate) would be lower for downward than for upward self-motion perception. Such measure only concerns the second phase after the begging of the visual motion, i.e., the latency for reporting self-motion perception. With both upward and downward self-motion conditions pooled the distribution of heart rate is a parametric one, this is the reason why the statistical comparisons have been conducted with the

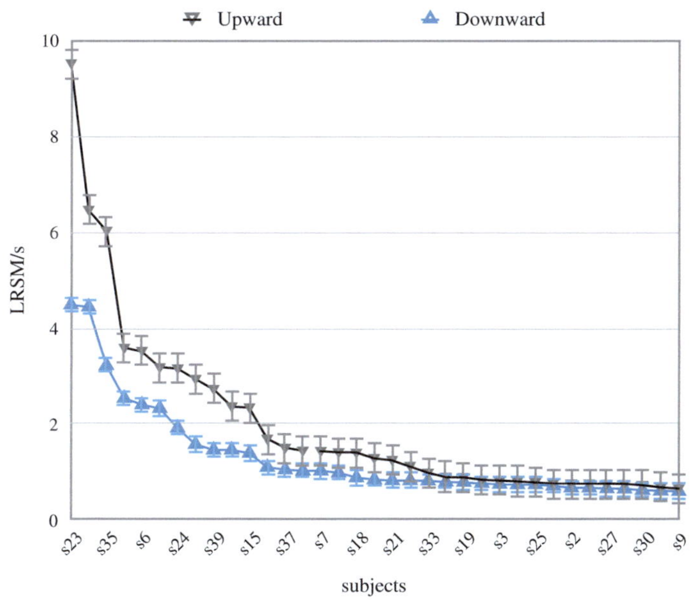

Fig. 2 Latency for reporting downward and upward self-motion

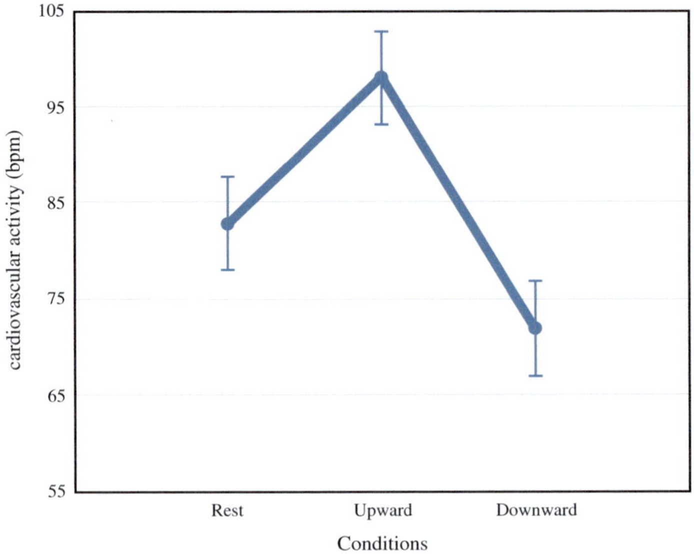

Fig. 3 Heart rate in vertical self-motion

student's test. Figure 3 presents the mean heart rate in the rest condition and in upward and downward self-motion conditions. The results have shown that compared to the rest condition, the mean heart rate is higher in the upward condition (student's test, $p < 0.001$) and lower in the downward condition (student's test, $p < 0.02$). The mean heart rate is lower in downward condition than in upward condition (student's test, $p < 0.001$).

4 Discussion

The results of the present study indicate that (1) the latency for reporting downward self-motion is shorter than the latency for reporting upward self-motion; (2) the cardiovascular responses measured by the heart rate is lower for the downward self motion than that the upward self-motion. These results are consistent with our hypotheses following which the intensity of visuo-vestibular conflict could influence the time for reporting self-motion but also the variation of the cardiovascular activity. Undeniably, the visuo-vestibular conflict refers to the fact that in self-motion perception, vestibular information indicates self-stationarity and the related visual information testifies self-motion. Given this situation Zacharias and Young [26] postulate the existence of a visually generated signal of reference that corresponds to the vestibular dynamics that would be expected if the observer was really in movement in space. In this context, the visual-vestibular conflict would correspond to the difference between the current dynamics of the vestibular information (self-stationarity) and the expected vestibular dynamic (self-motion).

Comparing latencies for reporting self-motion between sagittal and vertical axes, an inter-axis difference has been shown. More particular, in healthy adults and in gravitational environment, the latency for reporting self-motion is shorter for the vertical axis than for the sagittal axis [5]. This difference has been interpreted as determined by the variance magnitude of the visuo-vestibular conflict as this latter is more important on the sagittal axis than on the vertical axis. The present findings are not only consistent with the aforementioned studies but also with several studies following which the modification, reduction or attenuation of the visuo-vestibular interaction in patients in gravity conditions or in healthy participants in micro-gravity conditions modifies the latencies for reporting self-motion [16–19]. Contrary to the previous mentioned studies that have failed to demonstrate a significant intra-axis difference for reporting latencies on sagittal and vertical axes [5], the present data clearly demonstrate the existence of a significant intra-axis difference in latencies for reporting vertical self-motion. Namely, the latency for reporting downward self-motion is shorter than the latency for reporting upward self-motion. The difference between the aforementioned and the present study can be understood on the basis of technical disparities. In the former studies a peripheral visual environment, i.e., lamellar stimulation, was utilized, in the present study a visual environment, i.e., 3D pseudolamellar stimulation was produced via a HMD in central vision. In other words, the use of this enriched virtual environment with a full range of depth and inertial acceleration (as in the present study) could itself explain this difference. In the previous study the peripheral lamellar stimulation induced no asymmetry or reversed asymmetry between opposite directions (upward/downward vs. forward/backward), in the present study the difference between upward and downward directions is essentially due to participants with asymmetric self-motion navigation reflecting intra individual variability. Coherently, participants declared such asymmetric self-motion navigation at the end of the immersion. They felt they moved more easily downward than upward. Everything happens as if the central nervous system engages an asymmetric sensory weighting strategy of downward and upward self-motion perception by increasing or reducing the inter-sensory discordance. Our data are consistent with recent findings following which with constant gravitational acceleration acting in the downward direction, an asymmetric configuration occurs for upward and downward self-motion [21]. Expressly, under normal terrestrial conditions, both studies indicate that vertical self-motion is accomplished more rapidly when lined in the same direction as gravitational acceleration. In the absent of otolithic vestibular signal, i.e., in microgravity, the intra-axis asymmetry is rescind. Taken together, all the previous findings seem indicate that latencies' difference cannot only be confined to the inter-axis comparison but also affect the intra-axis comparison. Such data would indicate that with a constant gravitational acceleration acting in the downward direction, i.e., under normal terrestrial conditions, the latencies for reporting self-motion are shorter for vertical self-motion than sagittal self-motion and shorter for downward self-motion than for upward self-motion. These observations can be enriched by recent neuroimaging data underlying that the neural correlates of vertical self-motion perception (as linked to the gravitational field) activate a key cortex area receiving vestibular inputs: the PIVC parieto-insular vestibular cortex [27]. This cortical area, which is directly and indirectly associated with the neural activity of the occipito-temporo-parietal cortex [10–13] and with the frontal, temporal, parietal and prefrontal cortex [7–9] would also be associated with an internal model of gravity, i.e., an egocentric representation of the body in space [14, 28, 29].

The above considerations could account for the variations of the cardiovascular activity, i.e., the heart rate measured in our study. Actually, we have not only demonstrated that the autonomic cardiovascular response (i.e., the heart rate) is lower for the downward than for the upward self-motion. But that there is also a significant difference in cardiovascular activity between the rest condition and the upward condition. The cardiovascular activity is higher in upward self-motion condition than in rest condition. Namely, these results are consistent with our hypothesis claimed that the cardiovascular responses would be "vestibuloform" as they can be influenced by the otolithic saccular receptors. From experiments on animals and humans participants has demonstrated that inputs from vestibular otolith organs contribute to the control of heart rate during movement [30]. It follows that the intensity of the visuo-vestibular interaction along the vertical axis would also reshape cardiovascular activation depending on the directional condition (upward vs. downward). It is lower for downward self-motion that for upward self-motion. In other words, our data are clearly consistent with studies that have demonstrated that any reduction (because of the differential vestibular sensitivity) or loss of vestibular information, as it is the case in patients with unilateral or bilateral labyrinthine disease [24], provides an attenuation of the cardiovascular activation [31]. Similarly, it has been established that the development of motion sickness that is characterized by increased self-motion perception leads to the disintegration of autonomic nervous system balance. And this because, it is accompanied by an increase in sympathetic activity (and a decreased in parasympathetic activity). Analogously, the adaptation to motion sickness is accompanied by the recovery of autonomic nervous system balance [32]. In the same vein, significant changes in cardiorespiratory parameters occur during visually mediated illusory tilt and vertical self-motion. Such responses are consistent with the hypothesis that visuo-vestibular input contributes to the initial cardiovascular adjustment to a change in posture in humans [33]. However, it is not possible to determine, with the present studies, the precise mechanism that occurs but rather can only speculate that it plays an obligatory role in producing changes in cardiovascular autonomic activation during otolithic engagement in healthy adults.

5 Conclusion

Given the present findings, it can be concluded that during upward and downward self-motion perception, the engagement of vestibular saccular organs seems to contribute differently to latencies and cardiovascular activation depending on the direction of gravitational acceleration. Downward self-motion latencies (same direction acceleration) are shorter than upward self-motion latencies (opposite direction acceleration). In the same vein, cardiovascular autonomic activation, i.e., heart rate, is lower for downward self-motion than for upward self-motion. With that in mind, our findings provide evidence that visuo-vestibular interaction contributes to influence both latencies and cardiovascular variation in vertical self-motion perception. A top-down organisation associated to visuo-vestibular pathway along the vertical axis embodied to bodily self-consciousness, i.e., self-position and equilibrium, could afford a minimalistic neuromorphic basis in order to improve safe and reliable navigation of humanoid robots.

Acknowledgments To all the participants, the CNRS and the National Department of Education and Research.

References

1. Dichgans, J., Brandt, T.: Visual-vestibular interaction: effects on self motion perception and postural control. In: Held, R., Leibowitz, H.W., Teuber H.L. (eds.) Handbook of Sensory Physiology, vol. VIII, pp. 755–804. Springer, New York (1978)
2. Mergner, T., Becker, W.: Perception of horizontal self-motion: multisensory and cognitive aspects. In: Warren, R., Wertheim, A.H. (eds.) Perception and Control of Self-motion, pp. 219–263. Erlbaum, Hillsdale, NJ (1990)
3. Berthoz, A.: Le sens du mouvement. Odile Jacob, Paris (1997)
4. Howard, I.P.: The vestibular system. In: Boff, K.R., Kaufman, L., Thomas, J.P. (eds.) Handbook of Perception and Human Performance, vol. I, pp. 11-3 to 11-26. Wiley and Sons, New York (1986)
5. Giannopulu, I., Lepecq, J.C.: Linear vection chronometry along spinal and sagittal body-motion. Perception **27**, 363–449 (1998)
6. Giannopulu, I.: Contribution à la compréhension des représentations multimodales chez l'homme sain et chez des patients avec atteinte neuropsychologique: une perspective "lifespan". Habilitation à Diriger des Recherches en Sciences de la Vie et de la Santé-Neurosciences Cognitives, Paris VI (2011)
7. Bottini, G., Sterzi, R., Paulesu, E., Vallar, G., Cappa, S.F., Ermiono, F., Passingham, R.E., Frith, C.D., Frackowiak, R.S.J.: Identification of the central vestibular projections in man: a positron emission tomography activation study. Exp. Brain Res. **99**, 164–169 (1994)
8. Baudonnière, P.M., de Waele, C., Tran Ba Huy, P., Vidal P.P.: Vestibular evoked responses before and immediately after uni-lateral vestibular neurectomy in human. In: Collard, M., Jeannerod M, Christen Y (eds) The vestibular cortex. Irvinn, Strasbourg, pp 89–102, (1996)
9. de Waele, C., Tran Ba Huy, P., Diard, J.P., Freyss, G., Vidal, P.P.: Saccular dysfunction in Meniere's disease. Am. J. Otol. **20**, 223–232 (1999)
10. Straube, A., Brandt, T.: Importance of the visual and vestibular cortex for the self-motion perception in man (circularvection). Human Neurobiol. **6**, 211–218 (1987)
11. Büttner, U., Straube, A.: Ego and object-motion perception: where does it take place? Behav. Brain Res. **17**, 316–317 (1994)
12. Deutschländer, A., Bense, S., Stephan, T., Schwaiger, M., Dieterich, M., Brandt, T.: Rollvection versus linearvection: comparison of brain activations in PET. Human Brain Marring **21**(3), 143–153 (2004)

13. Becker-Bense, S., Buchholz, H. G., zu Eulenburg, P., Best, C., Bartenstein, P. Schreckenberger, M. and Dieterich, M.: Ventral and dorsal streams processing visual motion perception (FDG-PET study). BMC Neurosci. **16**, 13–81 (2012)
14. Giannopulu, I., Bertin, R.J.V., Brémond, R., Kapoula, Z., Espié, S.: Visual strategies in virtual and pre-recording environments. Adv. Transp. Stud. Int. J. Sect. B **14** (2008)
15. Napadow, V., Sheehan, J.D., Kim, J., Lacount, L.T., Park, K., Kaptchuk, T.J., Rosen, B.R., Kuo, B.: The brain circuitry underlying the temporal evolution of nausea in humans. Cereb. Cortex **23**(4), 806–813 (2013)
16. Cheung, B.S.K., Howard, I.P., Nedzelski, J.M., Landolt, J.P.: Circular vection about horizontal axes in bilateral labyrinthine-defective subjects. Acta Oto-laryngologica (Stockh) **108**, 336–344 (1989)
17. Wong, S.C.P., Frost, B.J.: The effect of visual-vestibular conflict on the latency of steady-state visually induced subjective rotation. Percept. Psychophys. **30**(3), 228–236 (1981)
18. Young, L.R., Shelhamer, M.: Weightlessness enhances the relative contribution of visually-induced self motion. In: Warren, R., Wertheim, A.H. (eds.) Perception and Control of Self-motion, pp. 523–538. Erlbaum, Hillsdale, NJ (1990)
19. Cheung, B.S.K., Howard, I.P., Money, K.E.: Visually-induced tilt during parabolic flights. Exp. Brain Res. **81**, 391–397 (1990)
20. Fluur, E.: The interaction between the utricle and the saccule. Acta Otolaryng **69**, 17–24 (1970)
21. De Saedeleer, C., Vidal, M., Lipshits, M., Bengoetxea, A., Cebolla, A.M., Berthoz, A., et al.: Weightlessness alters up/down asymmetries in the perception of self-motion. Exp. Brain Res. **226**, 95–106 (2013)
22. Pfeiffer, C., Serino, A., Blanke, O.: The vestibular system: a spatial reference for bodily self-consciousness. Front. Integr., Neurosci. **17**, 8–31 (2014)
23. Olufsen, M.S., Alston, A.V., Tran, H.T., Ottesen, J.T., Novak, O.V.: modeling heart rate regulation—Part I: Sit-to-stand versus head-up tilt. Cardiovasc. Eng. **8**(2), 73–87 (2008)
24. Yates, Y.B.J., Aoki, M., Burchill, P., Bronstein, A.M., Gresty, M.A.: Cardiovascular responses elicited by linear acceleration in humans. Exp. Brain Res. **125**, 476–484 (1999)
25. Wright, G.W.: Linear vection in virtual environments can be strengthened by discordant inertial input. 1157–1160. In: 31th Annual International Conference of the IEEE EMBS Minneapolis, Minnesota, USA, 2–6 Sept 2009
26. Zacharias, G.L., Young, L.R.: Influence of combined visual and vestibular cues on human perception and control of horizontal rotation. Exp. Brain Res. **41**, 159–171 (1981)
27. Indovina, I., Maffei, V., Pauwels, K., Macaluso, E., Orban, G.A., Lacquaniti, F.: Simulated self-motion in a visual gravity field: sensitivity to vertical and horizontal heading in the human brain. Neuroimage **71**, 114–124 (2013)
28. McIntyre, J., Zago, M., Berthoz, A., Lacquaniti, F.: Does the brain model Newton's laws? Nat. Neurosci. **4**, 693–694 (2001)
29. Indovina, I., Maffei, V., Bosco, G., Zago, M., Macaluso, E., Lacquaniti, F.: Representation of visual gravitational motion in the human vestibular cortex. Science **308**, 416–419 (2005)
30. Yates, B.J., Bolton, P.S., Macefield, V.G.: Vestibulo-sympathetic responses. Compr Physiol. **4** (2), 851–887 (2014)
31. Ray, C.A., Monahan, K.D.: Aging attenuates the vestibulosympathetic reflex in humans. Circulation **26**, **105**(8), 956–961 (2002)
32. Hu, S., Grant, W.F., Stern, R.M., Koch, K.L.: Motion sickness severity and physiological correlates during repeated exposures to a rotating optokinetic drum. Aviat. Space Environ. Med. **62**, 308–314 (1991)
33. Wood, S.J., Reschke, M.F., Sarmiento, L.A., Clement, G.: Tilt and translation motion perception during off-vertical axis rotation. Exp. Brain Res. **182**, 365–377 (2007)

Series Elastic Actuation for Assistive Orthotic Devices: Case Study of Pneumatic Actuator

A. Ortlieb, J. Olivier, M. Bouri and H. Bleuler

Abstract Wearable assistive robotics is a modern field where intelligent actuated systems work in collaboration with the body to replace a lost limb, to enhance performances (e.g. carrying load, walking, running, jumping) or to train or rehabilitate specific activities. Wearability (e.g. weight, bulkiness) and power are the two main competing characteristics of most assistive wearable devices. Energy efficient actuation systems with high power density per mass and volume are thus preferred. The biological muscle-tendon solution is very interesting for energy storage and generation of efficient cyclic patterns. The present study investigates on the capacity to replicate these biological properties using series elastic actuator (SEA) based on pneumatic cylinder technology. While classic SEA designs are composed of electric actuator in series with steel springs, pneumatic actuators are intrinsically compliant due to the compressibility of the fluid. The study starts by presenting an experimental approach for characterizing the elastic behavior of a pneumatic cylinder actuation targeting the assistance of the hip flexion. Results are then confronted to measurements of lower limb joints' stiffness observed during walking to identify the suitability of the solution with the targeted application..

Keywords Wearable assistive robotics · Series elastic actuator · Pneumatic cylinder · Walking assistive orthosis

1 Introduction

Wearable assistive robotics is a promising field with multiple applications in different domains. Assistive devices can provide support to people with muscle weakness, spinal cord injury (SCI) or post stroke neuromotor disorders for example.

A. Ortlieb (✉) · J. Olivier · M. Bouri · H. Bleuler
Laboratory of Robotic Systems, Swiss Federal Institute of Technology (EPFL), Lausanne, Switzerland
e-mail: amalric.ortlieb@epfl.ch

P. Wenger et al. (eds.), *New Trends in Medical and Service Robots*,
Mechanisms and Machine Science 39, DOI 10.1007/978-3-319-30674-2_9

They can also enhance the performance of healthy persons by contributing to activities requesting specific forces or activities subject to muscular injuries. Wearable devices need to meet challenging constraints on mechanical design. The actuation technology is very important to meet specifications on high dynamic performances combined to low weight of the device and low bulkiness. Bio-inspired solutions of series elastic actuators (SEA) are seen as one of the possible well adapted technology [1]. Numerous works have studied designs based on SEA to assist different activities. First developments were motivated in the field of legged robots about the 1980s [2] and led to advanced design of linear electric actuator in series with coil springs (e.g. Robinson et al. [3], Hutter et al. [4]). In the field of assistive devices, Pratt et al. proposed a Knee orthosis to enhance capabilities that is based on a similar SEA technology [5]. Veneman et al. also developed an electric SEA technology based on coil springs to assist the knee joint [6]. Kong et al. proposed a rotary SEA using a spiral spring coupled with an electric motor and applied it to both joints of an ankle-knee orthosis [7]. Recent works proposed rotary electric SEA for gait rehabilitation with the particularity of using specifically designed spring elements (e.g. [8, 9]). Grimmer et al. interestingly compared different serial and parallel configurations of springs with one actuator for the assistance of the ankle flexion [10]. They identified that double SEA are better in terms of low energy consumption and small peak power compared to single SEA or a combination of parallel and series elastic actuator. This solution is bio-inspired as it is similar to a whole muscle and antagonist muscle mechanism. Such a system allows to dynamically adjust the joint stiffness while also controlling the motion by moving the point of equilibrium.

Double SEA solutions are generally composed of two electric motors coupled with coil springs (E-SEA) [6, 11] or of two antagonistic pneumatic muscles (PM-SEA) [12–15]. Pneumatic cylinders, seems not to have been addressed in this field as an SEA solution as far as authors know. However double-acting pneumatic cylinders (PC-SEA) have the advantage of combining both actuators plus compliance in a single unit. Thus it can reduce both the bulkiness and potentially the weight of the actuator. Note that the elastic behavior of pneumatic solution is achieved through the compressibility of the gas and can be controlled by modulating the gas pressure in each chamber of the cylinder.

Different pros and cons between electric and pneumatic SEA can be discussed. First, E-SEA needs a high reduction between the motor and the spring element which affects the efficiency of the system. For PC-SEA, the actuator is in direct contact with the output, however the motion piston is a source of important friction. Another aspect is the power source, air can be stocked with high pressure or in other forms in a large tank (e.g. diving tank), or it can be generated by small compressors such as diaphragm pumps which works on battery. Basically, electric power source such as batteries are more mature with lighter and safer technology compared to pneumatic power source. A final aspect is the range of elastic properties, in E-SEA, the compliance is made by a spring that can be designed with few restrictions on material and shape, thus the range of stiffness is almost unlimited. For a PC-SEA, the compliance is limited to the gas properties and also to parameters such as cylinder diameter, range of pressure or cylinder length.

This last aspect is at the center of the current study, where it is proposed to characterize the elastic behavior of a pneumatic cylinder and then to confront the results with the properties of lower limb joints stiffness during level walking. Final discussion will inspect whether PC-SEA could be adapted for applications regarding lower limb assistance.

2 Problem Description and Materials

The chapter covers first the physics of double acting pneumatic cylinders in passive mode to highlight the elastic behavior of the system and identify the key parameters. The second section presents the mechanism designed to perform lower limb assistance of the hip or knee joint using a PC-SEA.

2.1 *Physics of PC-SEA*

Double acting pneumatic cylinder (PC-SEA, see Fig. 1) are composed of two chambers on each side of the piston. The difference of gas pressure in both chambers generates an output force from the actuator. In order to control this force, a pressure source and sink are connected through distributors to each chamber and allow to increase/decrease pressure into them. PC-SEA can also be transformed into a passive system by blocking any flow from/to the chambers. In analogy, it corresponds to locking both motors in the case of an E-SEA. This configuration will be used in this study to evaluate the elastic properties of a PC-SEA. Figure 1 presents

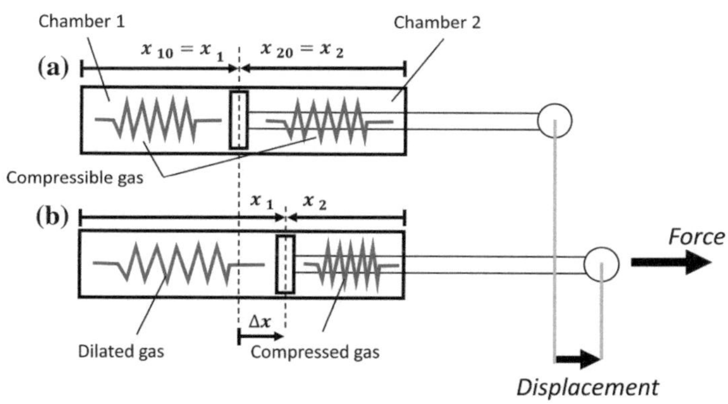

Fig. 1 Illustration of a pneumatic cylinder and its elastic reaction to an external force. **a** Cylinder at equilibrium without load. **b** Cylinder under a given force

passive PC-SEA at position of equilibrium (a) and its reaction under an external force (b) highlighting the compliant behavior.

In the following, the development leading to the expression of the elastic properties of a PC-SEA is described. Starting with the thermodynamics, the fluid of interest in this study being air and due to the non-insulation of the cylinder, the fluid compression/dilatation is assumed to be isothermal. Thus the expression of the state of each chamber of the cylinder at any time can be written as:

$$P_i \cdot V_i = cst \tag{1}$$

where P is the pressure and V the volume of a given chamber "i". Using the trivial relation between force and pressure and taking both chambers into consideration, the force exerted on the piston by the gas is expressed as:

$$P_1 \cdot S_1 - P_2 \cdot S_2 = F \tag{2}$$

where S_i represents the surface of the piston oriented towards chamber i. and F. is the force transmitted through the piston. Note that S_1 and S_2 are not equal due to the presence of a rod on one side of the piston. The surface being constant along the piston stroke, a change in chamber volume depends only on the piston position noted x. Equation (1) can be then written:

$$P_i \cdot x_i = cst \tag{3}$$

Any chamber state can be expressed in function of the equilibrium state (P_{i0}, x_{i0}) such as:

$$P_i = \frac{P_{i0} \cdot x_{i0}}{x_i} \tag{4}$$

By combining Eqs. (2) and (4), an expression between force and position can be written as:

$$F = \frac{x_{10}}{x_1} P_{10} \cdot S_1 - \frac{x_{20}}{x_2} P_{20} \cdot S_2 \tag{5}$$

Introducing the piston displacement Δx. which is identical for each chamber:

$$\Delta x = x_{10} - x_1 = -x_{20} + x_2 \tag{6}$$

Equation (5) can finally be rewritten as follows, where the force depends directly on the displacement.

$$F = \frac{x_{10}}{x_{10} - \Delta x} P_{10} \cdot S_1 + \frac{x_{20}}{x_{20} - \Delta x} P_{20} \cdot S_2 \tag{7}$$

Equation (7) highlights the non-linearity of the relation between the force and the displacement and also identifies all the parameters contributing to the elastic properties of PC-SEA: the equilibrium position and equilibrium pressure, and the surface of the piston. In the following, an optimized experiment will be presented to identify a simplified model of the elastic behavior of a PC-SEA.

2.2 *Rotary PC-SEA Mechanism (RPC-SEA)*

In order to propose an active solution to assist lower limb motions, a crank mechanism using a PC-SEA was designed (see Fig. 2). Dimensions were optimized to satisfy high torques, low bulkiness and a range of motion of 120°. The final system is composed of a 50 mm bore diameter double acting cylinder (SMC CG3) with a stroke of 200 mm. All three pivot joints are realized by ball bearings and the structure is made of aluminium. The length of the lever measures 100 mm, such that with a pressure source of 0.4 MPa (4 bar) and a sink at 0.1 MPa (1 bar), maximal torques range from 30 to 60 Nm depending on the position. Specifications on source pressure were made based on typical diaphragm pump nominal capacity and torques requirements were defined based on joint hip and knee peaks during level walking or stairs climbing [16–18].

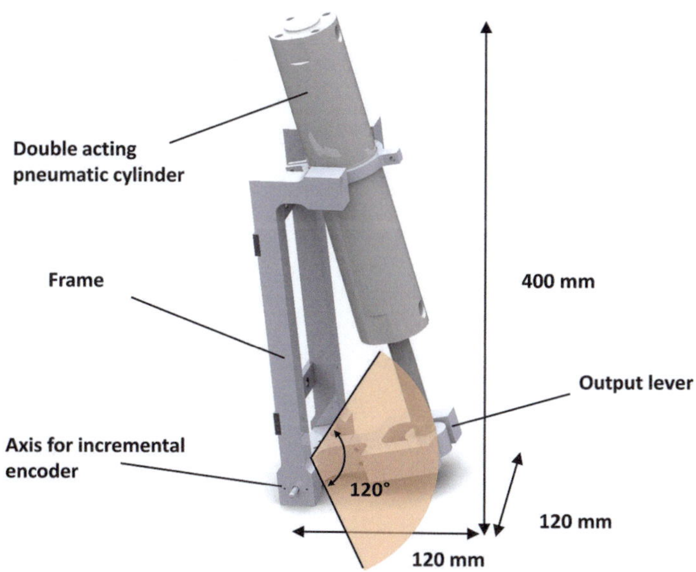

Fig. 2 Presentation of the RPC-SEA mechanism designed for lower limb assistance of the hip, where the frame can be fastened to the trunk and the output lever linked to the thigh of the wearer

In terms of wearability, the whole system with an aluminium structure weights 2.4 kg (cylinder alone: 1.42 kg) for maximal dimensions about $400 \times 120 \times 120\ \text{mm}^3$. Note that both weight and bulkiness can be largely reduced by increasing the source pressure or by reducing the torque requirements.

3 Methods

The expression of the stiffness of PC-SEA as presented by Eq. (7) appears highly non-linear. Moreover, the RPC-SEA mechanism adds a supplementary degree of non-linearity to the problem. In order to define a simplified model of the stiffness i.e. the relation between force and displacement, an experimental identification is realized based on a parametric model. This model can be written based on Eq. (7) where pressure contributes linearly to the stiffness but not the terms related to the position of equilibrium and the actual position. The parametric infinite model takes the form:

$$\Gamma_{out} = P_0 \cdot \sum_{m=0}^{\infty} \sum_{n=0}^{\infty} b_{mn} \cdot \alpha_0^m \cdot \Delta\alpha^m \tag{8}$$

where Γ_{out} is the torque exerted by the cylinder, b_{mn} are the parametric coefficients to be identified, P_0 is the pressure at equilibrium under no load which is simplified to be equal in both chambers, α_0 is the angular position at equilibrium under no load and $\Delta\alpha$ is the angular displacement (see Fig. 4, where $\Gamma_{\text{M}} = -\Gamma_{\text{out}}$).

The experiment comports three factors, one linear and two non-linear. A Box-Behnken design [19] is used to optimize the number of samples. This design is presented in Fig. 3 and is composed of 13 samples. Details about the factors and the response of the experiment are described in the following:

Angular position without load: The angular position α_0 (see Fig. 4) without load on the system is measured with an incremental encoder (Avago HEDR-5xxx

Fig. 3 Illustration of the three factors Box-Behnken design of the experiment

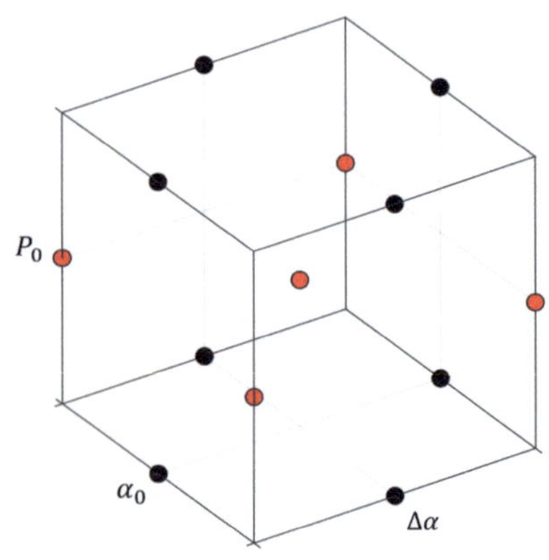

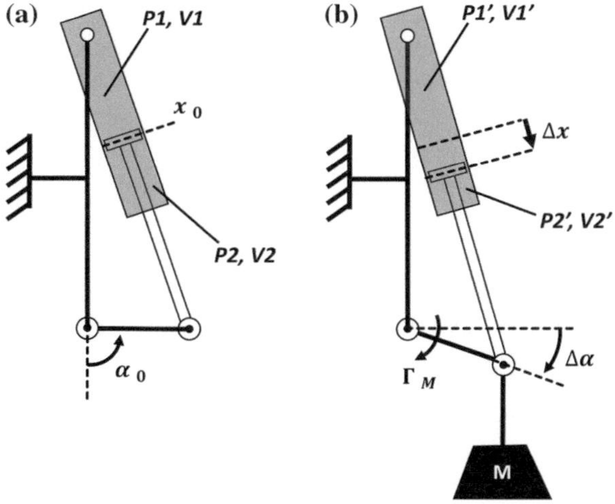

Fig. 4 Representation of the RPC-SEA system with experimental conditions: **a** System at equilibrium under no load. **b** System under constant load of mass M. With P and V respectively the pressure and volume state in both cylinder's chambers, x_0 and Δx the piston initial position and displacement, α_0 and $\Delta\alpha$ the joint angular position and displacement and Γ_M the torque applied on the joint by the added mass

3000 pulse/rev.). The three positions selected are about 60°, 100° and 140° which correspond respectively to a piston position of 1/4, 1/2 and 3/4 of the cylinder length.

Pressure without load: The pressures at rest in both chambers are measured using pressure sensors (SMC PSE530). Without load, pressure in both chambers are similar with a difference smaller than 1 %. P_0 is taken as the average pressure from both chambers. The sample of values retained are 1 bar, 2 bar and 3 bar (respectively 0.1, 0.2 and 0.3 MPa).

Displacement: The displacement $\Delta\alpha$ is measured by the difference of position between the loaded and unloaded case, each time at steady state. The displacement is generated only in one direction (see Fig. 4).

Response: The torques applied to the system are defined by different loads that are hanged at the lever end. The load torque Γ_M is calculated by projecting the force, due to the gravity, perpendicularly to the lever orientation. Three loads of 4, 10 and 18 kg are used for the experiment.

Finally a reference parametric model limited to the second order for m and n (see Eq. (8)) is used. This model contains 10 coefficients and can be written:

$$\begin{aligned}\Gamma_{out} = cst + b_{00}P_0 + b_{10}\alpha_0 P_0 + b_{01}\Delta\alpha P_0 + b_{11}\alpha_0\Delta\alpha P_0 + b_{20}\alpha_0^2 P_0 \\ + b_{02}\Delta\alpha^2 P_0 + b_{21}\alpha_0^2\Delta\alpha P_0 + b_{12}\alpha_0\Delta\alpha^2 P_0 + b_{22}\alpha_0^2\Delta\alpha^2 P_0 + \xi\end{aligned} \quad (9)$$

where cst is also called the intercept or the offset depending on the field and ξ represents the error. The method used to evaluate the coefficients b_{mn} and the intercept of any model is the least square linear regression which minimizes the error between the measurements and the model function. Two incremental approaches are proposed to reduce the complexity of Eq. (9): the forward selection and the backward elimination. The forward selection starts with the simplest model (i.e. the intercept) and evaluates which term from Eq. (9) correlates best with the measurements based on an F-statistics, each terms are evaluated at each steps and the algorithm stops as soon as the next step does not significantly improve the model (i.e. the p-value from the F-statistics is bigger than 5 %). The backward elimination works similarly but it starts with full model from Eq. (9) and reduces the model at each iteration based on the term with the poorest F-statistics. More details about the statistical materials can be found in [20, 21].

The experiment is conducted as followed: in a first phase, the unloaded system is brought to the chosen state (P_0, α_0) (see a in Fig. 4), then the defined mass is added while in/out valves of the cylinder are closed and displacement ($\Delta\alpha$) is recorded (see b in Fig. 4). The experiment is repeated 13 times with the different conditions defined by the Box-Behnken design (see Fig. 3).

The claimed hypothesis of the study is that the biological muscle-tendon actuation benefits from an optimized energy efficiency by using a passive compliant behavior coupled with actuation to adjust the stiffness. In order to evaluate the locomotion strategies and the range of stiffness found in human joints, kinematics and kinetics from the walking activity are observed. Hip, knee and ankle flexion data during walking are extracted from the observation of Winter [16] and Ounpuu [17]. Curves presenting joint torques in function of the angular positions are extracted in order to observe phases with static elastic properties. Results are presented in next section, starting with the characterization of the pneumatic actuator.

4 Results

4.1 RPC-SEA Elastic Properties

The simplified models resulting from the forward selection and backward elimination process are presented in respectively Eqs. (10) and (11). Both resulting models are composed of 4 terms including the intercept.

$$\Gamma_{out\_f} = cst + b_{01}\Delta\alpha P_0 + b_{02}\Delta\alpha^2 P_0 + b_{03}\Delta\alpha^3 P_0 + \xi \tag{10}$$

$$\Gamma_{out\_b} = cst + b_{11}\alpha_0\Delta\alpha P_0 + b_{02}\Delta\alpha^2 P_0 + b_{21}\alpha_0^2\Delta\alpha P_0 + \xi \tag{11}$$

Values and statistics from both linear regressions are presented in Tables 1 and 2, where data about the coefficient estimate, the sum of squares (SS), the degree of freedom (DF), the F-statistics and the p-value can be found. Curves of the response torque in function of the different factors are illustrated in Fig. 5 for model (10) and in Fig. 6 for model (11). The R^2 (fraction of variability in the data explained by the

Table 1 Results of the regression based on forward selection, model (10)

Term	Estimate	SS	DF	F	*p*
Constant	−0.92307	0.974	1		
$\Delta\alpha P_0$	−0.59705	164.27	1	380.82	1.12e-08
$\Delta\alpha^2 P_0$	−0.01279	12.688	1	29.414	0.000419
$\Delta\alpha^3 P_0$	−0.00022	2.9538	1	6.8474	0.027959
Residuals	–	3.8823	9		

Table 2 Results of the regression using model (11)

Term	Estimate	SS	DF	F	*p*
Constant	−1.376		1		
$\alpha_0 \Delta\alpha P_0$	−0.012572	131.9	1	1655.7	1.62e-11
$\Delta\alpha^2 P_0$	−0.005370	15.98	1	200.5	1.85e-07
$\alpha_0^2 \Delta\alpha P_0$	6.159e-05	81.17	1	1018.5	1.43e-10
Residuals	–	0.717	9		

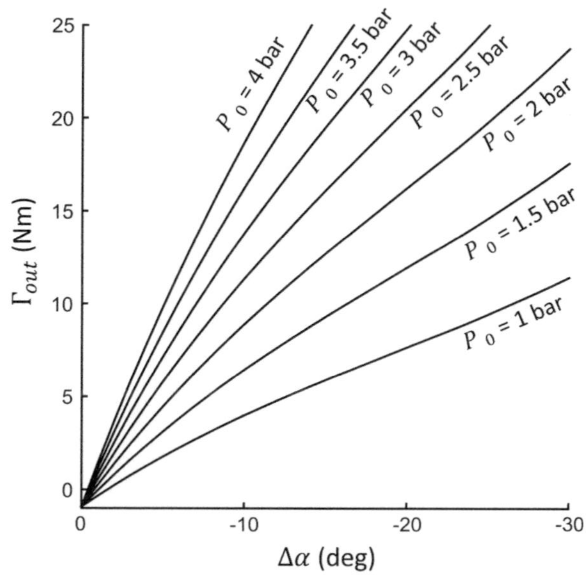

Fig. 5 Evolution of the response torque in function of the angular displacement and the zero-pressure for model (10)

model) shows a better regression of the data for model (11) with a value of 0.998 versus a value of 0.988 for model (10). Model (11) is selected for further use as the best expression of the elastic property of the passive RPC-SEA.

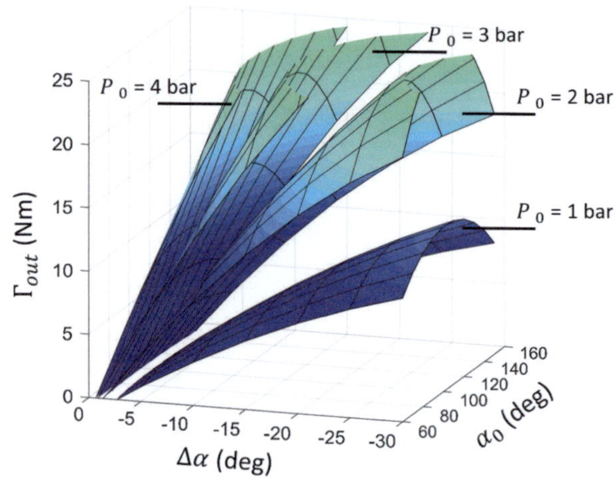

Fig. 6 Curves of the response torque in function of the three factors: the displacement, the zero-position and the zero-pressure for model (11)

4.2 *Joints Properties During Walking*

Curves of the hip, knee and ankle joints torque in function of the angular position are illustrated in Fig. 7 and Fig. 8 based on the data taken respectively from the measurements of Winter [16] and Ounpuu [17]. Average weight of subjects performing the experiment are about 70 kg.

If small differences between results from Winter and from Ounpuu can be observed, the graphs highlight that for every joint there exists important phases where the position-torque relation is quasi-linear. This indicates periods of constant stiffness where joints are used passively. The values of the stiffness during these phases are summarized for the different joints in Table 3.

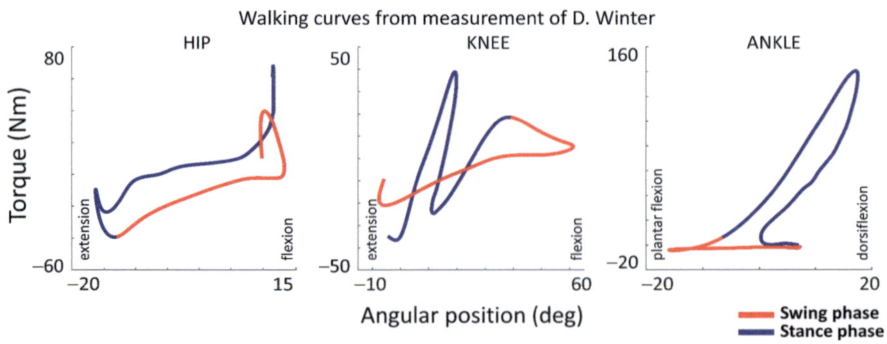

Fig. 7 Hip, knee and ankle torque in function of joint position for one gait cycle during walking based on measurement from Winter [16]

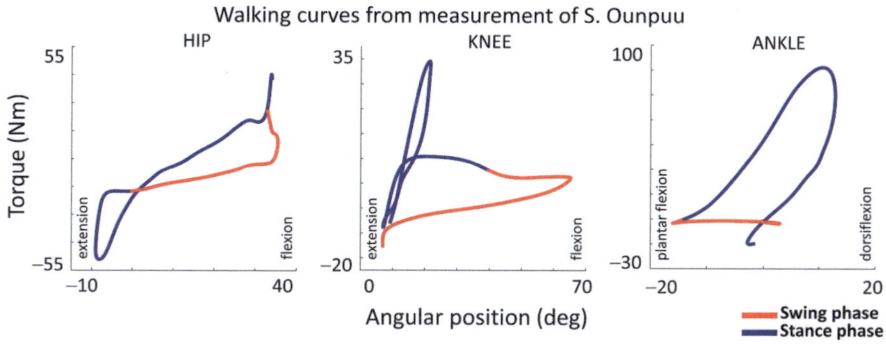

Fig. 8 Hip, knee and ankle torque in function of joint position for one gait cycle during walking based on measurement from Ounpuu [17]

Table 3 Stiffness of the joints during walking

Joint	Source	Stiffness (Nm/°)		
		Stance 1	Stance 2	Swing
Hip	Winter	1.31	–	1.47
	Ounpuu	1.20	3.80	0.40
Knee	Winter	4.09	1.78	0.38
	Ounpuu	3.40	–	0.21
Ankle	Winter	6.5	–	0.07
	Ounpuu	3.99	–	0.07

Table 4 Stiffness of the pneumatic actuator in Nm/°

Stiffness (Nm/°)		Initial pressure P_0 (MPa)				
		0.1	0.2	0.3	0.4	0.5
Angular displacement (°)	10	0.74	1.50	2.25	3.00	3.74
	30	0.96	1.92	2.89	3.85	4.81
	50	1.18	2.35	3.53	4.71	5.89

Joints stiffness range from 1.2 to 6.5 Nm/° during stance and from 0.07 to 1.47 Nm/° during swing. In comparison, Table 4 below express the stiffness of the RPC-SEA relatively to the initial pressure P_0 and the angular displacement about a mean zero-position α_0 of 100°.

Pneumatic actuator stiffness range from 0.74 to 5.89 Nm/° with pressures from 0.1 to 0.5 MPa. Joints' stiffness during walking are thus in a similar range during stance and smaller during the swing phase compared to the RPC-SEA.

5 Discussion

This study performed a precise characterization and simplification of the elastic behavior of an RPC-SEA mechanism. The high non-linearity of the system has been modeled by a four terms parametric model using an experimental approach with a Box-Behnken design to reduce the number of measurements. Two approaches, i.e. the forward selection and the backward elimination, have been used to optimize the complexity of the model. The main factors influencing the RPC-SEA stiffness for a given design were identified as being the pressure with a proportional effect, the equilibrium position and the displacement from that position.

In order to evaluate the adequacy of the RPC-SEA performances in comparison to the application of walking assistance, the hip, knee and ankle stiffness range were analyzed based on the kinetic and kinematic patterns measured by Winter [16] and Ounpuu [17]. Figures 7 and 8 shows how the joint torques evolve in function of the joint positions and illustrate the fact that locomotion uses only a few number of stiffness states during walking. The control has thus the advantage of being largely simplified compared to a position control following a dynamic trajectory. Results showed that the designed pneumatic actuator has a similar range of stiffness compared to the ones obtained from the joints' kinetics with a range of pressure from 0.1 to 0.5 MPa.

The current study demonstrated the adequacy of the RPC-SEA mechanism used as a series elastic actuator for assisting walking motions of the hip, knee and ankle joints. It highlighted also the strategy of bio-inspired solutions with maximization of the energy efficiency and reduction of the control complexity as each joint can be controlled by a reduced number of states (about three) for each gait cycle.

Acknowledgments Authors want to thank the ASRIM (Association Suisse Romande et Italienne contre les Myopathies) and the FSRMM (Fondation Suisse de Recherche sur les Maladies Musculaires) for supporting this work. A particular thanks is addressed to Anil Kodiyan who contributed in the design and assembly of the setup.

References

1. Pratt, G.A., Williamson, M.M.: Series elastic actuators. In: 1995 IEEE/RSJ International Conference on Intelligent Robots and Systems 95. "Human Robot Interaction and Cooperative Robots", Proceedings, vol. 1, pp. 399–406 (1995)
2. Raibert, M.H.: Legged Robots that Balance. MIT Press (1986)
3. Robinson, D.W., Pratt, J.E., Paluska, D.J., Pratt, G.A.: Series elastic actuator development for a biomimetic walking robot. In: 1999 IEEE/ASME International Conference on Advanced Intelligent Mechatronics, 1999. Proceedings, pp. 561–568 (1999)
4. Hutter, M., Remy, C.D., Hoepflinger, M.A., Siegwart, R.: High compliant series elastic actuation for the robotic leg ScarlETH. In: Proceedings of the International Conference on Climbing and Walking Robots (CLAWAR) (2011)

5. Pratt, J.E., Krupp, B.T., Morse, C.J., Collins, S.H.: The RoboKnee: an exoskeleton for enhancing strength and endurance during walking. In: 2004 IEEE International Conference on Robotics and Automation, 2004. Proceedings. ICRA'04, vol. 3, pp. 2430–2435 (2004)
6. Veneman, J.F., Ekkelenkamp, R., Kruidhof, R., van der Helm, F.C.T., van der Kooij, H.: A series elastic- and bowden-cable-based actuation system for use as torque actuator in exoskeleton-type robots. Int. J. Robot. Res. **25**(3), 261–281 (2006)
7. Kong, K., Bae, J., Tomizuka, M.: Control of rotary series elastic actuator for ideal force-mode actuation in human–robot interaction applications. IEEE/ASME Trans. Mechatron. **14**(1), 105–118 (2009)
8. Lagoda, C., Schouten, A.C., Stienen, A.H.A., Hekman, E.E.G., van der Kooij, H.: Design of an electric series elastic actuated joint for robotic gait rehabilitation training. In: 2010 3rd IEEE RAS and EMBS International Conference on Biomedical Robotics and Biomechatronics (BioRob), pp. 21–26 (2010)
9. Sergi, F., Accoto, D., Carpino, G., Tagliamonte, N.L., Guglielmelli, E.: Design and characterization of a compact rotary Series Elastic Actuator for knee assistance during overground walking. In: 2012 4th IEEE RAS EMBS International Conference on Biomedical Robotics and Biomechatronics (BioRob), pp. 1931–1936 (2012)
10. Grimmer, M., Eslamy, M., Gliech, S., Seyfarth, A.: A comparison of parallel- and series elastic elements in an actuator for mimicking human ankle joint in walking and running. In: 2012 IEEE International Conference on Robotics and Automation (ICRA), pp. 2463–2470 (2012)
11. Martinez-Villalpando, E.C., Weber, J., Elliott, G., Herr, H.: Design of an agonist-antagonist active knee prosthesis. In: 2nd IEEE RAS EMBS International Conference on Biomedical Robotics and Biomechatronics, 2008. BioRob 2008, pp. 529–534 (2008)
12. Tondu, B., Boitier, V., Lopez, P.: Naturally compliant robot-arms actuated by McKibben artificial muscles. In: 1994 IEEE International Conference on Systems, Man, and Cybernetics, 1994. Humans, Information and Technology, vol. 3, pp. 2635–2640 (1994)
13. Ariga, Y., Pham, H.T.T., Uemura, M., Hirai, H., Miyazaki, F.: Novel equilibrium-point control of agonist-antagonist system with pneumatic artificial muscles. In: 2012 IEEE International Conference on Robotics and Automation (ICRA), pp. 1470–1475 (2012)
14. Sawicki, G.S., Ferris, D.P.: A pneumatically powered knee-ankle-foot orthosis (KAFO) with myoelectric activation and inhibition. J. NeuroEng. Rehabil. **6**(1), 23 (2009)
15. Beyl, P., Knaepen, K., Duerinck, S., Damme, M.V., Vanderborght, B., Meeusen, R., Lefeber, D.: Safe and compliant guidance by a powered knee exoskeleton for robot-assisted rehabilitation of gait. Adv. Robot. **25**(5), 513–535 (2011)
16. Winter, D.A.: Kinematic and kinetic patterns in human gait: variability and compensating effects. Hum. Mov. Sci. **3**(1–2), 51–76 (1984)
17. Ounpuu, S.: The biomechanics of walking and running. Clin. Sports Med. **13**(4), 843–863 (1994)
18. Costigan, P.A., Deluzio, K.J., Wyss, U.P.: Knee and hip kinetics during normal stair climbing. Gait Posture **16**(1), 31–37 (2002)
19. Ferreira, S.L.C., Bruns, R.E., Ferreira, H.S., Matos, G.D., David, J.M., Brandão, G.C., da Silva, E.G.P., Portugal, L.A., dos Reis, P.S., Souza, A.S., dos Santos, W.N.L.: Box-Behnken design: an alternative for the optimization of analytical methods. Anal. Chim. Acta **597**(2), 179–186 (2007)
20. Xu, L., Zhang, W.-J.: Comparison of different methods for variable selection. Anal. Chim. Acta **446**(1–2), 475–481 (2001)
21. Sutter, J.M., Kalivas, J.H.: Comparison of forward selection, backward elimination, and generalized simulated annealing for variable selection. Microchem. J. **47**(1–2), 60–66 (1993)

Sensory-Motor Anticipation and Local Information Fusion for Reliable Humanoid Approach

H.F. Chame and C. Chevallereau

Abstract The possibility of developing increasingly sophisticated robots, and the availability of cloud-connected resources, have boosted the interest in the study of real world applications of service robotics. However, in order to operate under natural or less structured conditions, and given the information processing bottleneck and the reactivity required for a secure execution of the task, it is desirable that the agent can exploit more efficiently the local information available, so that being more autonomous, and relying less on remote computation. This study explores a strategy for obtaining reliable approach tasks. It considers the anticipation of perception, by taking into account the statistical regularities and the information redundancies induced in the sensory-motor coupling. From an initial perception of the object assisted by remote computation, contextual features are defined for capturing bodily sensations emerging in the task. The observations based on proprioceptive and visual data are fused in a Bayesian network, which is in charge of assessing the saliency during the object approach, thus constituting a local discriminative processing of the object. The strategy proposed reduces dependency on context-free models of behavior, while providing an estimate on the degree of confidence in the progress of the task.

Keywords Cognitive robotics · Embodied cognition · Humanoid robotics · Ego-localization · Top-down visual attention · Robot vision

1 Introduction

Ubiquitous computing is now a reality, given the progresses in the fields of information technology and artificial intelligence. In everyday life we have access to various applications offered on mobile devices. Just to mention a few, we can obtain

H.F. Chame (✉) · C. Chevallereau
CNRS, IRCCyN, Ecole Centrale de Nantes, Nantes, France
e-mail: Hendry.Ferreira-Chame@irccyn.ec-nantes.fr

C. Chevallereau
e-mail: Christine.Chevallereau@irccyn.ec-nantes.fr

P. Wenger et al. (eds.), *New Trends in Medical and Service Robots*,
Mechanisms and Machine Science 39, DOI 10.1007/978-3-319-30674-2_10

information about a product from a captured image, or identify a song from an audio sample. In such applications, due to the computational limitations of the local device, the processing is performed remotely on dedicated servers, equipped with extensive knowledge data-bases and a vast computing power. The local device is simply in charge of running the client application, thus, ensuring the aspects related to the usability in the human-machine interaction.

From the success of ubiquitous computing, several efforts are currently directed to developing solutions to more challenging scenarios in heath-care, assistance, or service robotics. Hence, robot applications can share knowledge or be assisted by cloud-connected resources. In this sense, there are initiatives that focus on the definition of robot architectures (e.g. Vasiliu et al. [20]), that integrate distributed resources to the task, so mitigating specific constraints of the robot platform. In parallel, several research communities are engaged in the definition of ontologies for knowledge sharing, distributed learning, and the collection and reuse of information for practical applications (e.g. Waibel et al. [21]).

However, since robots take action on the environment, the safety aspect is particularly affected by the information processing bottleneck during remote computing. When moving, the agent would ideally not depend at all on remote resources, since the communication with the server can be interrupted. It would also have the least possible of top-down deliberation, since it must be reactive to unexpected disturbances. Thus, it has to be endorsed with autonomy in order to ensure the maximum local progress on the task.

In this study, inspired by the research on embodied cognition, we explore the emergency of information during the task. From a first-person perspective definition of the approach, and taking into account the redundancies and the statistical regularities induced in the sensory-motor coupling, we examine the possibility of exploiting the anticipation of multi-sensory, contextual, and more diversified evidence about the object. To this end, we study a Bayesian network structure for information fusion, to discriminate the saliency related to the object.

This paper is organized as follows. In Sect. 2 some related contributions from the cognitivist approach to artificial intelligence are discussed, and contrasted to the point of view of embodied cognition research, that considers the emergent aspects of behavior. In Sect. 3 the definition of the approach task is presented. In Sect. 4 the aspect of autonomy is tackled, where the design of the features and the structure of the Bayesian network are detailed. A case-study has been developed and conducted with the robot Nao, which is going to be discussed in Sect. 5. Finally, the conclusions are given in Sect. 6.

2 Related Work

Vision-based locomotion control is a challenging task for walking robots. Unlike natural beings, which are in possession of extremely sophisticated sensory organs, the vast majority of the research in robotic vision has been carried out with quite inferior equipment, usually employing general purpose cameras. Moreover, the body structure and the actuation system used is much less stable, fine, and accurate, when compared to the natural musculo-skeletal system. In view of such limitations, some studies (e.g., Lewis and Simo [12], and Michel et al. [14]) have resorted to capture information from extra-corporal sensory, for achieving higher quality observations. Unfortunately, robot motion may occlude the cameras thus compromising the solution. Furthermore, the generality of the solution is affected once the scene is adapted to the task.

On-board solutions have been attempted under the visual servoing (VS) framework (see Chaumette and Hutchinson [4] and Corke [6]), which relates variations on image features to the spatial instantaneous velocity of a flying (dismembered) camera. A study by Dune et al. [7] has considered a monocular vision task with the robot HRP2. Given the walk style of the robot, the solution involved the cancellation of the oscillatory contribution to the control signal (also called the *sway motion*). A work by Moughlbay et al. [15] has considered approaching tasks with the robot Nao. In both studies, in order to handle the image noise, the tracking technique by Comport et al. [5] was employed. The algorithm is based on the principle of *verification vision*, so it required of visual odometry, and a realistic 3D model of the object (e.g. to measure parts of the room).

Model-based navigation have been explored in the simultaneous localization and mapping (SLAM) research (see Thrun et al. [19]). Examples of contributions in the field are numerous. Just to mention a few, in the work by Hornung et al. [10], starting from a volumetric map of the environment, precise indoor localization is obtained by adapting a range sensor to the robot's head. A work by Oriolo et al. [16] considered building the map on-line by fusing proprioceptive, inertial, and visual information, within an extended Kalman filter. In general, map-based navigation has produced impressive results, but it has also received some criticism. According to Shapiro [18], EC researchers disagree with the premise that organisms must firstly represent the environment for then transversing it. Indeed, this would be inconvenient to unstructured or reactive situations. Moreover, from the practical point of view, map-based solutions present as a drawback requiring maintenance, where environmental changes must be systematically acknowledged.

The works discussed so far fall within the so-called cognitivist research paradigm of artificial intelligence, that addresses the problem of automation under a representational focus, in which the solution of the task is modeled explicitly. In the last decades a different perspective has been adopted through the multi-disciplinary research in embodied cognition (EC). Under the EC methodology behavior is viewed as a complex system, emerging from the interactions with the environment (Anderson [1], Hoffmann and Pfeifer [9]). Thus, knowledge representation is considered to be grounded in the physical coupling (Brooks [2]), so emergent behavior would be neither explicitly described nor planned in advance.

The analysis of the sensory-motor coupling in natural tasks, from a dynamic system perspective, constitutes a promising research direction that can provide more efficient, easier to implement, and robust solutions. In this sense, a work by Lungarella and Sporns [13] has explored the relation between sensory-motor coordination, body morphology, and information processing. The study reported that higher levels of information correlation occurred when actions and perceptions were coordinated. Moreover, sensory-motor coordination reduced the dimensionality of the information content, given the perceptual regularities induced in the task. From these results, the information emerging in the task, including the motor activity, the body configuration, and the visual saliency; can be exploited to anticipate the evolution of the object in the field of vision. Thus, reducing the dependency on intensive context-free computations for perceiving the object in the scene.

3 Task Definition

The on-board localization is obtained from the definition of a sensory ego-cylinder, that heuristically takes the z-axis perpendicular to the ground, under the assumption of motion over a plane surface. Figure 1a illustrates the frames defined in the study. The frame G is placed at the ground level between the feet of the robot, it corresponds to the origin of the ego-cylinder. The frame T is set at the center of mass of the robot. The frame C is placed at the camera location on the forehead. The transformation between the reference frames G, T, and C, depend on the current joint configuration q of the robot. They are obtained by the classical modeling approach (see Khalil and

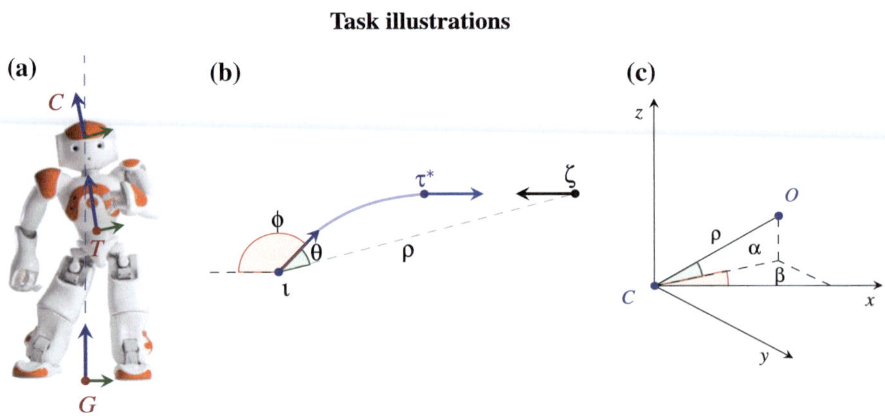

Fig. 1 **a** *Frontal* view of the task reference frames (camera C, trunk T, ground G). The z-axis is represented in *blue* and the y-axis in *green*. The x-axis goes towards the reader and is plotted as a *red dot*. Notice that the frames are not necessarily aligned. **b** *Upper* view of the task. The localization of the object is denoted by ζ. The *black dot* represents the object's center, the *black arrow* illustrates the direction of the projection on the motion plane of the mean normal direction to the tracked face of the object. The agent with the heading direction is represented in *blue*. A desired configuration in relation to the object is represented by τ^*. The trajectory followed to approach the object is illustrated in *light blue*. **c** Illustration of the look-at task. The position of the object center corresponds to O. After the head correction, the x-axis of the camera frame C will be aligned with the direction $\overline{CO}$

Dombre [11]), that considers the body as a set of interconnected serial structures departing from a common reference, which is taken as frame T.

As illustrated on Fig. 1b, the localization ζ of the object is represented by the four parameters

$$\zeta = \left[\rho\ \theta\ \iota\ \phi\right]^{\mathrm{t}}, \tag{1}$$

where ρ, θ, and ι are position components. Respectively, the distance, the azimuth, and the height of the center of the object. The parameter ϕ corresponds to the orientation of the object around the z-axis. It is estimated by the difference between the projection on the motion plane of the mean normal direction to the tracked face of the object, and the heading direction of the agent. The observation of the object's pose with respect to the camera frame C is obtained by defining a virtual oriented trapezoid, which delimits the image region containing the tracked face (see Fig. 2).

The task considered is the approach to a specific face of a static object, by walking on a plane, in a scene without obstacles. More specifically, starting from the knowledge of a desired ego-centric perception of the object, the agent has to autonomously return as close as possible to such state once disturbed. The behavior can be viewed as a regulation task where the control parameters include a 2D pose, which is defined with respect to a movable reference frame (on-board). Hence, the localization component ι is assumed to be constant. Formally, the approach error e expresses the desired configuration τ^* of the body (see Fig. 1b) in the actual egocentric perspective, such that

$$e = \left[\tau_{\rho^*}\ \tau_{\theta^*}\ \tau_{\phi^*}\right]^{\mathrm{t}}. \tag{2}$$

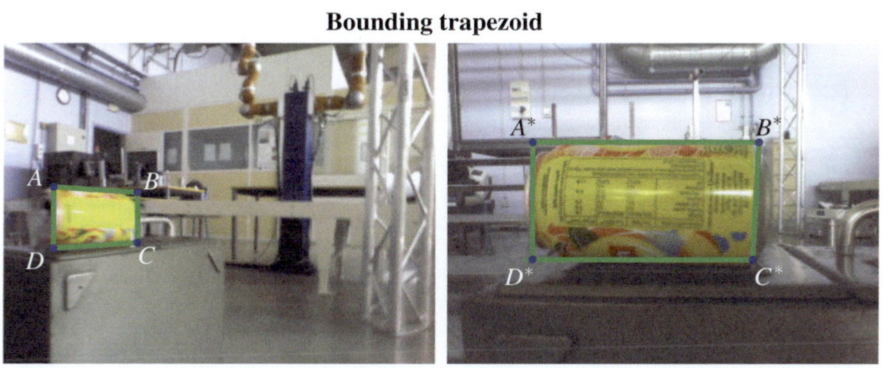

Fig. 2 The localization of the can is estimated by fitting the salient trapezoid to a rough geometric model of the object, which in this case is a cylinder. Notice that the lateral face of the can at the *left* is not salient. The observation of the approach error $\hat{e}$ (see Eq. (2)) is obtained from the spatial relation between the current view at the *left* and the desired view at the *right*

The solution of the task is based on the parallel execution of two motor behaviors: the walk and the look-at tasks. The former is in charge of steering the robot to ensure convergence toward the object. In order to take into account the aesthetics of motion, human walk is mimicked. That is, non-holonomic motion is used when human is far from the object, but holonomic motion is preferred when human is close enough to the goal. Thus, the Cartesian evolution of the walk task is described by

$$\begin{bmatrix} \dot{x} \\ \dot{y} \\ \omega \end{bmatrix} = \begin{bmatrix} \lambda(k_1\hat{e}_\rho) + \gamma(k_2\cos(\hat{e}_\theta)\hat{e}_\rho) \\ \gamma(k_3\sin(\hat{e}_\theta)\hat{e}_\rho) \\ \lambda(k_4\sin(\hat{e}_\theta - \hat{e}_\phi) + \hat{e}_\phi) + \gamma k_5\hat{e}_\phi \end{bmatrix}. \tag{3}$$

where $\dot{x}$ and $\dot{y}$ are the linear velocities, and ω is the angular velocity. The holonomic walk includes independent corrections along the 3 degrees of freedom, with different gains k_2, k_3, k_5. The non-holonomic walk does not include correction along the y-axis, since no lateral displacement is permitted. A correction along the walking direction is applied proportionally to the error distance $\hat{e_\rho}$ with gain k_1. The steering correction is chosen to direct the agent toward the object with gain k_4. The transition to the holonomic motion depends on the distance $\hat{e}_\rho$, such that $\lambda = 1/(1 + \exp(s_1(\hat{e}_\rho - s_2)))$, where s_1 is a proportional gain, and s_2 is the sensitive distance for the transition.

The look-at task is in charge of directing the view towards the object, thus maintaining it centered on the image. As illustrated in Fig. 1c, α and β are respectively the pitch and yaw angles of the Nao robot neck, that affect the pose of the camera frame C. The head motion is described by

$$\begin{bmatrix} \dot{\alpha} \\ \dot{\beta} \end{bmatrix} = \begin{bmatrix} \text{atan2}(l_\iota, \cos(l_\theta)\hat{\zeta}_\rho) \\ l_\theta \end{bmatrix}, \tag{4}$$

where l_θ and l_ι are the azimuth and the height correction desired, and $\hat{\zeta}_\rho$ is the observed distance to the object, expressed with respect to frame T.

4 Behavior Autonomy

As discussed earlier, the tasks in charge of the agent are moving toward the object and controlling the gaze direction. The available sources of information are the image acquired by the camera and the proprioceptive registry of the robot. The difficulty of the task consists in finding the object of interest on the image, by relying mostly on contextual representations. As illustrated in the diagram of Fig. 3, the idea is to provide the agent with an autonomous implementation of the behavior that can be continuously assessed. Thus, the agent would resort to remote services only when the level of confidence about the correctness of the task is low. For this, we will rely on the coupling between action and perception. The perception is based on the analysis of properties related to the image blobs (e.g. the area, the radio-aspect, and

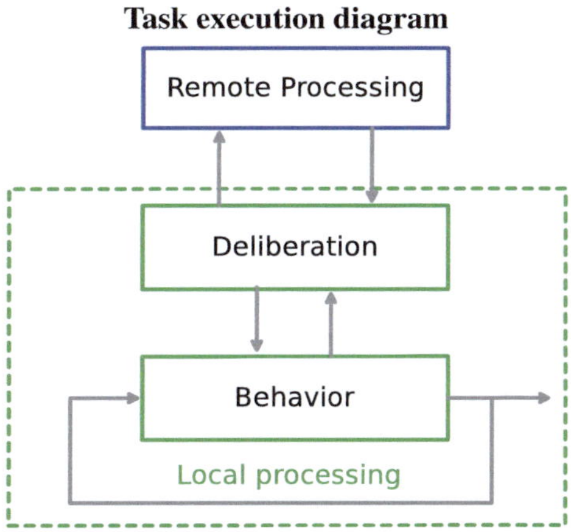

Fig. 3 The deliberative process evaluates the consistency of the autonomous local execution of the behavior. Once inconsistency is detected, remote processes are queried for support

the topology), which results from the color saliency. It is also based on the comparison of body postures, and the spatial relation between the agent and the object. The actions concern the motion control and a prediction of the localization, from the motion undertaken.

Table 1 details the definition of contextual features for assisting the object perception. The first two measurements are obtained from a particularly useful class of image features, which is known as moment (Corke [6]). For a binary image $B[x, y]$ the $(p+q)$th order moment is defined by

$$m_{pq} = \sum_{y=0}^{y_{\max}} \sum_{x=0}^{x_{\max}} x^p y^q B(x, y) \quad . \tag{5}$$

The radio-aspect F_3 is defined from the width and height of the minimum bounding-box (MBB) enclosing the blob, where the angle between the MBB's principal axis

Table 1 Saliency features

Expression	Description
$F_1 = (\frac{m_{10}}{m_{00}}, \frac{m_{01}}{m_{00}})$	Centroid
$F_2 = m_{00}$	Area
$F_3 = B_{height}/B_{width}$	Radioaspect, where B denotes the oriented bounding box
$F_4 = (\alpha, \beta)$	Posture, with α and β the pitch and yaw neck angles
$F_5 = v(S, s)$	Topology, where v attributes a 4-bit vicinity code according to the saliency set S around the blob s

and the image x-axis is $\gamma = 0.5(\text{atan}(2m_{11}/(m_{20} - m_{02})))$. The feature F_4 includes proprioceptive information from the instantaneous posture of the neck. The feature F_5 represents the topographic relation between the blobs, it is a descriptor of the presence of saliency at a four cardinal neighborhood.

The anticipation process involves a deterministic motion model, that assumes an ideal noise-free robot, moving at constant velocity $v = [\dot{x}, \dot{y}, \omega]^t$, along the time interval Δt. Thus, a prediction for the localization of the object $\breve{\xi}$ is obtained from the last observation available $\hat{\xi}$, and the expected displacement $m = v\Delta t$. Table 2 presents the definition of a set of features that relate the actual saliency to the anticipated information flow. Figure 4 illustrates the feature $\overline{F_1}$. In a periphery-to-center flow, information from salient regions (e.g., the blobs centroids) are projected to the sensory ego-space. Notice that among the features defined, some are not directly related to the motion of the agent, such is the case of $\overline{F_3}$ and $\overline{F_5}$.

The information fusion for the discriminative process is accomplished in a Bayesian network (BN), which is a directed acyclic graph, that represents the conditional probabilities of interconnected random variables. The BNs have been employed for diverse automatic diagnosing and recognition tasks (see Ertel [8]). In a BN a node is assumed to be conditionally independent from non-successors, given its parents. The joint probability $p(X_1, ..., X_n)$ of the nodes X_i is expressed by

$$p(X_1, \ldots, X_n) = \prod_{j=1}^{n} p(X_j | parents(X_j)). \tag{6}$$

Table 2 Anticipation features

Expression	Description
$\overline{F_1} = \lvert\sigma(F_1' - \breve{\xi})\rvert$	F_1' denotes the projection of the blob centroid in the ego-space, $\breve{\xi}$ is the predicted localization of the object, and σ weights the contribution of each component
$\overline{F_2} = 1 - \frac{F_2}{\left(\frac{\xi_\rho + m_\rho}{\xi_\rho}\right) F_{2(k-1)}}$	Relation between the actual blob's area F_2 and the simulated area from the expected motion m. Here $F_{2(k-1)}$ denotes the saliency during the last observation $\hat{\xi}$
$\overline{F_3} = \lvert F_{3(k)} - F_{3(k-1)}\rvert$	Difference between the current and the last detected radio-aspect
$\overline{F_4} = \lvert\check{F}_4 - \tilde{F}_4\rvert$	Difference between the simulated posture of the neck $\check{F}_4$, that would center the blob on the visual field, and the predicted attitude of the neck $\tilde{F}_4$
$\overline{F_5} = \sum_{i \in N} \delta(F_{5(k-1)i}, F_{5i})$	Estimate of the topographic relation through the Kronecker delta function $\delta(a, b)$. The neighborhood set is defined by $N = \{left, right, up, down\}$

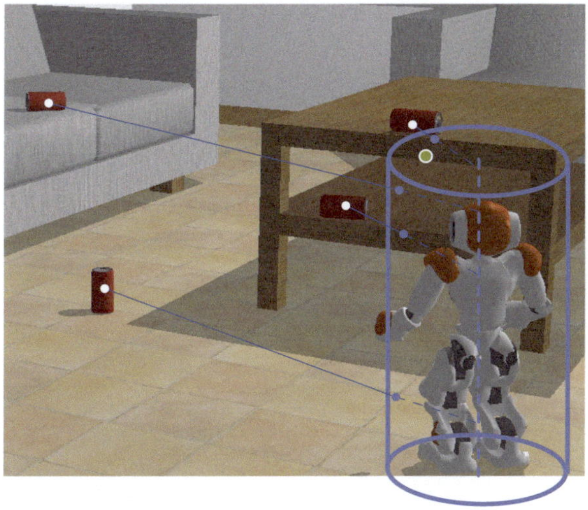

Fig. 4 The agent is approaching the *red can* on the *top* of the table. The *white dots* correspond to the *center* of the salient objects. The estimate on the distance to the blob center is unavailable during the saliency analysis, thus, the last observation $\hat{\zeta}_\rho$ is employed. The projection of the blobs in the ego-cylinder is represented by the *blue dots*, whereas the predicted localization is represented by the *yellow dot*

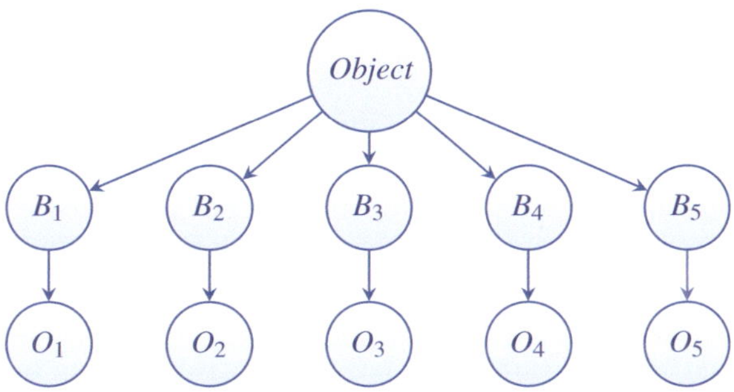

Fig. 5 Bayesian network for contextual information fusion

One important advantage of knowledge representation through BNs is that the information contained is directly understandable by humans, which facilitates doing future modifications (e.g. including new features, or more complex observations). As illustrated in Fig. 5, the structure of the network corresponds to a tree of height 2. The root node is a binomial random variable, which represents the probability that the blob saliency matches up with the object of interest. The intermediate nodes B_i are binomial random variables that represent the a posteriori probability of the features, given the observation of the object. This layer is included in order to simplify adjustments to the contribution of the features to the discriminative process. Probabilistic independence is assumed between the nodes B_i, which is also known as a *naive Bayes classifier*. The leaves O_i are multinomial random variables that represent the a posteriori probability of observing a particular intensity of $\overline{F_i}$, given B_i.

The tree can easily accommodate new features by horizontal expansion. The most likely blob s among the saliency set S is obtained by maximizing the expression

$$s = \text{argmax}_{s \in S} p(Object|B_i, O_i). \tag{7}$$

Thus, the BN can be used to classify the salience, while providing an estimate of the certainty in such classification. As we shall see in the case study, this information is of crucial importance to the deliberative process, once it has to decide whether or not resorting to remote processing.

5 Case Study

The case study included simulations of the task in Webots version 7.4.0, and a real approach task with the robot Nao. The robot is 58 cm tall, weighs 4.8 kg, has 25 degrees of freedom, and is equipped with a CMOS digital camera with a 58 degree field of view. The algorithms were implemented in the C++ programming language, and run under Ubuntu version 12.04.5 LTS. The vision processing was obtained with the support of the OpenCV library version 2.4.8. The Bayesian network implementation was provided by the dlib C++ Library version 18.13.

In the scenario considered the agent is expected to be assisted by remote resources. Thus, the first detection of the object, including the initial segmentation, and the virtual oriented trapezoid as seen from the desired configuration; are assumed to be provided remotely. This requirement was simulated in the study. The initial segmentation was manually provided through the GrabCut technique (Rother et al. [17]), and the desired pose was shown by demonstration (i.e. by placing the robot in front of the object). A color-based segmentation technique, defined under the Markof random field formalism, has been employed from our prior work (see Chame and Chevallereau [3]) for detecting the color saliency. The resulting algorithm presented a computational complexity $O(kn^2)$, where k is the maximum number of iterations allowed in the optimization process, and n is the number of pixels.

In the walk task the agent had to move to the desired location, and to stop once all the components of the observed localization error $\hat{e}$ (see Eq. 2) were smaller than a given threshold ϵ. The tolerance considered was a radial distance $\epsilon_\rho = 0.05$ meters (m), the bearing $\epsilon_\theta = 0.04$ radians (rad), and $\epsilon_\phi = 0.1$ rad for the orientation component. The walk primitive of the robot receives commands in position expressed in the Cartesian space. A motion request is sent by the walk task according to Eq. (3), under the assumption of constant velocity motion. The mean walk velocity was estimated to be around $\overline{v} = [0.022\ \text{m/s}, 0.04\ \text{m/s}, 0.106\ \text{rad/s}]^t$. Continuous motion was achieved by sending commands at regular time intervals. In order to prevent that unforeseen delays affect the fluidity of the walk, the actual displacement sent considered a larger delay (e.g. 1.5 times the expected value). Thus, a new command would be ideally sent before the routine could finish the previous one. If this would not be the case (e.g. due to losing the object, a program crash, etc.), the robot would stop moving after a while. This strategy ensured a fluid walk while keeping the safety aspects. For speeding up convergence, given the observation noise and the fact that the walk primitive is less precise in continuous motion, once the robot was nearly at the desired location (at $\hat{e}_\rho < 0.1$ m), the walk task switched to a step-by-step policy (i.e. a new correction was sent only after finishing the previous one).

The look-at task was also controlled in position. The correction of the head posture, through the actuation of the neck joints α and β, was obtained from Eq. (4) by assuming constant velocity motion. The tolerance $\epsilon = 0.03$ rad was admitted for convergence. The head posture is regulated independently from the walk. This means that the motions induced by the walk can affect the convergence of the look-at task, specially at slow turning of the head. Thus, a velocity profile of 4 rad/s was employed and convergence was obtained in few iterations.

The study of the anticipation process was based on the design of a controlled scene that contained a single salient object. The observation of the evidence was accomplished through the definition of data partitions, which were obtained from the statistical analysis of the information flow, as recorded by the agent. The Nearest Neighboor Method (see Ertel [8]) was employed to classify the observation $O_i \in \{0, 1, 2\}$, with 0 the lowest and 2 the highest intensity. A more complex task was then designed to evaluate the network performance. As illustrated in Fig. 6, various stimuli of the same kind were placed on the scene, where the agent had to approach a specific soda can. Despite stimuli were relatively close to each other, with the BN the agent was able to do the task autonomously (i.e. without remote assistance, as provided in Fig. 3) from different initial configurations, under different feedback delay profiles (between 100 and 2000 ms). Figure 7 shows a comparison of the performance of the network for two delay profiles. As noted, although the task was accomplished in both cases, at higher delay the network is less discriminative, since the anticipation is less consistent.

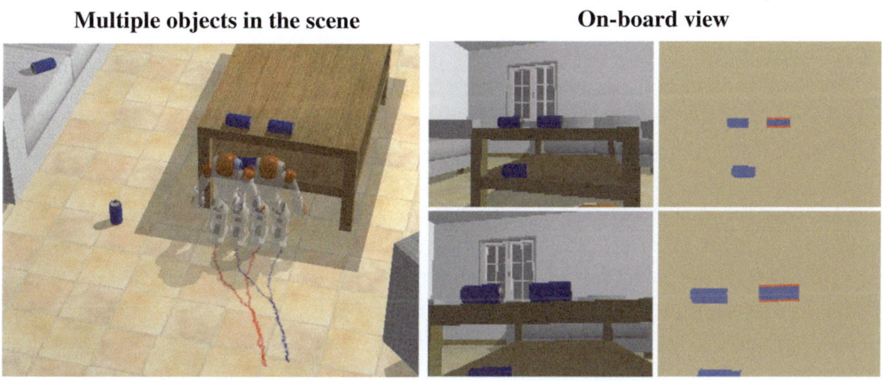

Fig. 6 On the *left* two trajectories followed are superimposed. Starting from the same position, the agent was required to approach a distinct can over the table. Some on-board views and their corresponding saliency are displayed on the *right*

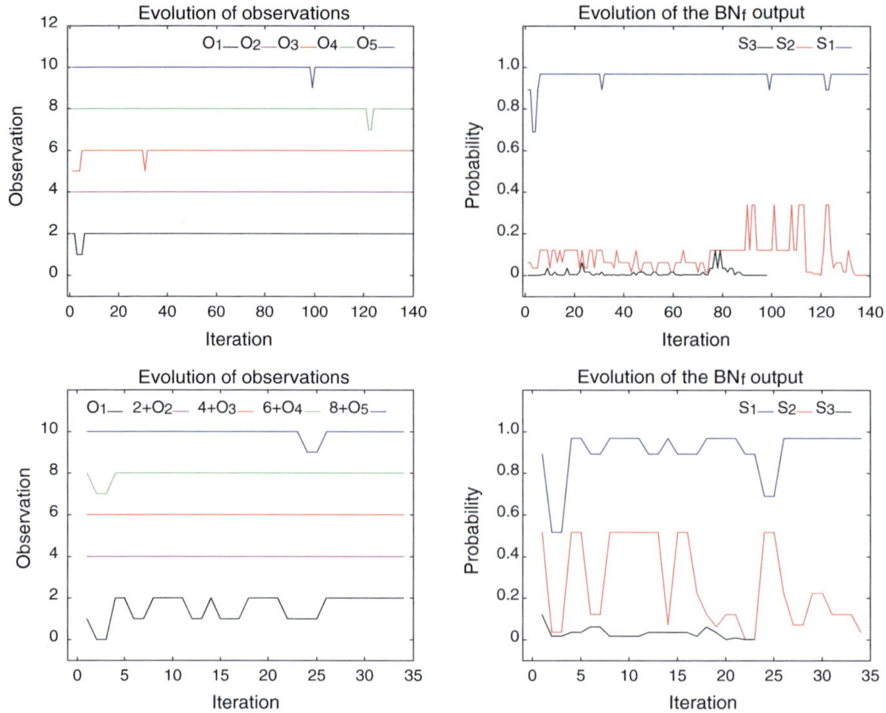

Fig. 7 Comparison of the network response with two delay profiles. The *upper row* presents the results for 300 ms delay. The bottom row presents the results for 1700 ms delay. The first column shows the evolution of the observations O_i (with 0 the lowest and 2 the highest intensity). The signal are shifted vertically for visualization, such that $O_i = 2(i-1) + O_i$. The second column shows the output of the network. The tracked can over the table is represented by s_1, and s_2 corresponds to the lateral neighbor (see Fig. 6). As it can be noted, the discriminative power of the network is reduced as the delay increases

Based on the simulation results we proceeded to do the experiment in the robotic lab of the IRCCyN, which is an unstructured environment, under natural and artificial illumination. As shown on Fig. 8, two colored tea cans were placed one beside the other at a distance around 4 cm, and the robot was required to approach one of them. Given the characteristics of the robot, the perceptive delay was set to 1700 ms, including at most two iterations for centering the object in the field of vision. The experiment was executed in two motion modalities. In the first one, a step-by-step approach was attempted, where the robot finished the motion before processing additional commands. In the second one, a continuous approach was adopted. The initial trials were conducted off-line, that is, the local deliberative module was disconnected (see Fig. 3), in order to evaluate the autonomous execution of the behavior. Thus, the network was allowed to select the most likely blob conforming to Eq. (7), regardless of the probability obtained. Under these conditions, the task was accomplished 7/10 times with step-by-step motion, and 5/10 times with continuous motion. Among the

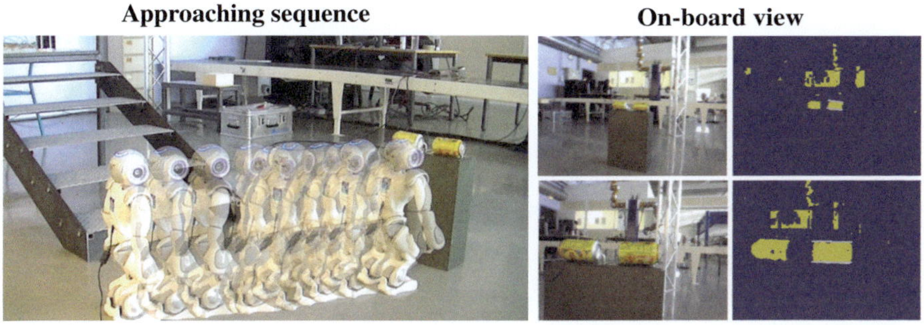

Fig. 8 Experimental task. The trajectory followed is shown on the *left*, whereas some on-board views and their corresponding color salience are shown on the *right*

reasons that affected the off-line execution of the task are: unexpected peaks on the feedback delay (e.g. the expected delay profile was occasionally exceeded in more than 2000 ms), irregular performance of the walk primitive, and momentary degradation on the color saliency detection.

Interestingly, the performance of the network in the off-line trials was very consistent, by yielding a chance $p_o < 0.5$ to blobs selected under degraded conditions. Therefore, it provided a reliable information about the degree of confidence on the task. Though, as shown in Fig. 7, at high delay profiles the discriminative power of the BN drops. Thus, the difference p_d between the two most likely candidates may be employed as an indicator of the actual discriminative power of the network. In a new set of trials on-line execution was attempted by activating the deliberative process. A tolerance $p_d > 0.2$ and $p_o > 0.6$ for the task reliability was set, so the deliberative process paused the behavior when the threshold was reached and waited for the user, who acting as the remote resource, selected the blob corresponding to the object. In the on-line execution of the experiment the task was accomplished all the times.

6 Conclusions

This study has focused on the problem of the autonomy of humanoid approach tasks. It has explored an efficient means of employing distributed resources, towards developing more realistic and robust applications for service robotics. Given the risks in the on-line implementation of the task, we concentrated our efforts in exploiting the emergence of contextual information, notably, the redundancies and the statistical regularities induced in the sensory-motor coupling. We examined the possibility of employing the anticipation of the information flow to assist a local, multi-sensory, perceptive process, thus reducing the dependency on context-free representations. In view of the stochastic difficulties inherent to the task, in the form of sensory noise, processing delays, and disturbances from the environment; we employed a Bayesian network structure to fuse information. The results obtained suggested that it is a convenient and easy-to-employ technique, which produces reliable information about the degree of confidence on the task. Such information is evaluated by a local deliberative process, that can resort to remote assistance in case the agent is no longer able to autonomously accomplish the task.

Acknowledgments This research has been funded by the Ecole Centrale de Nantes (ECN) and EQUIPEX ROBOTEX, France; and the CAPES Foundation, Ministry of Education of Brazil, Brasília - DF 700040-020, Brazil.

References

1. Anderson, M.: Embodied cognition: a field guide. Artif. Intell. **149**(1), 91–130 (2003). doi:10.1016/S0004-3702(03)00054-7
2. Brooks, R.A.: Cambrian Intelligence: The Early History of the New AI, 1st edn. A Bradford Book, Cambridge (1999)
3. Chame, H.F., Chevallereau, C.: Embodied localization in visually-guided walk of humanoid robots. ICINCO **2**, 165–174 (2014)
4. Chaumette, F., Hutchinson, S.: Visual servo control, part i: basic approaches. IEEE Robot. Autom. Mag. **13**, 82–90 (2006)
5. Comport, A., Marchand, E., Pressigout, M., Chaumette, F.: Real-time markerless tracking for augmented reality: the virtual visual servoing framework. IEEE Trans. Visual Comput. Graphics B **12**(4), 615–628 (2006). doi:10.1109/TVCG.2006.78
6. Corke, P.I.: Robotics, Vision and Control: Fundamental Algorithms in Matlab. Springer (2011)
7. Dune, C., Herdt, A., March, E., Stasse, O., Wieber, P.b., Yoshida, E.: Vision based control for humanoid robots. In: IROS Workshop on Visual Control of Mobile Robots (ViCoMoR) (2011)
8. Ertel, W.: Introduction to Artificial Intelligence. Springer, London (2011)
9. Hoffmann, M., Pfeifer, R.: The implications of embodiment for behavior and cognition: animal and robotic case studies (2012). arXiv:1202.0440
10. Hornung, A., Wurm, K., Bennewitz, M.: Humanoid robot localization in complex indoor environments. In: 2010 IEEE/RSJ International Conference on Intelligent Robots and Systems (IROS), pp. 1690–1695 (2010). doi:10.1109/IROS.2010.5649751
11. Khalil, W., Dombre, E.: Modeling, Identification and Control of Robots, 3rd edn. Taylor & Francis Inc, Bristol, PA, USA (2002)
12. Lewis, M.A., Simo, L.S.: Elegant stepping: a model of visually triggered gait adaptation. Connect. Sci. **11**(3–4), 331–344 (1999). doi:10.1080/095400999116287
13. Lungarella, M., Sporns, O.: Information self-structuring: key principle for learning and development. In: Proceedings of the 4th International Conference on Development and Learning, 2005, pp. 25–30 (2005). doi:10.1109/DEVLRN.2005.1490938
14. Michel, P., Chestnutt, J., Kuffner, J., Kanade, T.: Vision-guided humanoid footstep planning for dynamic environments. In: Proceedings of the IEEE-RAS Conference on Humanoid Robots (Humanoids'05), pp. 13–18 (2005)
15. Moughlbay, A., Cervera, E., Martinet, P.: Model based visual servoing tasks with an autonomous humanoid robot. In: Lee, S., Yoon, K.J., Lee, L. (eds.) Frontiers of Intelligent Autonomous Systems. Studies in Computational Intelligence, vol. 466, pp. 149–162. Springer, Berlin (2013). doi:10.1007/978-3-642-35485-4_12
16. Oriolo, G., Paolillo, A., Rosa, L., Vendittelli, M.: Vision-based odometric localization for humanoids using a kinematic ekf. In: 2012 12th IEEE-RAS International Conference on Humanoid Robots (Humanoids), pp. 153–158 (2012). doi:10.1109/HUMANOIDS.2012.6651513

17. Rother, C., Kolmogorov, V., Blake, A.: GrabCut—interactive foreground extraction using iterated graph cuts. ACM Trans. Graph. (SIGGRAPH) (2004)
18. Shapiro, L.: The embodied cognition research programme. In: Philosophy Compass 2(2), 338–346 (2007). doi:10.1111/j.1747-9991.2007.00064.x
19. Thrun, S., Burgard, W., Fox, D.: Probabilistic Robotics. The MIT Press, Cambridge (2005)
20. Vasiliu, L., Trochidis, I., Bussler, C., Koumpis, A.: Robobrain: a software architecture mapping the human brain. In: 2014 14th IEEE-RAS International Conference on Humanoid Robots (Humanoids), pp. 160–165 (2014). doi:10.1109/HUMANOIDS.2014.7041353
21. Waibel, M., Beetz, M., Civera, J., D'Andrea, R., Elfring, J., Galvez-Lopez, D., Haussermann, K., Janssen, R., Montiel, J., Perzylo, A., Schiessle, B., Tenorth, M., Zweigle, O., van de Molengraft, R.: Roboearth. Robot. Autom. Mag. IEEE **18**(2), 69–82 (2011). doi:10.1109/MRA.2011.941632

On the Design of the Exoskeleton Arm with Decoupled Dynamics

V. Arakelian, Y. Aoustin and C. Chevallereau

Abstract This paper focuses on the design of a 2-DOF exoskeleton arm with decoupled dynamics. The goal is to simplify the controller design by reducing the effects of complicated manipulator dynamics. The added epicyclic gear train allows the optimal redistribution of kinetic energy, which leads to the linearization and decoupling of the dynamic equations. The determination of the parameters of the added links is based on eliminating coefficients of nonlinear terms in the manipulator's kinetic and potential energy equations. The suggested design methodology is illustrated by simulations carried out using the software ADAMS.

Keywords Exoskeleton arm · Multibody system · Dynamic equations · Decoupling · Balancing · Epicyclic gear train

1 Introduction

It is known that the exoskeleton arm dynamics are highly coupled and nonlinear. The complicated dynamics results from varying inertia, interactions between the different joints, and nonlinear forces such as Coriolis and centrifugal forces. Nonlinear forces cause errors in position response at high speed, and have been shown to be significant even at slow speed [1]. Thus, improving the positioning accuracy of the exoskeleton arm via dynamic decoupling is suitable for their further improvement.

The decoupling of dynamic equations of robot mechanisms has attracted researchers' attention and different solutions have been proposed. They can be

V. Arakelian (✉) · Y. Aoustin · C. Chevallereau
IRCCyN, 1 Rue de La Noë, BP 92101, 44321 Nantes Cedex 03, France
e-mail: vigen.arakelyan@irccyn.ec-nantes.fr

V. Arakelian
Department of Mechanical and Control Systems Engineering, I.N.S.A. Rennes, 20 avenue des Buttes de Coësmes CS 14315, 35043 Rennes, France

P. Wenger et al. (eds.), *New Trends in Medical and Service Robots*,
Mechanisms and Machine Science 39, DOI 10.1007/978-3-319-30674-2_11

mentioned by three principal trends: (a) the decoupling of dynamic equations via actuator relocation, i.e. by the kinematic decoupling of motion when the rotation of any link is due to only one actuator [2–10] or via decoupling of kinematic chains [11–15]; (b) the decoupling of dynamic equations via optimum inertia redistribution [16–26]; (c) the decoupling of dynamic equations via added links [27–30]. The modification of the manipulator structure to achieve high-quality dynamic performance is a new promising tendency in the robot design and it is to pursue the development of new robot mechanisms which can be modeled accurately with little difficulty.

This paper proposes a new design concept, which allows the dynamic decoupling of exoskeleton arms by using epicyclic gears.

2 Design of the Decoupled 2-DOF Exoskeleton Arm

To understand better the suggested design concept let us first consider the dynamic equations for a planar exoskeleton arm with two degrees of freedom shown in Fig. 1.

They can be written as

$$\begin{bmatrix} \tau_1 \\ \tau_2 \end{bmatrix} = \begin{bmatrix} D_{11} & D_{12} \\ D_{21} & D_{22} \end{bmatrix} \begin{bmatrix} \ddot{\theta}_1 \\ \ddot{\theta}_2 \end{bmatrix} + \begin{bmatrix} D_{111} & D_{122} \\ D_{211} & D_{222} \end{bmatrix} \begin{bmatrix} \dot{\theta}_1^2 \\ \dot{\theta}_2^2 \end{bmatrix} + \begin{bmatrix} D_{112} & D_{121} \\ D_{212} & D_{221} \end{bmatrix} \begin{bmatrix} \dot{\theta}_1\dot{\theta}_2 \\ \dot{\theta}_1\dot{\theta}_2 \end{bmatrix} + \begin{bmatrix} D_1 \\ D_2 \end{bmatrix} \tag{1}$$

with $D_{11} = m_1 l_{AS1}^2 + m_2 l_1^2 + m_2 l_{BS2}^2 + 2m_2 l_1 l_{BS2} \cos\theta_2 + I_{S1} + I_{S2}$; $D_{12} = D_{21} = m_2 l_{BS2}^2 + m_2 l_1 l_{BS2} \cos\theta_2 + I_{S2}$; $D_{22} = m_2 l_{BS2}^2 + I_{S2}$; $D_{111} = 0$; $D_{122} = -m_2 l_1 l_{BS2} \sin\theta_2$; $D_{211} = m_2 l_1 l_{BS2} \sin\theta_2$; $D_{222} = 0$; $D_{112} = D_{121} = -m_2 l_1 l_{BS2} \sin\theta_2$; $D_{212} = D_{221} = 0$; $D_1 = (m_1 l_{AS1} + m_2 l_1) g \cos\theta_1 + m_2 g l_{BS2} \cos(\theta_1 + \theta_2)$; $D_2 = m_2 g l_{BS2} \cos(\theta_1 + \theta_2)$.

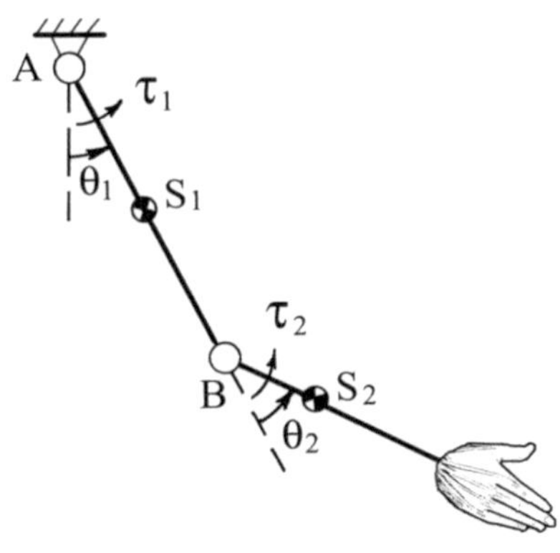

Fig. 1 An exoskeleton arm with two degrees of freedom

where l_1 are the length of link 1; θ_1 is the angular displacement of link 1 relative to the base; θ_2 is the angular displacement of link 2 relative to link 1; $\dot{\theta}_1$ is the angular velocity of link 1 relative to the base; $\dot{\theta}_2$ is the angular velocity of link 2 relative to link 1; m_1, m_2 are the masses of links 1 and 2; l_{AS_1} is the distance between the centre of mass S_1 of link 1 and joint centre A; l_{BS_2} is the distance between the centre of mass S_2 of link 2 and joint centre B, I_{S1} is the axial moment of inertia of link 1 relative to the centre of mass S_1 of link 1; I_{S2} is the axial moment of inertia of link 2 relative to the centre of mass S_2 of link 2; g is the gravitational acceleration.

There are two intrinsic problems involved in Eq. (1) regarding the manipulator dynamics: complexity and nonlinearity. The proposed design methodology described bellow will eliminate both the complexity and the nonlinearity.

The proposed exoskeleton arm differs from the traditional scheme by the fact that an epicyclic gear train is included between links 1 and 2 (Fig. 2).

In this design concept, gear 2′ is connected with link 2 of the exoskeleton arm. The epicyclic gear train with sun gear 1′ and epicyclic gears 3′ and 3″ is introduced between links 1 and 2 of the exoskeleton.

Let us rewrite the Lagrangian of the manipulator with the added links:

$$L = K - P = \sum_{i=1}^{4} K_i - \sum_{i=1}^{4} P_i = 0.5\left(m_1 V_{S1}^2 + m_2 V_{S2}^2 + m_3 V_{S3}^2 + m_4 V_{S4}^2\right) + 0.5\left[I_{S1}\dot{\theta}_1^2 + I_{S2}(\dot{\theta}_1 + \dot{\theta}_2)^2 + I_{S3}(\dot{\theta}_2 + \dot{\theta}_3)^2 + I_{S4}(\dot{\theta}_2 + \dot{\theta}_4)^2\right] - \sum_{i=1}^{4} P_i \quad (2)$$

where, $\dot{\theta}_3$ and $\dot{\theta}_4$ are the angular velocities of links 3 and 4.

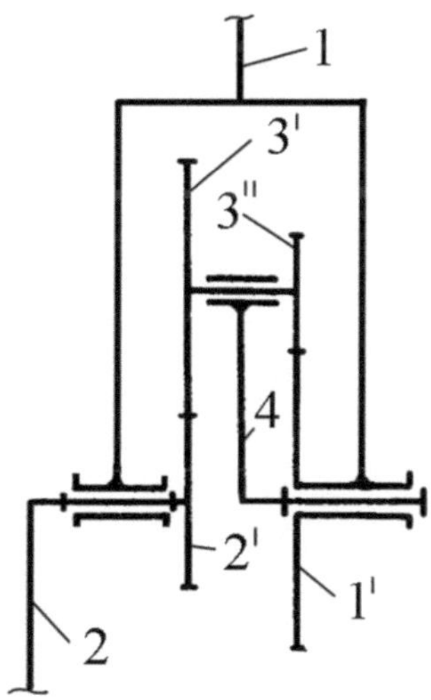

Fig. 2 The epicyclic gear train added between links 1 and 2

The static balancing of the exoskeleton arm leads to the condition $\sum_{i=1}^{4} P_i = 0$ and taking into consideration that the epicyclic gear train is symmetric regarding to the principal rotating axis, we obtain

$$L = 0.5\left[\left(m_1 l_{AS1}^2 + I_{S1} + m l_1^2\right)\dot{\theta}_1^2 + I_{S2}(\dot{\theta}_1 + \dot{\theta}_2)^2 + I_{S3}(\dot{\theta}_1 + \dot{\theta}_3)^2 + I_{S4}(\dot{\theta}_1 + \dot{\theta}_4)^2\right] \quad (3)$$

where m is the mass of link 2 with epicyclic gear train.

Now, let us consider the transmission ratio in the epicyclic gear train:

$$\frac{\dot{\theta}_2}{\dot{\theta}_4} = 1 - \frac{Z_{3'} Z_{1'}}{Z_{2'} Z_{3''}} \quad (4)$$

where, $Z_{1'}, Z_{2'}, Z_{3'}$ and $Z_{3''}$ are the number of teeth of the corresponding gears.

Now, let us suggest that $Z_{3'} = 2Z_{2'}$ and $Z_{1'} = Z_{3''}$, which leads to the condition:

$$\dot{\theta}_2 = -\dot{\theta}_4 \quad (5)$$

With regard to the angular velocity of the planetary gear, we obtain

$$\dot{\theta}_3 = 2\dot{\theta}_4 = -2\dot{\theta}_2 \quad (6)$$

Introducing (5) and (6) into (3), we get

$$L = 0.5\left[\left(m_1 l_{AS1}^2 + I_{S1} + m l_1^2\right)\dot{\theta}_1^2 + I_{S2}(\dot{\theta}_1 + \dot{\theta}_2)^2 + I_{S3}(\dot{\theta}_1 - 2\dot{\theta}_2)^2 + I_{S4}(\dot{\theta}_1 - \dot{\theta}_2)^2\right] \quad (7)$$

The obtained equation can be rewritten as:

$$L = 0.5\left(k_1\dot{\theta}_1^2 + k_2\dot{\theta}_2^2 + k_3\dot{\theta}_1\dot{\theta}_2\right) \quad (8)$$

where, $k_1 = m_1 l_{AS1}^2 + m l_1^2 + I_{S1} + I_{S2} + I_{S3} + I_{S4}$; $k_2 = I_{S2} + 4I_{S3} + I_{S4}$ and $k_3 = 2(I_{S2} - 2I_{S3} - I_{S4})$.

Thus, if $k_3 = 0$, i.e. $I_{S2} = 2I_{S3} + I_{S4}$, we obtain $L = 0.5\left(k_1\dot{\theta}_1^2 + k_2\dot{\theta}_2^2\right)$ and consequently $\tau_1 = k_1\ddot{\theta}_1$ and $\tau_2 = k_2\ddot{\theta}_2$.

It should be noted that the epicyclic gear train provides very compact construction with high transmission ratio, which is a design advantage of the suggested decoupling technique.

In order to evaluate the performance of the suggested design concept let us consider an illustrative example.

3 Numerical Simulations

For illustration of the suggested decoupling approach, simulations using ADAMS software have been carried. The exoskeleton arm parameters with decoupled dynamic equations are the following: $m_1 = 2\,\mathrm{kg}$, $m_2 = 8\,\mathrm{kg}$, $I_{S1} = I_{S2} = 0.1\,\mathrm{kg\,m^2}$, $l_{AS1} = 0.1\,\mathrm{m}$, $l_{BS2} = 0$ (taking into account that the epicyclic gear train is mainly a balanced system), $I_{S3} = 0.03\,\mathrm{kg\,m^2}$, $I_{S4} = 0.04\,\mathrm{kg\,m^2}$ (i.e. $I_{S2} = 2I_{S3} + I_{S4}$).

To better show the dynamic decoupling of motion equations the following input laws have been chosen: $\theta_1 = 60t$ and $\theta_2 = \sin(2\pi t)$ with $0 \leq t \leq 1s$. Figure 3 shows

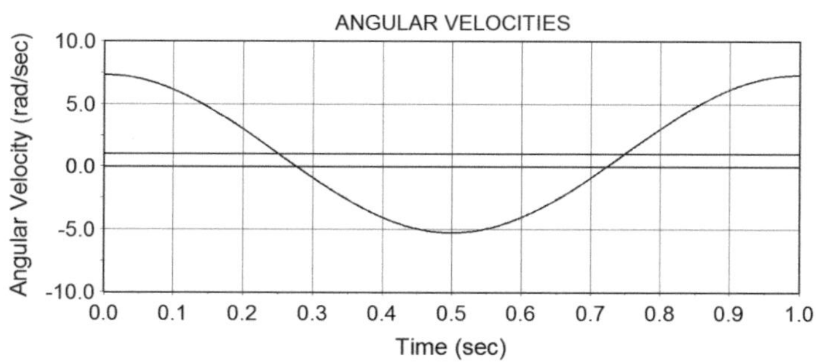

Fig. 3 Angular velocities of input links

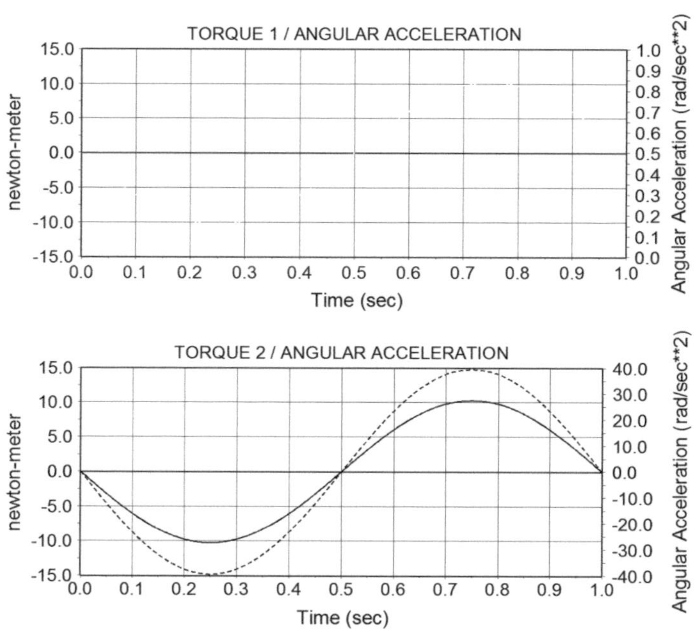

Fig. 4 Actuator torques (*solid line*) and angular accelerations (*dashed line*) for decoupled exoskeleton arm

the angular velocities of input links. Thus, the angular accelerations are $\ddot{\theta}_1 = 0$ and $\ddot{\theta}_2 = -4\pi^2 \sin(2\pi t)$.

Figure 4 shows the simulations results obtained by using ADAMS software, i.e. the variations of the input torques and accelerations. We can see that the dynamic decoupling of motion equations are carried, i.e. $\tau_1 = k_1\ddot{\theta}_1$ and $\tau_2 = k_3\ddot{\theta}_2$. Indeed, the first torque is cancelled and the second torque is the following: $\tau_2 = 0,26 \cdot [-4\pi^2 \sin(2\pi t)]$ (N).

4 Conclusions

In order to increase the accuracy of high-speed mechanical systems the nonlinear dynamic control algorithms have been developed. However, taking into account the permanent tendency to decrease the price of robotic systems, the price of implementation of a complete dynamic control on the industrial practice is still high. In the case of the reproduction of the trajectory in the Cartesian space by large number of given points is a laboriousness task requiring relatively long time of computation. Therefore, in many cases, the reduction (or cancellation) of coupling and nonlinearity in the manipulators, is necessary.

This paper introduced a new design concept for the linearization and decoupling of dynamic equations of exoskeleton arms. It is achieved by adding to the initial architecture of the exoskeleton an epicyclic gear train. The determination of the parameters of the added gears is based on eliminating coefficients of nonlinear terms in the manipulator's kinetic and potential energy equations. After such a redistribution of masses the actuator torque in each driven joint becomes a linear function of its angular acceleration.

Acknowledgments This work is supported by the Pays de la Loire Region, the Project LMA and "Gérontopôle Autonomie Longévité" of the Pays de la Loire Region.

References

1. Brady, M., Hollerbach, J. Xl., et al.: Robot Motion: Planning and Control. MIT Press, Cambridge (1983)
2. Artobolevskii I.I., Ovakimov A.G.: One property of a matrix describing the structure of a manipulator drive, Transactions of the USSR Academia of Sciences, vol. 230, (in Russian, see English version in http://adsabs.harvard.edu/abs/1976DoSSR.230..298A) (1976)
3. Belyanin P.N., et al.: Mechanical arm. U.S. Patent 4259876, 7 Apr 1981
4. Youcef-Toumi K.: Analysis, Design and Control of Direct-Drive Manipulators. Ph.D thesis, Massachusetts Institute of Technology, Department of Mechanical Engineering (1985)
5. Youcef-Toumi K., Asada, H.: The design of arm linkages with decoupled and configuration-invariant inertia tensors: Part II: Actuator relocation and mass redistribution. In: Proceedings of 1985 ASME, Winter Annual Meeting, Miami, pp. 153–161 (1985)

6. Korendyasev A.L., et al.: Manipulation Systems of Robots. Moscow, Mashinostroyenia, 782p. (1989)
7. Minotti, P.: Découplage dynamique des manipulateurs: propositions de solutions mécaniques. Mech. Mach. Theor. **26**(1), 107–122 (1991)
8. Youcef-Toumi, K.: Analysis and design of manipulators with decoupled and configuration-invariant inertia tensors using remote actuation. Trans. ASME J. Dyn. Syst. Meas. Contr. **114**(June), 204–212 (1992)
9. Chug, Y.-H., Gang, J.-G., Lee, J.-W.: The effect of actuator relocation on singularity, Jacobian and kinematic isotroy of parallel robots. In: Proceedings of the 2002 IEEWRSJ International Conference on Intelligent Robots and Systems EPFL, Lausanne, Switzerland, October 2002, pp. 2147–2153 (2002)
10. Vukobratovic, K.M., Stokic, D.M.: Contribution to the decoupled control of large-scale mechanisms. Automatica, pp. 9–21 (1980)
11. Glazunov, V.: Design of decoupled parallel manipulators by means of the theory of screws. Mech. Mach. Theor. **45**(2), 239–250 (2010)
12. Briot, S., Arakelian, V., Guegan, S.: PAMINSA : a new family of partially decoupled parallel manipulators. Mech. Mach. Theor. **44**(2), 425–444 (2009)
13. Carricato, M., Parenti-Castelli, V.: On the topological and geometrical synthesis and classification of translational parallel mechanisms. In: Proceedings of the 11th World Congress in Mechanism and Machine Science, Tianjin, China, 2004, pp. 1624–1628 (2004)
14. Kong, X., Gosselin, C.M.: A class of 3-DOF translational parallel manipulator with linear input–output equations. In: Workshop on Fundamental Issues and Future Research for Parallel Mechanisms and Manipulators, Quebec City, Quebec, Canada, 2002, pp. 25–32 (2002)
15. Gosselin C.M., Kong X., Foucault, S., Bonev, I.A.: A fully decoupled 3-DOF translational parallel mechanism. In: PKM International Conference, Chemnitz, Germany, 2004, pp. 595–610 (2004)
16. Asada, H., Youcef-Toumi K.: Decoupling of manipulator inertia tensor by mass redistribution. In: Proceedings of the Design Engineering Technical Conference, Cambridge, October, ASME Paper 84-DET-40 (1984)
17. Youcef-Toumi, K., Asada H.: The design of open-loop manipulator arms with decoupled and configuration-invariant inertia tensors. In: Proceedings of the IEEE Conf. on Robotis and Automation (ICRA'84), San Francisco, pp. 2018–2026 (1986)
18. Youcef-Toumi, K., Asada H.: The design of arm linkages with decoupled and configuration-invariant inertia tensors: Part I: open kinematic chains with special drive mechanisms. In: Proceedings of 1985 ASME, Winter Annual Meeting, Miami, pp. 145–152 (1985)
19. Yang, D.C.H., Tzeng S.W.: Simplification and linearization of manipulator dynamics by design. In: Proceedings of the 9th Applied Mechanics Conference, Kansas City, Missouri, 28–30 Oct 1985
20. Yang, D.C.H., Tzeng, S.W.: Simplification and linearization of manipulator dynamics by the design of inertia distribution. Int. J. Robot. Res. **5**(3), 120–128 (1986)
21. Youcef-Toumi, K., Asada, H.: The design of open-loop manipulator arms with decoupled and configuration-invariant inertia tensors. Trans. ASME J. Dyn. Syst. Meas. Contr. **109**, 268–275 (1987)
22. Abdel-Rahman, T.M., Elbestawi, M.A.: Synthesis and dynamics of statically balanced direct-drive manipulators with decoupled inertia tensors. Mech. Mach. Theor. **26**(4), 389–402 (1991)
23. Park, H.S., Cho, H.S.: General design conditions for an ideal robotic manipulator having simple dynamics. Int. J. Robot. Res. **10**(1), 21–29 (1991)
24. Minotti, P., Pracht, P.: Design of robots driven by linear servo systems. Robotica **10**, 361–368 (1992)
25. Filaretov, V.F., Vukobratovic, M.K.: Static balancing and dynamic decoupling of the motion of manipulation robots. Mechatronics **3**(6), 767–782 (1993)

26. Arakelian, V., Dahan, M.: Equilibrage optimal des mécanismes pour manipulateurs. In: Acts du 12e Congrès Français de Mécanique, Strasbourg, 4–8 Septembre, vol. 4, pp. 373–376 (1995)
27. Zhang, Y., Gruver, W.A., Gao, F.: Dynamic simplification of three degree of freedom manipulators with closed chains. Robot. Auton. Syst. **28**(4), 261–269 (1999)
28. Coelho, T.A.H., Yong, L., Alves, V.F.A.: Decoupling of dynamic equations by means of adaptive balancing of 2-dof open-loop mechanisms. Mech. Mach. Theor. **39**(8), 871–881 (2004)
29. Moradi, M., Nikoobin, A., Azadi, S.: Adaptive decoupling for open chain planar robots. Sci. Iranica: Trans B, Mech. Eng. **17**(5), 376–386 (2010)
30. Arakelian, V., Sargsyan, S.: On the design of serial manipulators with decoupled dynamics. Mechatronics **22**(6), 904–909 (2012)

Assisting Control of Forces in Laparoscopy Using Tactile and Visual Sensory Substitution

Thomas Howard and Jérôme Szewczyk

Abstract It is widely recognized that despite its many benefits, the ergonomics of laparoscopic surgery lead to severe perceptual distortions for the surgeon. In particular, interaction forces at the instrument tip are masked by interfering forces at the trocar and distorted due to a lever effect around the insertion point. This leads to improper control of tool-tip interaction forces, increasing the risk and occurrence of intra-operative injuries, unnecessary trauma to healthy tissue and suture breakage. Here, we propose an experiment aimed at determining the efficacy and usability of cutaneous vibrotactile and/or visual feedback of tool-tip interaction forces in assisting a surgeon in controlling fine interaction forces. 16 novice subjects performed force-reach and -hold tasks in a laparoscopic setting under provision of 9 forms of feedback (visual, 4 variants of vibrotactile feedback, and their combinations). Feedback increased precision (up to 85.8 % reduction in error when aiming for a target force), repeatability (up to 84 % reduction in spread of aiming errors), speed of reaching a target force (up to 18-fold increase in speed of reaching a target force at equal accuracy) and reduced force drift over time (>68 % reduction in cumulative deviation from a target force over a 20 s period). Results show best performance for visual feedback, with promising performance for pulsed vibrotactile feedback, allowing us to draw initial conclusions on the potential for using tactile feedback to represent interaction forces in laparoscopy and to gain insights into axes for its improvement.

Keywords Haptics · Laparoscopy · Force feedback · Sensory substitution · MIS

1 Introduction

Laparoscopic surgery (LS) is widely used to treat a variety of pathological conditions [4, 9, 14] boasting many advantages for the patient due to the reduced access trauma. However, the deteriorations in dexterity and perception stemming from the

T. Howard (✉) · J. Szewczyk
ISIR, CNRS, UMR 7222, INSERM, U1150, Agathe-ISIR, Sorbonne Universités, UPMC Univ Paris 06, 75005 Paris, France
e-mail: howard@isir.upmc.fr

P. Wenger et al. (eds.), *New Trends in Medical and Service Robots*, Mechanisms and Machine Science 39, DOI 10.1007/978-3-319-30674-2_12 manipulation of thin elongated instruments inserted into the abdomen through trocars coupled with vision from a 2-D endoscopic camera are the cause of sub-optimal performance on the part of surgeons [19]. This sometimes results in unnecessary complications [2, 3, 5, 15]. Among the most cited problems in LS, distorted and partially lost haptic perception of forces is a major cause for concern [10, 13, 16], prompting us to seek solutions for assisting surgeons in better controlling them.

Haptic perception of forces is also a major issue in robotically assisted minimally invasive surgery (RMIS), as teleoperation has only worsened the situation compared to LS, exacerbating the problem of excessive applied forces. An interesting overview of force feedback in RMIS is given by Weber et al. [17], who perform a meta-analysis of 21 studies comparing surgical task performance with and without force feedback. They conclude that force feedback has a moderate effect on accuracy, a strong beneficial effect on the control of average and peak forces and no effect on task completion times. However, technical difficulties in implementing force feedback for RMIS have prompted research in alternate methods for presenting force information, in particular through sensory substitution.

Both audio [1, 7, 8] and visual feedback in RMIS [7, 11] and LS (e.g. [18]) have proven effective in reducing mean and peak forces during suturing and tissue manipulation. However, implementing audio feedback in the operating room where ambient noise is high and it may impede communication remains challenging. Visual feedback requires a possibly distracting display alongside the endoscopic image, and increasing the already high visual cognitive load.

For this reason, tactile feedback has been considered as an option for displaying interaction forces, with the advantage of not competing with other important information passing through the same perceptual channel, and providing immediate, private and non-disruptive cues. To the best of our knowledge, most work on tactile feedback for LS has focussed on cutaneous feedback of grasping forces [12, 18] and tissue palpation forces [20] with promising results.

In the case of suture knot tying, there is great benefit to be obtained from better control of interaction forces at the tool-tip. Sutures are safe as long as they exceed a minimum thread tension when tied, ensuring good closure of the wound. On the other hand, excess suture thread tension leads to tissue damage or suture breakages and associated complications [18].

Here, we propose an experiment aimed at determining whether it is possible to represent tool-tip interaction forces through haptic and/or visual cues in a manner that is intuitively usable to better control them, seeking insight into the best form for representing forces. Subjects are asked to apply and hold pre-defined levels of suture thread tension under provision of visual and/or vibrotactile feedback.

Section 2 describes our experimental set-up and protocol. Results obtained are shown in Sect. 3 and subsequently discussed for each evaluation metric. Finally, general conclusions are drawn in Sect. 4 and axes for future work are outlined.

2 Materials and Methods

Our experiment focussed on the manipulation of a suture thread attached to the end of a laparoscopic instrument, with the aim of subjecting it to given levels of tension forces. 16 Subjects (10 male, 6 female, all novices in laparoscopy) performed a sequence of force reach and hold tasks for a selection of 10 feedback conditions.

2.1 Experimental Hardware

Subjects were placed in front of a laparoscopic trainer (EndoSim LaproTrain) containing a plate equipped with a force sensor with a fixture for holding a suture wire (3-0 gauge Braun Novosyn 90/10), as shown in Fig. 1 left. They manipulated standard laparoscopic forceps with the suture wire attached so as to avoid time losses associated with novices attempting to grasp a suture thread. Figure 1 left highlights the force sensor (ATI Nano17E 6-axis force/torque sensor, sensing range [0–12 N], force values acquired at 40 Hz) in yellow, the spring between the force/torque sensor and suture thread in blue and the suture thread in red. The role of the spring was to introduce a relatively low stiffness elastic component between the highly stiff wire and force sensor, mimicking the natural elasticity of tissue during suture knot tying or tissue manipulation. Subjects observed the scene on a 24" LCD monitor placed directly in front of them, and manipulated the laparoscopic forceps through a 5 mm trocar, observing the inside of the laparoscopic trainer as shown in Fig. 1 right. Loose white sheets were placed over the force/torque sensor and spring so as to minimize visual cues that could aid in assessing the thread tension. Vibrotactile feedback was provided using an ERM motor (Precision Microdrives PicoVibe 307-100, vibration intensity range [0–7 g] strapped to the inside of the subject's hand so as to simulate

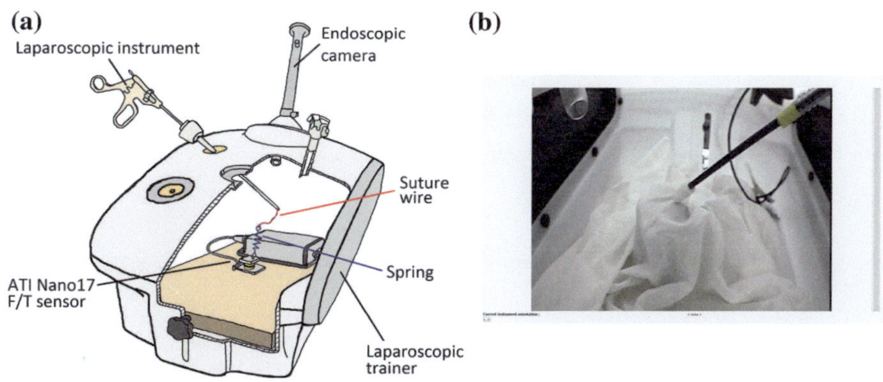

Fig. 1 **a** Experimental setup. **b** Endoscopic image as seen by the subject

integration of feedback to a LS tool handle. New feedback commands were generated at a frequency of 40 Hz, following the acquisition of the force data.

2.2 Feedback Conditions

Reference—No feedback (L): Subjects received no feedback about the suture thread tension $F_{tension}$ and relied solely on the visual information from the endoscope and natural tactile information from the instrument.

Visual feedback (V): Subjects received visual feedback about $F_{tension}$ in the form of a vertical bar-graph displayed next to the endoscopic image. The bar-graph displayed forces in the range [0–3 N]. We did not highlight the target force in any way. The feedback level as a function of $F_{tension}$ is shown in green in Fig. 2a.

Continuous vibrotactile (T): Subjects received tactile feedback about $F_{tension}$ through an ERM vibration motor. The tension force $F_{tension}$ was displayed through a linearly proportional variation of vibration amplitude (0–5.2 g), as shown in red in Fig. 2a.

Pulsed vibrotactile—fixed pulse length (Uf): The same vibration motor as for condition T displayed the suture tension F_t though series of vibration pulses at a fixed amplitude (3.4 g) and length (45 ms) with a spacing inversely proportional to the applied force varying between 525 and 15 ms, as shown in red in Fig. 2b.

Pulsed vibrotactile—varying pulse length and interval (Up): Identical set-up to Uf, however this time the length and spacing of the pulses were varied jointly in the

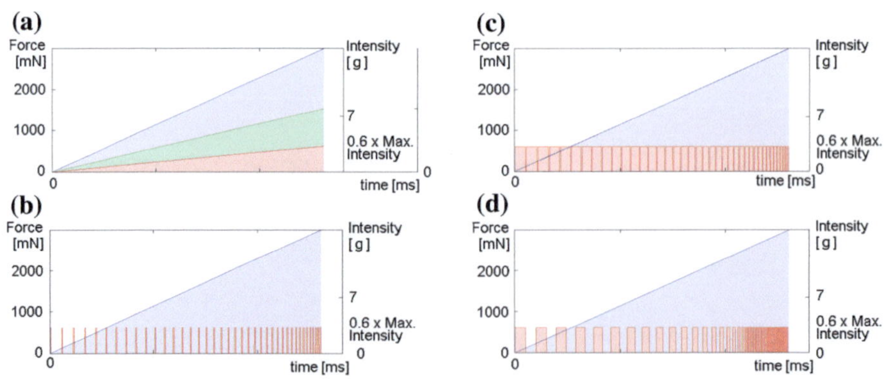

Fig. 2 Feedback levels depending on the magnitude of force to be displayed. From the *top left* to *bottom right*: **a** Visual (V) and continuous vibrotactile feedback (T). **b** Pulsed vibrotactile feedback (Uf). **c** Pulsed vibrotactile feedback (Uq). **d** Pulsed vibrotactile feedback (Up). The *blue curve* indicates the force magnitude, the *green curve* the associated bargraph heigh and the *red curve* the vibration intensity (Color figure online)

same manner as the spacing in Uf, always keeping spacing and length equal. The pattern of force encoding is shown in red in Fig. 2d.

Pulsed vibrotactile—fixed pulse interval (Uq): Identical set-up to Uf, however this time the pulse spacing was kept constant at 45 ms, and the pulse length was varied between 525 and 15 ms in inverse relation to the applied suture tension, as shown in red in Fig. 2c.

Vibrotactile and visual conditions (TV, UfV, UpV and UqV): These four conditions are identical to T, Uf, Up and Uq respectively, whereby we simultaneously provide visual feedback as in condition V.

2.3 Task

In chronological order, the task to be performed consisted of:

- **1 definition of a target force** between 1 and 3 N: Subjects pulled on the suture wire while receiving feedback corresponding to the given condition and pressed a button to define the current force as their target for the rest of the task (referred to as the actual target force F_{tgt} in the following). Subjects were under no time pressure to select a target force.
- **1 force reach task**, where the objective was to aim for the previously defined F_{tgt}, having changed the instrument's orientation (see Fig. 3) in order to minimize the impact of visual cues in the endoscopic image on assessment of F_t. The subjects pressed a button once they thought they had reached F_{tgt} (in the following, the force applied at the moment of this button press will be referred to as the estimated target force $F_{tgt,est}$).
- **1 force hold task**, where the objective was to hold $F_{tgt,est}$ for a duration of 20 s.

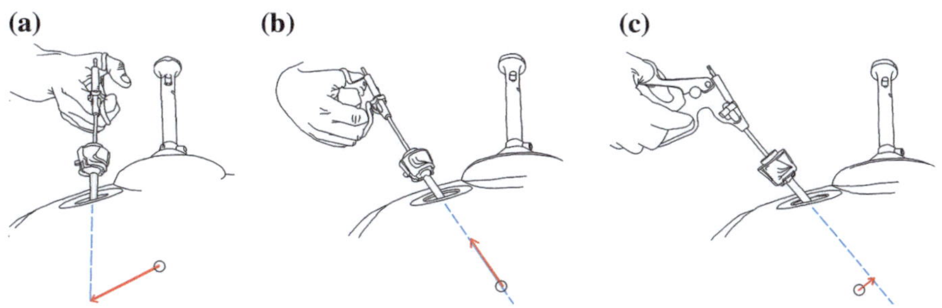

Fig. 3 Extreme cases of tool orientations when pulling on the suture wire. The *blue dotted line* shows the instrument axis, the *red arrow* the suture thread axis. From *left* to *right*: pulling on the wire using lever effect with instrument parallel to the saggital plane (**a**), directly pulling on the wire with intrument and wire aligned on the trocar axis (**b**), and pulling on the wire using lever effect with instrument parallel to the coronal plane (Color figure online)

- **3 force repeat tasks**, where the objective was once again to aim for F_{tgt} as precisely as possible, changing the instrument orientation every time. For this, the subject pressed a button to begin, pulled on the thread, and pressed the button again once F_{tgt} was thought to have been reached.

To keep the experiment duration manageable, subjects were assigned a randomized sequence of the conditions L, V, T, Uf, Up, Uq, and one of the four visual + tactile conditions (TV, UfV, UpV or UqV). For each condition, subjects performed two to three repeats of the task previously described. They were each given detailed instructions about the experimental sequence and manipulation of the laparoscopic instrument. Furthermore, they were briefed and given an example for each form of feedback prior to performing the task.

2.4 Evaluation Metrics

Mean distance to target (DTT): We calculated DTT as the mean of differences between F_{tgt} and $F_{tgt,est}$ for each force reach and force repeat task for each subject.

$$DTT_{Subject} = \frac{\sum_{i=1}^{N}(F_{tgt}(i) - F_{tgt,est}(i))}{N}[\text{mN}]$$

where $N = no.\ of\ force\ reaches + no.\ of\ force\ repeats$ performed by the subject.

Values close to 0 indicate higher aiming accuracy. Lower spread indicates greater repeatability. Dividing subject DTT for each condition by the subject's DTT for condition L highlights improvements (values < 1) or deteriorations (values > 1) from the provided feedback while compensating for differences in subject's natural capabilities in laparoscopic instrument manipulation.

Speed of aiming (SFR): We evaluated the speed of aiming at a target force for a given final accuracy.

$$SFR = \frac{1}{N}\sum_{i=1}^{N}\frac{F_{tgt}(i)}{(TCT(i) * |DTT(i)|)}[\text{s}^{-1}]$$

Larger values indicate lower DTT at equal reach speeds or higher reach speeds at equal DTT. We evaluate mean subject SFR for each condition divided by subject SFR in condition L to compensate for subject's natural capabilities in manipulating the laparoscopic instrument.

Mean error during force-hold task (FHE): FHE is the mean of differences between the subject's mean force applied during the force-hold task and $F_{tgt,est}$ from the initial force-reach task for a given condition:

$$FHE = \frac{1}{K}\sum_{i=1}^{K} F_{tgt,est}(i) - mean(F_{tension}(i))[\mathrm{mN}]$$

where K is the number of force-hold tasks performed by the subject.

Cumulative deviation (CD): CD is calculated as the mean of the integral of applied force over the duration of force hold tasks for a given feedback condition:

$$CD = \frac{1}{K}\sum_{i=1}^{K}(\sum_{j=1}^{duration\ of\ force\ hold} F_{tension}(i,j))[\mathrm{N\ s}]$$

This metric is representative of amplitude of oscillations around the target force and drift. Larger values indicate worse performance.

Drift angles: Mean drift for a given condition is calculated by fitting a line to the curve of applied force during the force-hold task and evaluating its slope (the drift angle—Dα—in [N/s]). Values further away from zero indicated a marked tendency to drift away from $F_{tgt,est}$. The sign of the drift angles also gives an indication of the direction of drift, with positive values indicating a tendency to apply more force over time and negative values indicating a tendency to reduce applied forces over time.

3 Results and Discussion

In the following, we present and discuss the main results obtained for the various evaluation metrics described earlier.

3.1 Precision and Repeatability of Reaching a Target Force

Figure 4a shows that providing feedback systematically reduces mean subject DTT (see Table 1 for subject mean DTT), all differences in means significant with at least $p < 0.05$.

The best performance is obtained for conditions V (81.77 % reduction in mean error over condition L, $p < 0.01$), TV (85.8 % reduction in mean error over condition L, $p < 0.01$), UpV (81.98 % reduction in mean error over condition L, $p < 0.01$) and UqV (83.23 % reduction in mean error over condition L, $p < 0.01$), with a systematic improvement of performance over condition L for all subjects. We believe the better performance obtained through visual feedback can be attributed to the fact that it not only provides information on the current force magnitude but also provides relative distances to the maximum and minimum levels of feedback at any given time, whereas the level of tactile feedback is harder to place on the range of possible feedback levels.

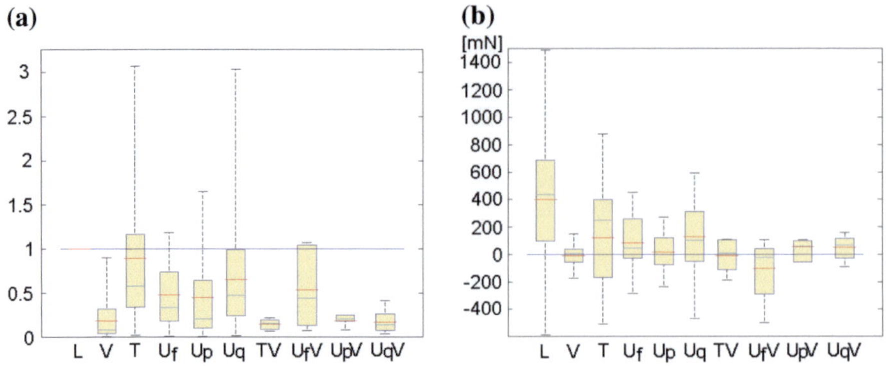

Fig. 4 **a** Mean distance to target for force reach and repeat tasks for each subject, divided by the subject's mean DTT in condition (L) [dimensionless]. Medians are indicated by the *light blue* and means by the *red horizontal lines*. **b** Mean DTT for each subject, grouped by condition [mN] (Color figure online)

Table 1 Mean subject DTTs for each condition [mN]

	L	V	T	Uf	Up	Uq	TV	UfV	UpV	UqV
Means	398.91	−8.996	121.64	82.94	15.58	127.57	−11.3	−102.1	52.16	51.02
SDs	531.79	197.6	375.21	307.54	253.2	309.87	118.45	204.9	293.96	81.85

Vibrotactile feedback alone leads to moderate improvements, with the best performance achieved for Uf (52.21 % reduction in mean error over L, improvements in >75 % of cases) and Up (55.07 % reduction in mean error over L, improvements in >75 % of cases), although in some rare cases, subjects did not succeed in performing better with them than with visual feedback alone. It seems that vibrotactile pulses yields higher sensitivity to changes than continuous vibration. Also, this difference could relate to greater user comfort when vibration was presented in short bursts. Indeed, condition T shows the worst performance of all tactile conditions, with improvements over L observed <75 % of the time.

In order to further analyse the effect of feedback on errors when aiming for predefined target forces, Fig. 4b shows the mean DTT values for each subject. In the absence of feedback, there is a marked tendency to not reach the predefined target force. This graph allows analysis of the effect of feedback on repeatability of aiming, shown by the spread of values for each condition (see Table 1 for CD means and standard deviations (SD)). Improvements in mean errors generally hold true for spread, with the best repeatability obtained for conditions V (62.8 % reduction in SD over condition L), Up (52.4 % reduction in SD over condition L), TV (77.7 % reduction in SD over condition L) and UqV (84.7 % reduction in SD over condition L). Conditions Uf and UpV yield moderate improvements in spread (42.2 % and 44.7 % reduction in SD over condition L respectively) while the remaining conditions yield only very slight improvements.

In terms of precision, there seems to be no great use in combining visual and tactile feedback (except for the improvement between UqV and Uq, $p < 0.05$), as the combination is either detrimental to performance or the tactile feedback is clearly ignored in favour of the visual feedback. The only positive impact that can be noted is a slight improvement in terms of repeatability, which can probably be attributed to the redundancy of information.

3.2 Speed of Reaching a Target Force

Feedback significantly increases SFR at identical DTT ($p < 0.05$) except for conditions T, UpV and UqV (Fig. 5). Table 2 sums up the mean values for each condition.

The best improvements are obtained for conditions V (18.23-fold increase in mean SFR), TV (18.34-fold increase in SFR) and UfV (13.34-fold increase in SFR). Conditions Uf, Up and UqV yield moderate improvements (4.55-fold, 3.92-fold and 5.52-fold increase in SFR). The significantly better performance for condition V over all tactile conditions (all differences in means significant at $p < 0.01$) can be attributed to additional available information we discussed earlier as well as the higher speed of the information delivery. Pulsed vibrotactile feedback requires a certain number of pulse cycles to convey the feedback level, whereas a bargraph provides the same information instantaneously.

If this were the only factor at play, we should expect good performance from condition T. However, the observed bad performance is largely attributable to the low

Table 2 Subject means for speed of reaching a target force for a given DTT, relative to subject's performance in condition L [dimensionless], against subject mean TCT in each condition [s]

	L	V	T	Uf	Up	Uq	TV	UfV	UpV	UqV
SFR	1	18.23	2.12	4.55	3.92	2.71	18.34	13.34	2.90	5.52
TCT [s]	7.08	7.26	6.77	10.02	9.77	8.71	8.96	9.92	6.75	6.77

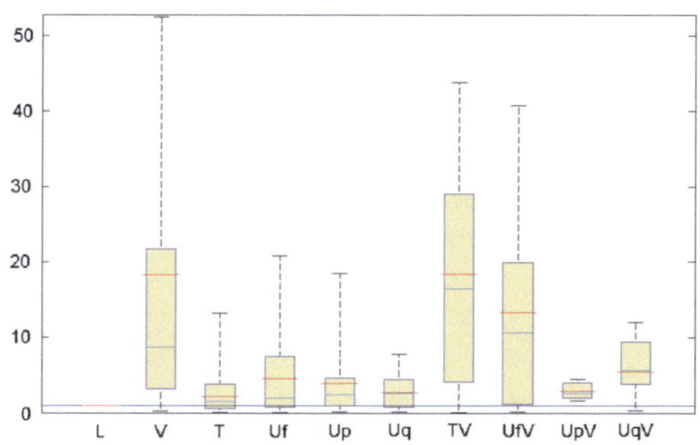

Fig. 5 Mean subject speed of reaching a target force (SFR) for a given DTT, relative to subject's performance in condition L [dimensionless]

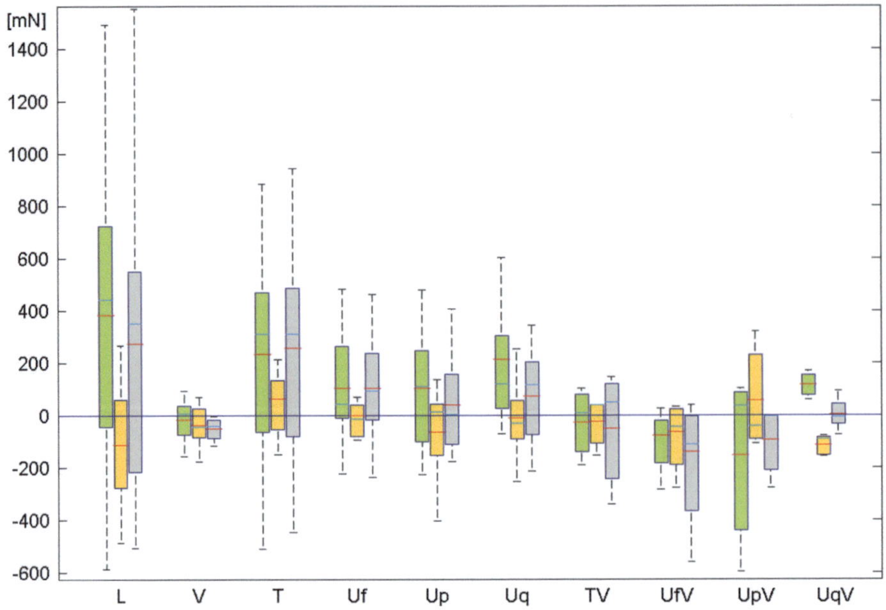

Fig. 6 Mean subject FHE (*yellow boxplot*), against subject DTT from the inital force reach task (*green boxplot*), and the resulting error (DTT + FHE), *grey boxplot* (Color figure online)

accuracy in condition T due to the poor clarity of the feedback. This conclusion is supported by the TCTs for the force reach and repeat tasks, which are not significantly different for conditions L, V and T (see Table 2).

3.3 Quality of Holding a Target Force

3.3.1 Mean Error

In the absence of feedback, FHE are large and subject to great spread. Condition V yields low FHE (35.3 mN mean error) but performs on par with pulsed vibrotactile conditions (no significant differences), with Uf and Uq performing moderately better (0.05 mN and 10.72 mN respectively) (Fig. 6). However, the bad performance of Uf in terms of DTT leads to an overall poor precision (when comparing mean force during force hold and the actual target force).

Table 3 Subject mean force hold error (FHE) [mN]

	L	V	T	Uf	Up	Uq	TV	UfV	UpV	UqV
FHE	−111.6	−35	63.9	0.1	−62.8	−10.7	−23.7	−63.7	58	−111.5
FHE + DTT	273.2	−49.6	256.2	102.2	40.3	75	−48.5	−138.2	−94	4.1

It would seem that tactile feedback performs comparatively well to visual feedback when it comes to avoiding drift from a given value, with an edge to pulsed vibrotactile feedback Uf. Continuous vibrotactile feedback is of little use in this task, with significantly worse FHE than all other tactile feedback conditions and the visual feedback condition (Table 3).

Combining visual and tactile feedback yields no significant benefit over visual or tactile feedback alone. Surprisingly, condition UqV leads to significantly worse performance, which could be due to the feedback not combining in an intuitive manner. Indeed, subjects tended to report difficulties in using Uq alone, which could account for a disturbing effect when combined with visual feedback that also demands the subject's attention. Combined feedback TV yields performance on par with condition V, leading us to believe that subjects ignored the tactile component of the combined feedback in favour of the visual feedback.

3.3.2 Drift and Cumulative Deviation

As expected, the absence of feedback yields the highest CD, due to a marked tendency to drift from $F_{tgt,est}$, with a tendency to increase the applied force over time (70 % of upward drifts against 30 % of downward drifts) and a large spread and amplitude of Dαs.

Visual feedback is more effective at reducing drift amplitude than tactile feedback alone, though not significantly. Concerning tactile feedback alone, the best performance is achieved for conditions Uf and Up (significantly outperforming T and Uq at $p < 0.1$).

All combined visual and tactile conditions significantly reduce drift and bring the mean Dαs close to 0 N/s (equal tendency to increase and decrease force over

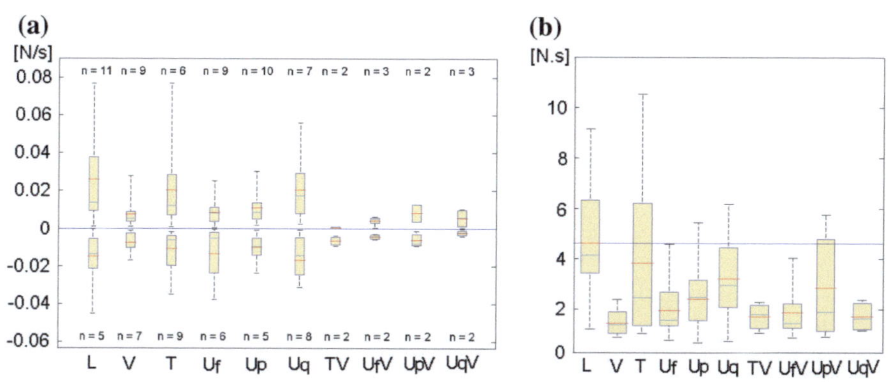

Fig. 7 **a** Subject mean drift angles Dα for force hold task [N/s]. The Dαs are separated depending on the drift direction (*upwards* or *downwards*), with the number of observations for each being shown so as to give an idea of the distribution of drift directions. **b** Subject mean cumulative deviation (CD) [N s]

Table 4 Subject mean drift angles ($D\alpha$) [N/s] and cumulative deviations (CD) [N s]

L	V	T	Uf	Up	Uq	TV	UfV	UpV	UqV
Dα (Up)	0.03	0.008	0.02	0.009	0.011	0.021	0.0004	0.004	0.008	0.006
Dα (Down)	−0.015	−0.008	−0.011	−0.013	−0.01	−0.017	−0.007	−0.004	−0.006	−0.002
CD	4.61	1.44	3.81	1.94	2.41	3.20	1.72	1.88	2.85	1.73

time, lowest means and spreads of $D\alpha$ values), highlighting a major benefit from combined visual and tactile feedback. In particular, condition TV shows a significant improvement over both conditions V and TV ($p < 0.05$).

Figure 7 right shows the mean cumulative deviation from the target force for subjects during the force hold task (mean values in Table 4). The lowest CD are obtained for condition V (68.8 % reduction in CD when compared to condition L, $p < 0.01$, 100 % of improvements over L), closely followed by conditions Uf (57.9 % reduction in CD when compared to condition L, $p < 0.01$), TV (62.7 % reduction in CD when compared to condition L, $p < 0.01$), UfV (59.2 % reduction in CD when compared to condition L, $p < 0.01$) and UqV (62.5 % reduction in CD when compared to condition L, $p < 0.01$). None of the differences in performance between V, Uf, TV, UfV and UqV are significant.

This shows that despite the results obtained from comparison of FHE, visual feedback and its combination with tactile feedback tends to slightly improve performance when it comes to staying close to a target over time. This can probably be attributed to the speed of delivery of the visual information when compared to the tactile information as we already mentioned in Sect. 3.2. Once again, when observing performance for TV, it becomes clear than the tactile component was ignored in favour of the visual feedback. Concerning UpV, the performance is worsened when compared to either of the individual forms of feedback, which may indicate a poor matching of the visual and tactile feedbacks which confused subjects.

Of the tactile feedback conditions, T (no significant difference to condition L) and Uq (difference in mean significant at $p < 0.1$) perform worst, which we believe is mainly attributable to the poor understandability of these forms of feedback.

4 Conclusion

In this paper, we describe an experiment aimed at evaluating feedback of tool-tip interaction forces in laparoscopy through haptic and/or visual cues. We compared four forms of vibrotactile feedback, on-screen visual feedback via a bar-graph and their combinations.

Providing no feedback yielded the worst overall performance for precision (strong tendency to not reach the target force, very large errors and low repeatability), speed (slowest for reaching a target force with a given accuracy) and constancy of holding a given force over time (strong tendency to increase the applied force over time, strong oscillations of force and large errors), in line with literature results on forces in LS.

Visual feedback yielded the best performance overall. Precision and repeatability when aiming at a target force were better than those achieved through tactile feedback, and on par with or better than those achieved for combined visual and tactile feedback. Visual feedback significantly outperformed tactile feedback in terms of speed. When holding a force, it effectively allowed for reduction and correction of drift, with comparable performance to the best of tactile feedback. We believe the overall better performance of visual feedback to be due to additional information provided by the bar-graph when compared to the vibrotactile feedback as well as the comparatively higher speed of delivery of the information to the user. Vibrotactile feedback moderately improved precision. It was shown to be effective in reducing mean force errors and their spread and moderately increasing task execution speed. Concerning the quality of holding a force, the best performance in terms of drift and error reduction were achieved through pulsed vibrotactile feedback. Vibrotactile feedback involving continuous or near-continuous vibration was usually outperformed by pulsed feedback, probably due to greater user comfort.

Condition TV yielded the best results in terms of precision and speed of task execution, outperforming either T or V individually. Conditions UfV, UpV and UqV yielded significant improvements over no feedback without reaching those achieved with TV, and not necessarily better than visual feedback alone, though they outperformed pulsed vibrotactile feedback alone. Concerning holding of a target force over time, combined tactile and visual feedback led to comparable errors with V and the best performance from tactile feedback alone, but usually significantly reduced drift when compared to V and tactile feedback alone respectively. It seems that pulsed vibrotactile feedback in some cases acted as a disturbance when combined with visual feedback, possibly because of discrepancies between their respective information delivery speeds.

Despite the better performance of visual feedback, these results are encouraging for the use of vibrotactile feedback in communicating force information in LS. Indeed, vibrotactile feedback clearly improves performance over no feedback and retains the advantage that it may prove effective in keeping visual cognitive load for surgeons manageable, though this remains to be investigated.

This study suffers from a few limitations, first of which being that subjects were not familiar with laparoscopy. An evaluation of the best performing forms of feedback in actual suturing trials with laparoscopic surgeons will be required. For practical reasons, the task did not take into account grasping of the thread or needle, which may impact behaviour, especially when using tactile feedback. Surgical suture knot tying is also usually a bi-manual task, so it remains to be seen whether this changes behaviour with regards to the use of feedback with implications for its design. Finally, there was no requirement to focus attention on the endoscopic image, leading to low ecological validity and likely skewing results in favour of visual feedback. Discussion with subjects showed that in conditions with visual feedback, they barely paid attention to the endoscopic image, focussing mainly on the bar-graph. We plan to address these limitations in future experiments expanding on our present work.

Acknowledgments This work was supported by French state funds managed by the ANR within the Investissements d'Avenir programme (Labex CAMI) under reference ANR-11-LABX-0004.

References

1. Bark, K., et al.: In vivo validation of a system for haptic feedback of tool vibrations in robotic surgery. Surg. Endosc. **27**, 656–664 (2013)
2. Dankelman, J., et al.: Human reliability and training in minimally invasive surgery. Minim. Invasive Ther. Allied Technol. **12**, 129–135 (2003)
3. Deziel, D.J., et al.: Complications of laparoscopic cholecystectomy: a national survey of 4,292 hospitals and an analysis of 77,604 cases. Am. J. Surg. **165**, 9–14 (1993)
4. Ding, J., et al.: Hand-assisted laparoscopic surgery versus open surgery for colorectal disease: a systematic review and meta-analysis. Am. J. Surg. **207**, 109–119 (2014)
5. Joice, P., et al.: Errors enacted during endoscopic surgery—a human reliability analysis. Appl. Ergon. **29**, 409–414 (1998)
6. Kitagawa, M., et al.: Analysis of suture manipulation forces for teleoperation with force feedback. Lecture Notes in Computer Science, vol. 2488, pp. 155–162 (2002)
7. Kitagawa, M., et al.: Effect of sensory substitution on suture manipulation forces for surgical teleoperation. Stud. Health Technol. Inf. **98**, 157–163 (2004)
8. Kitagawa, M., et al.: Effect of sensory substitution on suture-manipulation forces for robotic surgical systems. J. Thorac. Cardiovasc. Surg. **129**, 151–158 (2005)
9. Memon, M.A., et al.: Laparoscopic appendicectomy the current status. Ann. Roy. Coll. Surg. Engl. **79**, 393–402 (1997)
10. Nisky, I., et al.: Perception of stiffness in laparoscopy–the fulcrum effect. Stud. Health Technol. Inf. **173**, 313–319 (2012)
11. Reiley, C.E., et al.: Effects of visual force feedback on robot-assisted surgical task performance. J. Thorac. Cardiovasc. Surg. **135**, 196–202 (2008)
12. Schoonmaker, R.E., et al.: Vibrotactile feedback enhances force perception in minimally invasive surgery. In: Human Factors and Ergonomics Society 50th Annual Meeting, pp. 1029–1033 (2006)
13. Sjoerdsma, W., et al.: Force transmission of laparoscopic grasping instruments. Minim. Invasive Ther. Allied Technol. **6**, 274–278 (1997)
14. Tan, H.J., et al.: Population level assessment of hospital based outcomes following laparoscopic versus open partial nephrectomy during the adoption of minimally invasive surgery. J. Urol. **191**, 1231–1237 (2014). Friction dynamics of trocars. Surg. Endosc. **21**, 1338–1343 (2007)
15. Van Der Voort, M., et al.: Bowel injury as a complication of laparoscopy. Br. J. Surg. **91**, 1253–1258 (2004)
16. Vinatier, D., et al.: What can the operator actually feel when performing a laparoscopy ? Surg. Endosc. **19**, 95–100 (2004)
17. Weber, B., et al.: The effects of force feedback on surgical task performance: a meta-analytical integration. In: Auvray, M., Duriez, C. (eds.) Haptics: Neuroscience, Devices, Modeling and Applications. Lecture Notes in Computer Science, pp. 150–157. Springer, Berlin (2014)
18. Westebring-van der Putten, E.P.: A Sense of Touch in Laparoscopy (Dissertation) (2011). ISBN: 9789051550719
19. Xin, H., et al.: Laparoscopic surgery, perceptual limitations and force: a review. In: First CSCBC (2006)
20. Zhou, M., et al.: Force perception threshold varies with experience in minimally invasive surgery. In: IEEE SMC, pp. 2228–2232 (2007)

A Dual-User Teleoperation System with Adaptive Authority Adjustment for Haptic Training

Fei Liu, Arnaud Lelevé, Damien Eberard and Tanneguy Redarce

Abstract This paper presents a shared control based dual-user teleoperation haptic training system. The main contribution is an Adaptive Authority Adjustment (AAA). The authority is determined on-line according to the trainee's behavior performance. An evaluation method is introduced based on an adaptive virtual boundary, which results into a time-varing dominance factor. An overruling function is set upstream to solve some specific cases. The system is modeled and controled in port-Hamiltonian form for passivity preserving. Experiments are conducted for validation.

Keywords Dual-user teleoperation · Port-Hamiltonian · Adaptive Authority Adjustment (AAA) · Shared control

1 Introduction

Medical robotics have received a great deal of attention for the past decades [18]. As an important part of this field, bilateral teleoperation systems which enable the execution of a remote task by providing haptic feedback, find useful applications such as Minimally Invasive Surgery (MIS) [17] and medical training systems [8]. Indeed, MIS requires skilled and trained staffs as it requires precision, dexterity and reliability for the surgeon who is penalized by a limited observation and operation field (shaking cameras, reduced field of view, visual interruptions, ...). Simulation based training is progressively extending the classical medical hands-on training [1] but for complex training cases, it is useful to work on a simulated environment with

F. Liu (✉) · A. Lelevé · D. Eberard · T. Redarce
Université de Lyon, INSA de Lyon, Laboratoire Ampère (UMR 5005), F-69621 LYON, France
e-mail: fei.liu@insa-lyon.fr

A. Lelevé
e-mail: arnaud.leleve@insa-lyon.fr

D. Eberard
e-mail: damien.eberard@insa-lyon.fr

T. Redarce
e-mail: tanneguy.redarce@insa-lyon.fr

P. Wenger et al. (eds.), *New Trends in Medical and Service Robots*,
Mechanisms and Machine Science 39, DOI 10.1007/978-3-319-30674-2_13

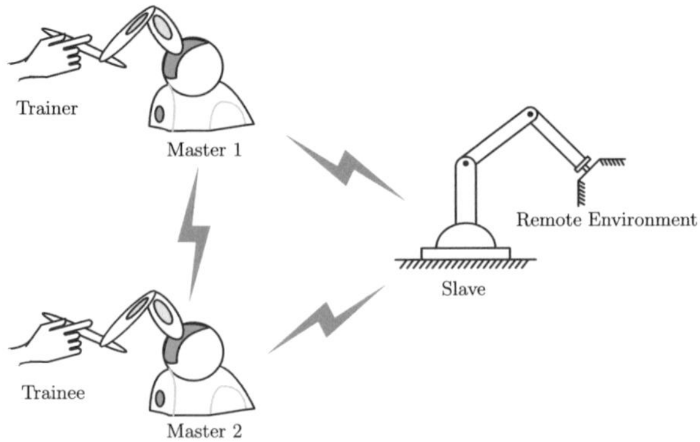

Fig. 1 A dual-user training system

a mentor who can make demonstrations and to bring real-time corrections to the trainee's motions.

Dual-user teleoperation systems have been proposed to fulfill the purpose of supervised haptic training. This kind of system is an extension of the traditional bilateral teleoperation system, which features two users working collaboratively and simultaneously on a shared remote environment. A typical dual-user training system is shown in Fig. 1.

Several architectures have been proposed for the dual-user teleoperation system. The *Shared Control* based structure has been mostly developed in [2, 3, 7, 9]. The main idea of this architecture is to share the control authority of each user over the slave robot according to a dominance factor ($\alpha \in [0, 1]$). When $\alpha = 1$ (resp. 0), the trainer (resp. trainee) has full authority on the trainee's (resp. trainer's) device and the slave. When $0 < \alpha < 1$, both users share the slave control with a dominance (over the other user) which is function of α. The control authority shared between the users is chosen according to their relative level of skills and experiences.

For the haptic training application, it is important to design a system enabling adaptive authority adjustment. During a given training task, the authority of the trainee over the slave should be adjusted adaptively according to his performances. This allows the trainer to focus on the task without having to manually manage the authority factor when the trainee deviates from the right motion. In any case, the trainer still holds the rights to reset the trainee's authority during the training progress, even when the trainee shows skillfulness.

This kind of system requires for Online Authority Adjustment (OAA) behaviors without disturbing the stability and performance. At the same time, an online motion measure of the trainee's skill level which adapts the control authority should be provided. We found that only a few papers are concerned with this issue. In [13], the control authority is adaptively adjusted according to the trainee's expertise. But it requires to specify a maximum desired level of authority of the trainee over the task at first. As a matter of fact, the trainer cannot alter this desired level during training progress. In [14], the shared control authority is managed using a time-varying dominance factor. However, the proposed method necessitates a bounded first-derivative for the dominance factor $\alpha(t)$. This involves that it should be pre-designed as a derivable function. Both of the two aforementioned methods constrains the cases of emergency when the authority needs to be changed suddenly.

In this paper, our main contribution is to incorporate the Adaptive Authority Adjustment (AAA) into a shared control based dual-user teleoperation system. The passivity of the system is ensured by port-Hamiltonian approach. The outline of this paper is as follows: next section introduces the dual-user architecture we based our work on. Sect. 3 defines the AAA while Sect. 4 shows experimentation results before our conclusions.

2 Shared Control Based Dual-user Teleoperation

In this section, we introduce a shared control based teleoperation, as shown in Fig. 2. The system is modeled within port-Hamiltonian framework.

2.1 *Port-Hamiltonian Approach*

The port-Hamiltonian framework is an energetic based generalization of the standard Hamiltonian mechanics. The port-Hamiltonian approach allows to keep track of the energy flows in the dynamic behaviors with its energetic structure, which is favorable in the modeling process. From the view of control, one of the advantages of such approach is that the Hamiltonian function, which is usually formed as Lyapunov

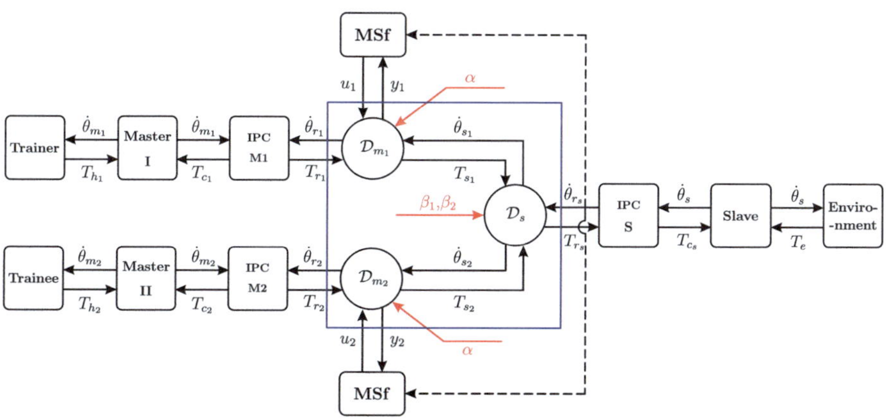

Fig. 2 The global scheme of shared control based dual-user teleoperation system. The structure inside the solid square line is the shared control based architecture

function explicitly appears in the dynamics of the system [5]. The most common representation of a port-Hamiltonian system is the following:

$$\begin{cases} \dot{x} = [J(x) - R(x)]\dfrac{\partial H}{\partial x} + g(x)u \\ y = g^T(x)\dfrac{\partial H}{\partial x} \end{cases} \tag{1}$$

where $x \in \mathbb{R}^n$ is the state and $H(x) : \mathbb{R}^n \to \mathbb{R}$ represents the Hamiltonian function; $J(x) = -J^T(x)$ is a skew-symmetric matrix representing Dirac structure, $R(x) = R^T(x) \geq 0$ specifies the energy dissipation, $g(x)$ is a matrix representing the way that the power is exchanged through the power ports formed by input-output pair (u, y) between the system and its environment.

Port-Hamiltonian approach has been applied for bilateral system modeling and controlling in [12, 16]. The intrinsically passive controller (IPC) is proposed, which is passive regardless the characteristics and parameters. This provides a natural robustness and leaves freedom to tune its parameters for performance. In our architecture, we reuse the IPC controllers as our local compliance controller.

2.2 Shared Control Based Architecture

In this study, a one degree of freedom (rotation) system is modeled. The main concept of shared control is to introduce a dominance factor. We use *Dirac* structure, which keeps the power balance (see [11]), for authority management. Three Dirac structures are inserted between the IPC controllers, named $\mathcal{D}_{m_1}$, $\mathcal{D}_{m_2}$ and $\mathcal{D}_s$. In order to achieve our control goal, three dominance factors $\alpha, \beta_1, \beta_2 \in [0, 1]$ are adopted. As the efforts (forces) and flows (velocities) follow power-conserving interconnection (skew-symmetric representation, see [11]), the behavior of these Dirac structures is passive and lossless. The $\mathcal{D}_{m_1}$, $\mathcal{D}_{m_2}$ and $\mathcal{D}_s$ in input-output matrix are given by,

$$\begin{aligned}
\mathcal{D}_{m_1} &: \begin{pmatrix} \dot{\theta}_{r_1} \\ T_{s_1} \\ y_1 \end{pmatrix} = \begin{pmatrix} 0 & \alpha & 1-\alpha \\ -\alpha & 0 & 0 \\ \alpha - 1 & 0 & 0 \end{pmatrix} \begin{pmatrix} T_{r_1} \\ \dot{\theta}_{s_1} \\ u_1 \end{pmatrix} \\
\mathcal{D}_{m_2} &: \begin{pmatrix} \dot{\theta}_{r_2} \\ T_{s_2} \\ y_2 \end{pmatrix} = \begin{pmatrix} 0 & 1-\alpha & \alpha \\ \alpha - 1 & 0 & 0 \\ -\alpha & 0 & 0 \end{pmatrix} \begin{pmatrix} T_{r_2} \\ \dot{\theta}_{s_2} \\ u_2 \end{pmatrix} \\
\mathcal{D}_{s} &: \begin{pmatrix} \dot{\theta}_{s_1} \\ \dot{\theta}_{s_2} \\ T_{rs} \end{pmatrix} = \begin{pmatrix} 0 & 0 & \beta_1 \\ 0 & 0 & 1-\beta_2 \\ -\beta_1 & \beta_2 - 1 & 0 \end{pmatrix} \begin{pmatrix} T_{s_1} \\ T_{s_2} \\ \dot{\theta}_{rs} \end{pmatrix}
\end{aligned} \tag{2}$$

The relationship between α and β_1, β_2 are defined as,

$$\beta_1 = \begin{cases} \alpha, & \alpha = 1, 0 \\ 1, & 0 < \alpha < 1 \end{cases} \qquad \beta_2 = \begin{cases} \alpha, & \alpha = 1, 0 \\ 0, & 0 < \alpha < 1 \end{cases} \tag{3}$$

Thus, we obtain three modes by changing the dominance factor α: training mode ($\alpha = 1$), guidance mode ($0 < \alpha < 1$) and evaluation mode ($\alpha = 0$). Notice that the modulated flow source **MSf** is associated with a velocity signal which is equal to $\dot{\theta}_{rs}$.

2.3 Passivity

As shown in Fig. 2, in oder to analyze the close-loop passivity, the dual-user system can be divided into several parts. Both users and the environment could be considered with passive behaviors, which is a common assumption in the literature. The master and the slave robot are physically passive. The IPC controllers are intrinsically passive. The shared control based architecture is passive due to the power-conserving composition of three *Dirac* structures. As long as the modulated flow sources **MSf** keep passive behaviors, the passivity of close-loop dual-user teleoperation system is preserved.

Proposition 1 *The modulated flow sources* ***MSf*** *hold passive behaviors: i.e.,* $\exists$ *finite constant* $d \in \mathbb{R}$ *s.t.*

$$\int_0^t u_1^T y_1 + u_2^T y_2 \,\mathrm{dt} \le d^2 \quad \forall t \ge 0 \tag{4}$$

i.e., maximum generated energy from the ***MSf*** *is bounded.*

Proof Let us first denote the generated energy at time t from **MSf** by integrating Eq. 2 as,

$$\begin{aligned} \int_0^t u_1^T y_1 + u_2^T y_2 \,\mathrm{dt} &= \int_0^t (1-\alpha) T_{r_1}^T \dot{\theta}_{r_s} + \alpha T_{r_2}^T \dot{\theta}_{r_s} \,\mathrm{dt} \\ &= \int_0^t -T_{r_1}^T \dot{\theta}_{r_1} - T_{r_2}^T \dot{\theta}_{r_2} + T_{r_s}^T \dot{\theta}_{r_s} \,\mathrm{dt} \end{aligned} \tag{5}$$

Considering the subsystem of masters (or slave) with the corresponding IPC controller, which is passive, there exists a finite constant $c_i, \in \mathbb{R}$, s.t.

$$\int_0^t T_{h_1}^T \dot{\theta}_{m_1} + T_{r_1}^T \dot{\theta}_{r_1} \mathrm{dt} \geq -c_1^2 \quad \forall t \geq 0$$
$$\int_0^t T_{h_2}^T \dot{\theta}_{m_2} + T_{r_2}^T \dot{\theta}_{r_2} \mathrm{dt} \geq -c_2^2 \quad \forall t \geq 0 \tag{6}$$
$$\int_0^t T_e^T \dot{\theta}_s - T_{r_s}^T \dot{\theta}_{r_s} \mathrm{dt} \geq -c_3^2 \quad \forall t \geq 0$$

Suppose that the operators and the environment define passive mappings, i.e., $\exists$ finite constant $k_i \in \mathbb{R}$ s.t.

$$\int_0^t -T_{h_1}^T \dot{\theta}_{m_1} \mathrm{dt} \geq -k_1^2 \quad \forall t \geq 0$$
$$\int_0^t -T_{h_2}^T \dot{\theta}_{m_2} \mathrm{dt} \geq -k_2^2 \quad \forall t \geq 0 \tag{7}$$
$$\int_0^t -T_e^T \dot{\theta}_s \mathrm{dt} \geq -k_3^2 \quad \forall t \geq 0$$

By combining Eqs. 5, 6 and 7, we can straightforward prove the passive behavior of **MSf** in Eq. 4, that is:

$$\int_0^t u_1^T y_1 + u_2^T y_2 \mathrm{~dt} \leq c_1^2 + c_2^2 + c_3^2 + k_1^2 + k_2^2 + k_3^2 = d^2 \quad \forall t \geq 0 \tag{8}$$

Proposition 2 *The closed-loop system is passive regardless variation dominance factors $\alpha \in [0, 1]$.*

Proof Firstly, we consider the shared control based architecture. The three Dirac structures form a lossless architecture which can be easily concluded. The energy stored inside them is always zero. Then, by denoting the Hamiltonian function of each subsystem at masters and slave sides (in Port-Hamiltonian framework) with H_{m_1}, H_{m_2}, H_s. Considering energy generated by **MSf** as internal stored part, we set the close-loop energy function as,

$$\begin{aligned} \frac{\mathrm{d}}{\mathrm{d}t} V(t) &= \frac{\mathrm{d}H_{m_1}}{\mathrm{d}t} + \frac{\mathrm{d}H_{m_2}}{\mathrm{d}t} + \frac{\mathrm{d}H_s}{\mathrm{d}t} + u_1^T y_1 + u_2^T y_2 + 0 \\ &= -T_{h_1}^T \dot{\theta}_{m_1} - T_{h_2}^T \dot{\theta}_{m_2} - T_e^T \dot{\theta}_s - P_{m_1} - P_{m_2} - P_s \end{aligned} \tag{9}$$

where P_{m_1}, P_{m_2}, P_s are the dissipated power at each subsystem.

Since the close-loop energy function has no relationship with the dominance factors α, β_1, β_2, and according to the condition for passivity of a switched system given by [4], we confirm the conclusion of Proposition 2.

3 Adaptive Authority Adjustment

In this section, we introduce the Adaptive Authority Adjustment (AAA), which adapts in real-time the authority according to the behavior performances of the trainer.

3.1 Adaptive Virtual Boundary

The virtual boundary is the maximum allowed distance between both master positions. It is used to guide the trainee through the right trajectory. The trainee can move his device freely inside the boundary. The virtual boundary is defined as:

$$d_{\theta_m} = (\theta_{m_1} - \theta_{m_2})^2 \leq B \tag{10}$$

where B defines the maximum allowed distance between the trainer and the trainee. We take the form of B specified in [13], as a function of the adaptive dominance factor (see the following section). That is,

$$B = B_0 - k_b ln(\alpha_a + \epsilon) \tag{11}$$

where B_0 is the maximum allowed distance when the trainer gets full control, i.e. $\alpha_a = 1$. The $ln(\cdot)$ function enables a non-linear behavior which results in the decreasing of the boundary as the trainee gets qualified (i.e. $\alpha = 0$). k_b is a tuning gain and ϵ is a very small value to avoid the zero argument case for $ln(\cdot)$, i.e. when $\alpha_a = 0$.

As soon as the condition given in Eq. (10) is violated, a virtual torque will be generated, defined as follows:

$$T_v = -k_v(\theta_{m_1} - \theta_{m_2}) \tag{12}$$

where k_v acts as a virtual stifness. Notice that in our architecture, this torque won't be transmitted back to the trainee (which is different from [13]), but used as a criterion for evaluation of the expertise of the trainee.

3.2 Adaptive Dominance Factor

The adaptive dominance factor refers to α_a, which determines the shared control authority based on the expertise of the trainee. The worse the trainee performs, the higher virtual torque T_v is generated. Therefore, we make use of T_v as an evaluation index. α_a is defined as follows:

$$\alpha_a = 1 - e^{-\frac{T_v^2}{2\cdot(T_0)^2}} \tag{13}$$

where T_0 is a task based parameter. It is straightforward to conclude that α ranges from 0 to 1, which represents expertise of the trainee ranges from inexperienced to professional.

It is worth to note that the control authority can be switched to any expected value online by the trainer, denoted by α_o. We call this is the **overrule** function. The final decision of α is:

$$\alpha = \begin{cases} \alpha_a, \text{overrule} = \text{False} \\ \alpha_o, \text{overrule} = \text{True} \end{cases} \tag{14}$$

4 Experiment

In order to validate our proposed architecture with Adaptive Authority Adjustment method, we conducted the following experiments. The dual-user teleoperation platform is shown in Fig. 3.

Two Sensable® PHANTOM Omni devices (only their first joints) were employed as the two masters operated by the trainer and the trainee. The devices' kinematic and dynamic parameters are available in [10]. The slave system and control software were implemented using Matlab Simulink. A simulated one d.o.f. joint robot (with mass M_s and f_s friction coefficient) was set up for the virtual slave. The master IPC controllers adopt the form proposed in [15]. Note that we applied a different form of IPC controller for the slave, for the purpose of fitting reverse causality interaction with two masters. The explicit equations of the master controllers can be found in [15]. The one of the slave IPC controller can be obtained in the same way. The AAA parameters are selected as:

$$B_0 = 0.05\ \text{rad},\ \ k_b = 0.01\ \text{rad},\ \ k_v = 10\ \text{N} \cdot \text{m/rad},\ \ T_0 = 0.707\ \text{N} \cdot \text{rad} \tag{15}$$

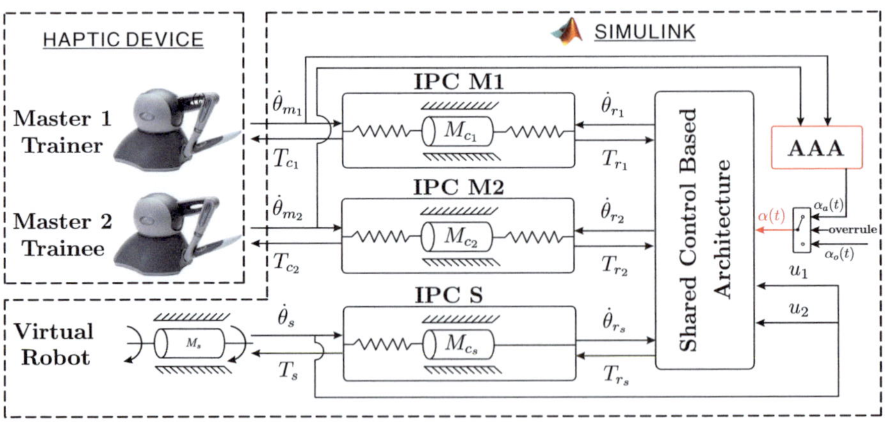

Fig. 3 The experiment setup

4.1 AAA Behavior

In the first experiment, we conducted an Adaptive Authority Adjustment. The training goal of this experiment was to move the slave device at target position located at angle 0.3 rad. A virtual obstacle (which may represent a human bone) is set at angle 0.5 rad. The obstacle model is:

$$T_w = \begin{cases} 0, & \theta_s < 0.5 \text{ rad} \\ -k_w(\theta_s - 0.5), & \theta_s \geq 0.5 \text{ rad} \end{cases} \tag{16}$$

where $k_w = 10\ \text{N} \cdot \text{m/rad}$ is the obstacle stiffness and θ_s is the slave robot's joint angle. The hand torques are estimated with a Nicosia observer described in [6]. The tracking of positions and hand/environment torques are shown in Fig. 4. The experiment time is separated into nine phases, i.e. A-I, given as Table 1.

In Fig. 4, we can check that the phase A corresponds to the training mode. The authority is overruled by the trainer with $\alpha_o = 1$. The trainer guides the trainee and the slave to the target position. The authority is set to the trainee during phase B. But due to unskilled behavior of the trainee, the slave does not reach the target position. Then, the trainer tries to lead the slave to the right position in phase C. The virtual boundary narrows down. There is a variation of authority during this period. The authority of the trainee over the slave reduced to around 0.4 based on the adaptive distance evaluation method, i.e. Eq. (13). Both the trainer and the trainee feel a torque on their hands during this period. In phase D, the full authority is given back to the trainee again. But he leads the slave beyond the target position. The trainer tries to revise the position by moving his device back a little. But it takes no effect since the trainee is still inside the virtual boundary. Under such cases, the overrule behavior could be adopted to set an expected authority. In this experiment, the overrule authority is set to 1 in phase E. The trainer guides the slave to the right position. In phase F, the trainee gets another chance to perform the task, but this time he leads his device to the virtual obstacle. The slave contacts the obstacle at time 50.9 s. Afterwards,

Table 1 The experiment phases

Phase	A	B	C	D	E	F	G	H	I
α	1	0	[0,1]	0	1	0	[0,1]	≈ 1	0
β_1	1	0	1	0	1	0	1	1	0
β_2	1	0	0	0	1	0	0	0	0
α_a	0	0	[0,1]	0	1	0	[0,1]	≈ 1	0
α_o	1	0	0	0	1	0	0	0	0
Mode	T	E	G	E	T	E	G	G	E
Wall contact	N	N	N	N	N	N	**Y**	N	N
Overrule	**Y**	N	N	N	**Y**	N	N	N	N

Mode: T = Training, G = Guidance, E = Evaluation
Wall contact: Y = Yes, N = No Overrule: Y = Yes, N = No

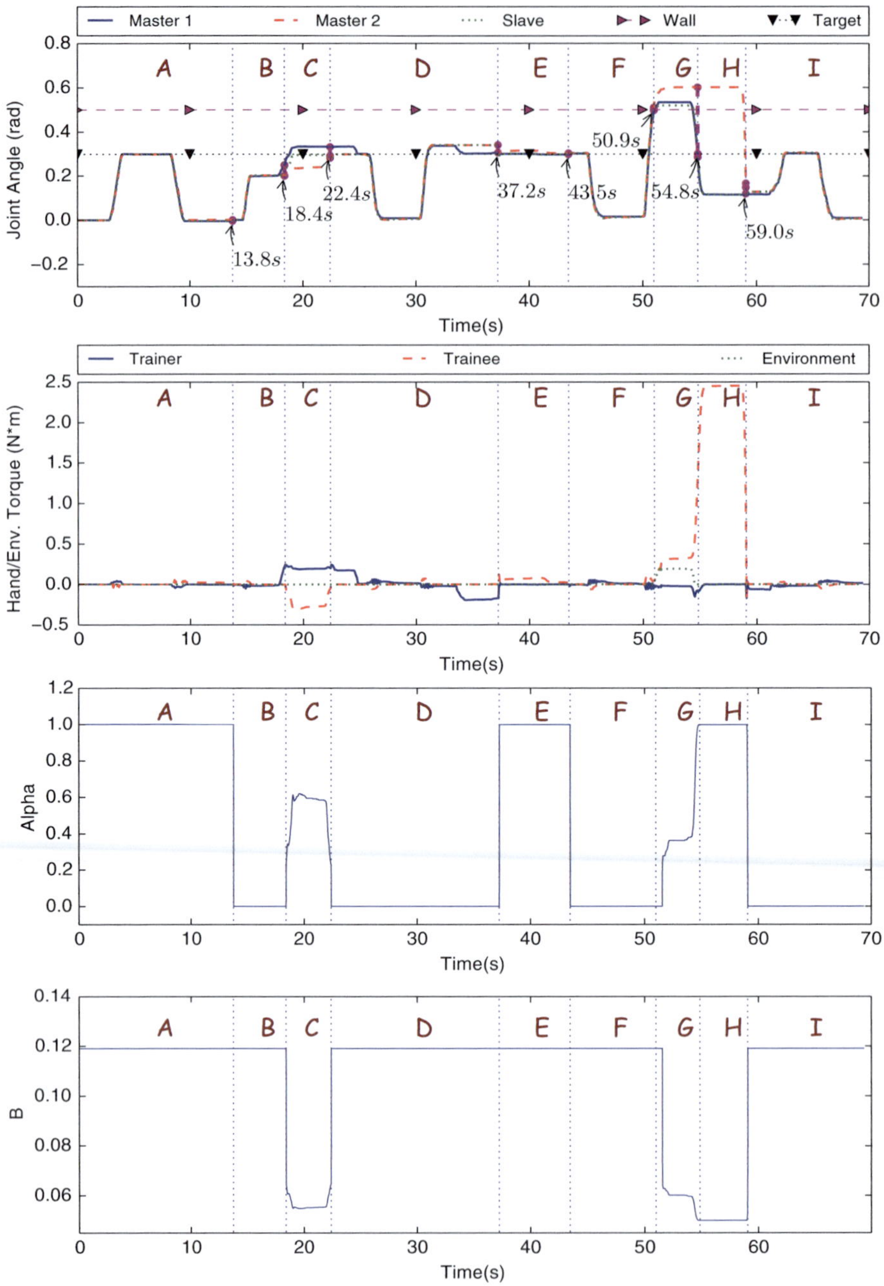

Fig. 4 Positions and torques tracking with variations of authority and virtual boundary

the trainer pulls the slave to the opposite direction, to get a certain level of authority. He almost gets full control at time 54.8 s. The slave mainly follows the trainer. The trainee feels a bigger resistance torque, that informs him the wrong behavior. After releasing his device, he gets full authority again. At last, he leads the slave to the target position and finishes the task in phase I.

4.2 *Transparency*

It is worth to explore the force details during the wall contact cases. The transparency is an important issue in teleoperation problems, which indicates whether the user feels the environment properly. In our last experiment, both of the trainer and the trainee experienced a weighted torque (due to shared value of α) compared with the one generated by the obstacle (i.e., T_w) in phase G.

In this experiment, all the configurations keep the same as previously. The result is shown in Fig. 5

The experiment is divided into two phases A and B. During the first phase A, the trainee guides the slave to the obstacle, and gets into contact with it at time 3.3 s. Then, the trainee continues his motion in depth until 0.6 rad. From the torque track-

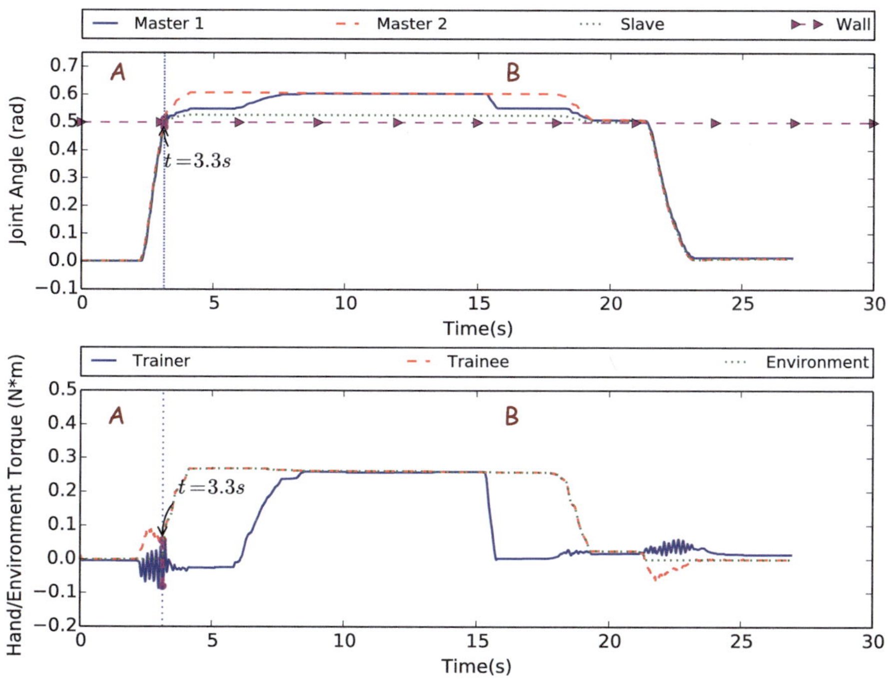

Fig. 5 Positions and torques tracking

ing, we could conclude the trainee experiences full obstacle feedback torque. But the trainer doesn't feel it. Afterwards, the trainer tries to move his device towards the same position as the trainee. Then, both the trainer and the trainee feel a full reaction torque generated by the environment, which indicates good transparency.

5 Conclusions

In this paper, we designed a shared control based dual-user teleoperation system with Adaptive Authority Adjustment (AAA). The adaptive virtual boundary and adaptive dominance factor are introduced for evaluation of the trainee's behavior performance. The authority is adaptively determined base on this evaluation. An overrule function is brought forward to respond some specific cases. The stability of the system is ensured by an energetic modeling which guarantees the passivity of the system while the authority parameters evolve in time. The experiments revealed a good performance and transparency. Future work will extend the number of degrees of freedom and involve time delays.

Acknowledgments The authors acknowledge the financial support of the China Scholarship Council (CSC) Scholarship.

References

1. Fairhurst, K., Strickland, A., Maddern, G.J.: Simulation speak. J. Surg. Educ. **68**(5), 382–386 (2011)
2. Ghorbanian, A., Rezaei, S., Khoogar, A., Zareinejad, M., Baghestan, K.: A novel control framework for nonlinear time-delayed dual-master/single-slave teleoperation. ISA Trans. **52**(2), 268–277 (2013)
3. Khademian, B., Hashtrudi-Zaad, K.: Shared control architectures for haptic training: performance and coupled stability analysis. Int. J. Robot. Res. **30**(13), 1627–1642 (2011)
4. Mahapatra, S., Zefran, M.: Stable haptic interaction with switched virtual environments. In: Proceedings of IEEE International Conference on Robotics and Automation (ICRA), pp. 1241–1246 (2003)
5. Maschke, B., van der Schaft, A.: Port controlled hamiltonian systems: modeling origins and system theoretic properties. In: Proceedings of the Third Conference on Nonlinear Control Systems (NOLCOS) (1992)
6. Nicosia, S., Tomei, P.: Robot control by using only joint position measurements. IEEE Trans. Autom. Control **35**(9), 1058–1061 (1990)
7. Nudehi, S., Mukherjee, R., Ghodoussi, M.: A shared-control approach to haptic interface design for minimally invasive telesurgical training. IEEE Trans. Control Syst. Technol. **13**(4), 588–592 (2005)
8. Panait, L., Akkary, E., Bell, R., Roberts, K., Dudrick, S., Duffy, A.: The role of haptic feedback in laparoscopic simulation training. J. Surg. Res. **156**(2), 312–316 (2009)
9. Razi, K., Hashtrudi-Zaad, K.: Analysis of coupled stability in multilateral dual-user teleoperation systems. IEEE Trans. Robot. **30**(3), 631–641 (2014)

10. Sansanayuth, T., Nilkhamhang, I., Tungpimolrat, K.: Teleoperation with inverse dynamics control for phantom omni haptic device. In: 2012 Proceedings of SICE Annual Conference (SICE), pp. 2121–2126 (2012)
11. Schaft, A.J.V.d.: L2-Gain and Passivity Techniques in Nonlinear Control. Springer (1996)
12. Secchi, C., Stramigioli, S., Fantuzzi, C.: Control of Interactive Robotic Interfaces: A Port-Hamiltonian Approach. Springer (2007)
13. Shahbazi, M., Atashzar, S., Patel, R.: A dual-user teleoperated system with virtual fixtures for robotic surgical training. In: 2013 IEEE International Conference on Robotics and Automation (ICRA), pp. 3639–3644 (2013)
14. Shahbazi, M., Talebi, H., Patel, R.: Networked dual-user teleoperation with time-varying authority adjustment: a wave variable approach. In: 2014 IEEE/ASME International Conference on Advanced Intelligent Mechatronics (AIM), pp. 415–420 (2014)
15. Stramigioli, S.: Modeling and IPC Control of Interactive Mechanical Systems: A Coordinate-Free Approach. Springer (2001)
16. Stramigioli, S., van der Schaft, A., Maschke, B., Melchiorri, C.: Geometric scattering in robotic telemanipulation. IEEE Trans. Robot. Autom. **18**(4), 588–596 (2002)
17. Tavakoli, M., Patel, R., Moallem, M.: Haptics For Teleoperated Surgical Robotic Systems. World Scientific (2008)
18. Taylor, R., Stoianovici, D.: Medical robotics in computer-integrated surgery. IEEE Trans. Robot. Autom. **19**(5), 765–781 (2003)

Strategy to Lock the Knee of Exoskeleton Stance Leg: Study in the Framework of Ballistic Walking Model

Y. Aoustin and A.M. Formalskii

Abstract The paper aim is to show theoretically the feasibility and efficiency of a passive exoskeleton for human carrying a load. Human is modeled using a mathematical model of a planar bipedal five-link anthropomorphic mechanism. This mechanism consists of a trunk and two identical legs; each leg consists of a thigh and shin with point-foot. The exoskeleton is considered also as a five-link anthropomorphic mechanism. The shape and the degrees of freedom of the exoskeleton are identical to biped (to human). If the biped is equipped with an exoskeleton, then the links of this exoskeleton are attached to the corresponding links of the biped and the corresponding hip-, knee-, and ankle-joints coincide. We compare the walking of a biped alone (without exoskeleton) and of a biped equipped with exoskeleton; both models are with a load. A ballistic walking gait is designed in both cases. During the ballistic walking of the biped with exoskeleton the knee of the stance leg of the exoskeleton (and as a consequence of the biped) is locked. The locking can be realized in the knee of each leg of the exoskeleton by any mechanical brake device with no energy consumption. There are not any actuators in our exoskeleton. Therefore, we call it *passive* exoskeleton. The walking of the biped consists of alternating single- and double-support phases. In our study, the double-support phase is assumed as instantaneous. At the instant of this phase, the knee of the previous swing leg is locked and the knee of the previous stance leg is unlocked. Numerical results show that during the load transport the human with the exoskeleton spends less energy than human alone.

Keywords Human · Bipedal model · Passive exoskeleton · Ballistic walking · Instantaneous double support · Impulsive torque · Optimization

---

Y. Aoustin (✉)
L'UNAM, Institut de Recherche en Communications et
Cybernétique de Nantes, UMR 6597, CNRS, École Centrale de Nantes,
Université de Nantes, 1, rue de la Noë, BP 92101, 44321 Nantes, France
e-mail: Yannick.Aoustin@irccyn.ec-nantes.fr

A.M. Formalskii
Institute of Mechanics, Lomonosov Moscow State University,
1, Michurinskii Prospect, Moscow 119192, Russia
e-mail: formal@imec.msu.ru

P. Wenger et al. (eds.), *New Trends in Medical and Service Robots*,
Mechanisms and Machine Science 39, DOI 10.1007/978-3-319-30674-2_14

1 Introduction

Exoskeleton robots are integrated mechanical devices (mechanisms), which can be wearable and attached to the human body. Research in powered human exoskeleton devices began in the late 1960 s for military purposes, [1]. Hardiman, (Human Augmentation Research and Development Investigation) was an enormous powered exoskeleton (with mass 680 kg) to drastically increase the strength capabilities of the wearer, (approximately 25:1), see [2]. Vukobratovic and his associates at the Mihailo Pupin Institute in Belgrade in 1960 and 1970 s started with a passive device for measuring the kinematics of walking, see [3]. Then this work progressed to the development of powered pneumatic exoskeletons. The design of the exoskeletons is currently an important area of research in performance enhancement but also in rehabilitation robotics, injury prevention. They can enhance strength and endurance during locomotion of for example military, firemen or life savers with heavy load. The University of California, Berkeley in collaboration with Schilling Robotics, developed the exoskeleton *BLEEX*, see [4–6]. A person who is equipped with a *BLEEX* can carry a rucksack of mass 75 kg while walking at 0.9 m/s and can walk at speeds of up to 1.3 m/s. The mass of an exoskeleton depends on the actuators. For the second generation of the Berkeley exoskeleton, in part due to the implementation of electric actuation with a hydraulic transmission system, it is approximately 14 kg. Recently, Percro a fully actuated body extender to amplify the force of a human operator has been designed, realized and tested, see [7]. A lower limb exoskeleton is proposed in [8] etc. to assist persons with paraplegia. The relation between human and exoskeleton is also a complex task. Strausser and Kazerooni [9] proposed a Humanoid Machine Interface (HMI) for a mobile medical exoskeleton to allow the users to stand up, walk, and sit down independently. Current trends and major challenges in the development of assistance devices are discussed in [10].

Then the idea to limit the number of actuators is also explored. Through simulations van den Bogert, see [11], proved that an exoskeleton with passive elastic devices can reduce muscle force and metabolic cost of human in walking. As a consequence a quasi-passive exoskeleton concept has been developed at the Massachusetts Institute of Technology Media Laboratory, see [12]. The objective is to exploit the passive dynamics of human walking in order to create lighter and more efficient exoskeleton devices. There are not any actuators for adding power at the joints of the MIT exoskeleton. The quasi-passive elements of the exoskeleton, which are springs and variable dampers, have been chosen from an analysis of the kinetics and kinematics of human walking. Another quasi-passive exoskeleton has been designed at University of Delaware, Newark, see [13, 14] for the leg of a human subject. This gravity balancing exoskeleton, also does not use any motors, but through springs and a four bars mechanism is able to partially or fully unload the hip and knee joints from the gravity throughout the range-of-motion of the leg. Dariush, see [15] proposed a strategy for a partition between natural voluntary control by the central nervous system of human and artificial assist by the exoskeleton controller. In [16] a passive exoskeleton with artificial tendons is proposed. However, authors showed that the effect of the artificial tendons on the energy expenditure while walking is much lower than expected.

For a given assistance device with ballistic motions and impulsive impacts it is theoretically shown in [17] that an assistance at the level of hips only is a good compromise.

Despite all these remarkable contributions, devices are still relatively heavy wearable versus the weight of a human. They are efficient to balance a static payload, but some progresses are necessary to balance the reactive or dynamic effects of the payload. It is not yet demonstrated that an exoskeleton is more efficient to reduce the metabolic cost of transport than the load-carriage with a standard rucksack. The location and the number of actuators of an exoskeleton and its autonomy remain a difficult challenge.

The paper aim is to prove theoretically the feasibility and the efficiency of the passive exoskeleton with locked knee of its stance leg. The advantages of the passive exoskeleton are autonomy, lightness, and robustness. Such exoskeleton is autonomous and light because it does not contain any sources of energy and actuators.

A study is proposed in this paper, based on the ballistic movements in the single-support and impulsive torques in the double-support. The walking in the sagittal plane is studied. We consider the locking of the swing leg knee of the exoskeleton (and as a consequence of the biped) at the instant when this leg touches the support (becomes stance leg) and the unlocking of the knee of the stance leg at the instant when it leaves the support (becomes swing leg). The energy consumption of the impulses is calculated to explore the possibilities to reduce the energy consumption of a biped (human) with an exoskeleton.

Human motions comprise alternating periods of muscle activity and relaxation, and the double-support phase is relatively short with respect to the single-support phase. Then it is logical to consider the problem of purely ballistic swing phases and instantaneous double-support phases with impulsive inter-link torques. A similar statement of the problem is proposed by Formalskii [18–20], Mochon and McMahon [21], McGeer [22], and Aoustin and Formalskii [23]. Mathematically this statement of the problem is reduced to the boundary value problem with given boundary configurations of the biped.

We consider a 2D model of human to focus the attention to the transport of the payload during a walking. A planar anthropomorphic bipedal model is considered, with a torso, two identical legs without feet (with point-feet). Similar models are studied, for example, in [24, 25]. In the single-support phase, this model has five degrees of freedom and it is described by essentially nonlinear differential equations of tenth order. The mathematical model for the double support is quite different. Thus, the structure of the mathematical model changes during the alternating single- and double-support phases. This model would be too complex, if we take into account, for example, compliances, tendons, muscles etc. The exoskeleton has the same degrees of freedom, the same size and shape than the biped. The torso, thighs and shins of the exoskeleton are assumed strongly strapped to the torso, thighs and shins of human. In our study, the mass of the exoskeleton is also taken into account.

In this paper, initially we find a ballistic walking of the biped alone (with no exoskeleton) for the transport of a payload. The energy consumption of the biped is calculated. After, the biped equipped with the exoskeleton is studied. We find for this biped ballistic walking with the locked knee of the stance leg. Then we show that the energy consumption for the transport of the same payload is higher for the biped alone than for the biped equipped with the exoskeleton. This is the main contribution of the paper.

The impulsive control torques, which are applied in the inter-link joints between the neighboring single-support phases are described by delta-functions of Dirac. Our approach can be considered as asymptotic because it is not possible to realize these purely impulsive control torques.

The rest of the paper is organized as follows. Section 2 is devoted to the mathematical model of the biped with its walking assist device. The physical parameters of the system are presented here. The instantaneous double-support phase also is described shortly in this Sect. 2. Problem definition of the ballistic walking is given in Sect. 3. The boundary value problem to design ballistic swing motion is presented here. Three sub-phases of the double-support phase are described. The algebraic equations for each sub-phase are designed in this Sect. 3. The chosen effort cost functional for the impulsive control is described in Sect. 4. The results of simulation are shown in Sect. 5. Our conclusion and perspectives are offered in Sect. 6.

2 Mathematical Model of Biped with Exoskeleton

Here, we give physical parameters of the biped with the exoskeleton. Its mathematical model is developed. The modeling of the biped in double-support phase is described.

2.1 Physical Parameters of the Biped and Exoskeleton

For the five-link bipedal model shown in Fig. 1, we use the physical parameters from [19]. The whole mass of the biped is 75 kg, its height is 1.75 m. The distance between the knee joint and the center of mass for the shin is: $S_s = 0.324$ m, between the hip joint and the center of mass for the thigh: $S_t = 0.18$ m, between the hip joint and the center of mass for the trunk: $S_T = 0.386$ m (see Fig. 1b). The head mass is included in the trunk that its length is l_T. The shape and the degrees of freedom of the exoskeleton are identical to human. To simplify the mathematical model we assume that the links of the exoskeleton have the same positions of the centers of mass as the links of human. Thus the positions of the centers of mass of the human (biped) alone are identical to the positions of the centers of mass of the human (biped) with the exoskeleton. Table 1 gathers the masses, the lengths and the inertia moments for each link of the bipedal model and the walking assist device.

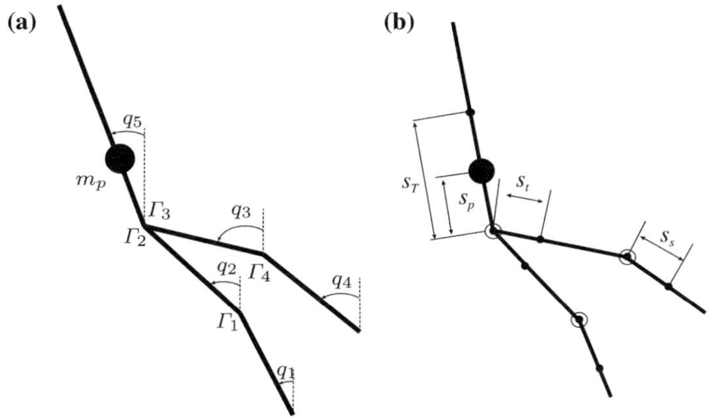

Fig. 1 **a** The kinematic model with its degrees of freedom and link frames of human and its exoskeleton. **b** Positions of the centers of mass of each link

Table 1 Physical parameters of the five-link biped and of the exoskeleton

	Mass (kg)	Length (m)	Inertia moment (kg m^2)	Center of mass (m)
Human shin	$m_s = 4.6$	$l_s = 0.55$	$I^s = 0.0521$	$s_s = 0.324$
Human thigh	$m_t = 8.6$	$l_t = 0.45$	$I^t = 0.75$	$s_t = 0.18$
Human trunk	$m_T = 48.6$	$l_T = 0.75$	$I^T = 11.3$	$s_T = 0.386$
Exoskeleton shin	$m_1 = 1.0$	$l_1 = 0.497$	$I^1 = 0.0260$	$s_s = 0.324$
Exoskeleton thigh	$m_2 = 2.0$	$l_2 = 0.41$	$I^2 = 0.0354$	$s_t = 0.18$
Exoskeleton trunk	$m_3 = 8.0$	$l_3 = 0.75$	$I^3 = 0.3817$	$s_T = 0.386$

In Fig. 1a notation m_p means mass of the payload, S_p means distance between the hip-joint and payload. In our calculations we use payload with mass $m_p = 40$ kg and distance $S_p = 0.1$ m.

2.2 *Mathematical Model*

Vector **x** of the generalized coordinates is such as

$$\mathbf{x} = [q_1, q_2, q_3, q_4, q_5, x, y]^{\mathsf{T}}.$$

Here angles q_1, q_2, q_3, and q_4 define the absolute orientation of the shin and thigh for both legs, see Fig. 1a. The absolute orientation of the trunk is defined through angular variable q_5. Cartesian hip-joint coordinates are indicated as x and y. Superscript $^\top$ means transposition.

The mathematical model of the biped with its walking assist device is:

$$\mathbf{A}(\mathbf{x})\ddot{\mathbf{x}} + \mathbf{h}(\mathbf{x}, \dot{\mathbf{x}}) = \mathbf{D}\boldsymbol{\Gamma} + \mathbf{J}_{\mathbf{r}_1}^\top \mathbf{r}_1 + \mathbf{J}_{\mathbf{r}_2}^\top \mathbf{r}_2, \tag{1}$$

Here $\mathbf{A}(\mathbf{x})$ is the 7×7 symmetric positive definite inertia matrix, $\mathbf{h}(\mathbf{x}, \dot{\mathbf{x}})$ is the 7×1 vector, which groups the centrifugal, Coriolis, and gravity forces. $\boldsymbol{\Gamma}$ is the 4×1 vector of the joint torques applied by human or by the brake devices of the exoskeleton. We consider the torques applied in the hip and knee joints. Vectors $\mathbf{r}_i$, with $i = 1, 2$, are the ground reactions applied in both point-feet. The size of these vectors is (2×1). $\mathbf{J}_{r_1}$ and $\mathbf{J}_{r_2}$ are the 2×7 Jacobian matrices.

The following constraint equations are correct when the front or/and rear leg is/are on the support

$$\mathbf{J}_{\mathbf{r}_i}\ddot{\mathbf{x}} + \dot{\mathbf{J}}_{\mathbf{r}_i}\dot{\mathbf{x}} = \mathbf{0} \qquad \text{for } i = 1 \text{ or/and } 2. \tag{2}$$

Because the vector of generalized coordinates is composed of absolute angle variables instead of joint variables we applied the principle of virtual work to calculate matrix $\mathbf{D}$ in equation (1), see [26]. Let us detail this calculation. The joint variables θ_i for $i = (1,\ 2,\ 3,\ 4)$ as functions of the generalized coordinates are:

$$\theta_1 = q_2 - q_1,\ \theta_2 = q_5 - q_2,\ \theta_3 = q_5 - q_3,\ \theta_4 = q_3 - q_4. \tag{3}$$

The virtual work δW_i of each torque Γ_i, applied to the corresponding joint with virtual variable $\delta\theta_i$, $(i = 1,\ 2,\ 3,\ 4)$ is described by equation:

$$\delta W_i = \Gamma_i \delta\theta_i = \Gamma_i \mathbf{D}_i^\top \delta\mathbf{x} \tag{4}$$

Then matrix $\mathbf{D}$ of the torques is: $\mathbf{D} = [\mathbf{D}_1, \mathbf{D}_2, \mathbf{D}_3, \mathbf{D}_4]$ with the following columns,

$$\mathbf{D}_i = \frac{\partial}{\partial \Gamma_i}\left(\frac{\partial \delta W}{\partial \delta\mathbf{x}}\right). \tag{5}$$

If the torques from human or exoskeleton are applied in these four joints (in the hip- and knee-joints), matrix $\mathbf{D}$ is:

$$\mathbf{D} = \begin{pmatrix} -1 & 0 & 0 & 0 \\ 1 & -1 & 0 & 0 \\ 0 & 0 & -1 & 1 \\ 0 & 0 & 0 & -1 \\ 0 & 1 & 1 & 0 \\ 0 & 0 & 0 & 0 \\ 0 & 0 & 0 & 0 \end{pmatrix} \tag{6}$$

The principle of virtual work can be also used to obtain matrices $\mathbf{J}_{\mathbf{r}_1}$ and $\mathbf{J}_{\mathbf{r}_2}$.

2.3 Modeling the Biped with the Exoskeleton in Double-Support Phase

During the biped's gait, an impact occurs at the end of a single-support phase, when the swing leg tip touches the ground. At the instant of impact, denoted by T, the double-support phase is assumed instantaneous. At the instant of the passive inelastic impact, the biped looses energy. Therefore, the velocity vector after the impact will not be the desired one, if the bearing surface is horizontal. Then for the next ballistic step the desired initial velocity vector will not be reached. As a consequence, a complete walking cyclic gait of the biped with its assist device cannot be realized on a horizontal surface without active torques. However, theoretically, "around" the instantaneous double-support it is possible to define impulsive torques in order to ensure the desired velocity jump; see Formalskii [19, 20], Hurmuzlu, and Chang [27]. In the next Section, it is shown how to calculate these impulsive torques.

3 Ballistic Swing Motion and Double-Support with Impulses: Problem Definition

During the ballistic swing motion of the biped with no exoskeleton, the torques in the joints are zero. In the single-support motion of the biped with the exoskeleton all torques are zero except the torque in the knee of the stance leg. This torque is developed to lock the knee by mechanical break. Therefore, we also call this motion as ballistic. The equations of the single-support ballistic motion of the biped with the exoskeleton and with no exoskeleton are described in this section. The relations to find control impulsive torques in the double-support phase are obtained from the general mathematical model (1), (2).

3.1 Single-Support Phase

In the single-support phase, the stance leg (let it be leg 1) is assumed that there is no sliding motion, no take-off. Furthermore, with a torque Γ_1, the exoskeleton carries out the locking of the knee of this stance leg by any mechanical brake (without any motor).

Let $\mathbf{x}(0)$ be the initial configuration of the biped at time $t = 0$. The final configuration of the biped in the single-support phase at the given time $t = T$ is noted $\mathbf{x}(T)$. In Fig. 2, both boundary configurations $\mathbf{x}(0)$ and $\mathbf{x}(T)$ are shown as side view. The left pose in Fig. 2 is initial configuration $\mathbf{x}(0)$, the right pose is terminal configuration $\mathbf{x}(T)$. Our biped is walking from left to right. Final configuration is similar to initial configuration with the legs swapped. Both legs are straightened in these boundary configurations, the torso is slightly inclined forward ($q_5(0) = -3°$). We assume, the

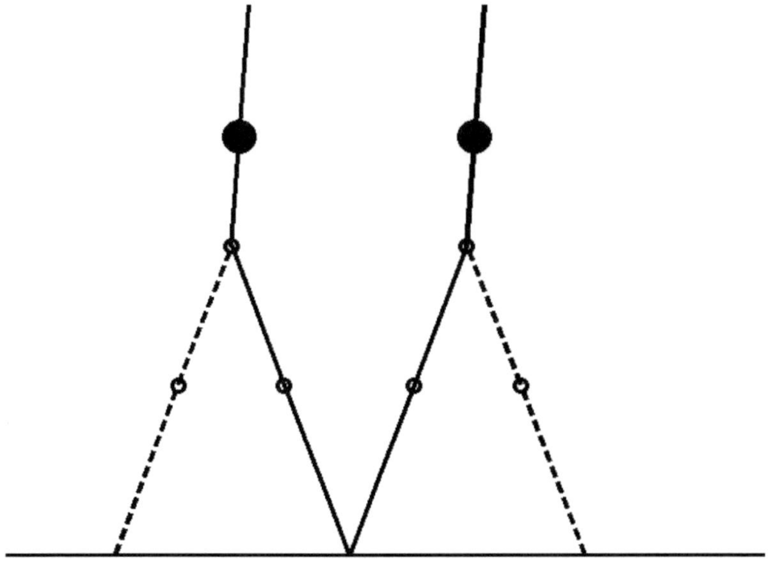

Fig. 2 Initial $\mathbf{x}(0)$ and final $\mathbf{x}(T)$ configurations of the biped (side view)

front and hind legs in the initial configuration are the stance and swing legs respectively. The stance leg is shown by solid line, the swing leg—by dashed line. Let L be the length of the step corresponding to a single-support. We consider a ballistic motion during the single-support phase with the torques provided through human null, $\mathbf{\Gamma}_i = 0$, with $i = 2,\ 3$ and 4. As a consequence, the matrix equation (1) for the ballistic motion becomes:

$$\mathbf{A}(\mathbf{x})\ddot{\mathbf{x}} + \mathbf{h}(\mathbf{x}, \dot{\mathbf{x}}) = \begin{bmatrix}\mathbf{D}_1 & \mathbf{D}_2 & \mathbf{D}_3 & \mathbf{D}_4\end{bmatrix} \begin{bmatrix} \Gamma_1 \\ \mathbf{0}_{3\times 1} \end{bmatrix} + \mathbf{J}_{\mathbf{r}_1}^{\top} \mathbf{r}_1, \tag{7}$$

with the constraint equation (2) for the stance leg tip fixed on the ground:

$$\mathbf{J}_{\mathbf{r}_1}\ddot{\mathbf{x}} + \dot{\mathbf{J}}_{\mathbf{r}_1}\dot{\mathbf{x}} = \mathbf{0}, \tag{8}$$

and with the constraint equation for the knee of the stance leg locked in the swing phase:

$$\mathbf{D}_1^{\top}\ddot{\mathbf{x}} = 0. \tag{9}$$

Notation $\mathbf{0}_{3\times 1}$ in equation (7) means the column with three zero-elements, $\mathbf{D}_1$ in (9) is the first column of the matrix $\mathbf{D}$, see (6). System (7)–(9) contains ten scalar equations with ten unknown variables: q_1, q_2, q_3, q_4, q_5, x, y, Γ_1, r_{1x}, and r_{1y}.

The ballistic single-support motion of the biped alone (with no exoskeleton) is described by matrix equations (7) and (8), but with all torques $\boldsymbol{\Gamma}_i = 0\,(i = 1, 2, 3, 4)$. In this case, matrix equation (7) becomes as follows:

$$\mathbf{A}(\mathbf{x})\ddot{\mathbf{x}} + \mathbf{h}(\mathbf{x}, \dot{\mathbf{x}}) = \mathbf{J}_{\mathbf{r}_1}^{\mathsf{T}} \mathbf{r}_1, \tag{10}$$

The stance leg of the biped alone is not locked; therefore condition (9) must be omitted. But equation (8) is still valid. The numerical values of the parameters in matrices $\mathbf{A}(\mathbf{x})$, $\mathbf{h}(\mathbf{x}, \dot{\mathbf{x}})$ and $\mathbf{J}_{\mathbf{r}_i}$ $(i = 1, 2)$ of course are different for the mathematical models of the biped with exoskeleton and with no exoskeleton.

To design the ballistic motion of the biped with the exoskeleton in the single-support phase, it is necessary to find the solution $\mathbf{x}(t)$ of the matrix equations (7)–(9) with the given boundary conditions $\mathbf{x}(0)$ and $\mathbf{x}(T)$. We have to find the initial velocity vector $\dot{\mathbf{x}}(0)$ such that solution $\mathbf{x}(t)$, starting from the given initial configuration $\mathbf{x}(0)$ with the velocity vector $\dot{\mathbf{x}}(0)$, reaches the given final configuration $\mathbf{x}(T)$ at the given time T. Unknown velocity vector $\dot{\mathbf{x}}(0)$ for the biped with the exoskeleton must satisfy condition $\mathbf{D}_1^{\mathsf{T}}\dot{\mathbf{x}}(0) = 0$.

The given boundary conditions $\mathbf{x}(0)$ and $\mathbf{x}(T)$ are chosen such that the positions of the biped with its exoskeleton are similar to human configurations. The formulated above boundary value problem can be numerically solved using a Newton method with vector $\dot{\mathbf{x}}(0)$ unknown. The motion of the biped is admissible, if the vertical component of the ground reaction in the stance leg is positive (directed upwards), if the swing leg moves over the ground for $0 < t < T$, and if the swing leg bends the knee forward. We check these constraints after solving the boundary value problem—*a posteriori*. The ground reaction $\mathbf{r}_1$ and the torque $\boldsymbol{\Gamma}_1$ developed by brake device are calculated during solving this boundary value problem with matrix equations (7)–(9).

After solving the boundary value problem, the vector of the initial velocities $\dot{\mathbf{x}}(0)$ is known. We denote it by $\dot{\mathbf{x}}^a$. If the initial conditions $\mathbf{x}(0)$, $\dot{\mathbf{x}}^a$ are known, then by integration of the system (7)–(9) the vector of the terminal velocities $\dot{\mathbf{x}}(T)$ can also be found. We denote it by $\dot{\mathbf{x}}^b$.

3.2 *Structure of Double-Support Phase*

Similarly to [20, 28] or [23] let us consider the current ballistic motion on the stance leg 1 and the following ballistic motion on the stance leg 2. Let the final velocity vector $\dot{\mathbf{x}}^b$ of the current ballistic swing motion and the initial velocity vector $\dot{\mathbf{x}}^a$ of the next ballistic swing motion be known from the solution of the boundary value problem[1] and the numerical integration of the matrix equations (7)–(9). Let us

[1]Therefore there is a permutation operation between $\dot{\mathbf{x}}^a$ and the solution of the boundary value problem to take into account the exchange of the role of both legs.

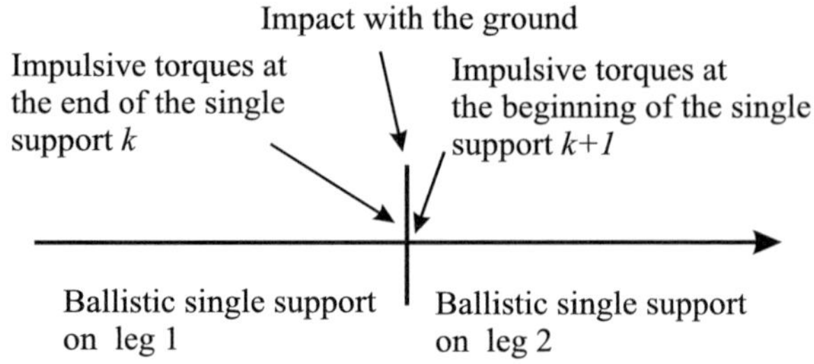

Fig. 3 Decomposition of the instantaneous double-support phase; see [20, 28], or [23]

consider the instantaneous double-support phase between two neighboring single-support phases (see Fig. 3).

We divide this instantaneous double-support phase into *three* instantaneous sub-phases and investigate them. Let us apply the impulsive torques in the joints with the vectors of the magnitudes $\mathbf{I}^-(I_1^-, I_2^-, I_3^-, I_4^-)$ and $\mathbf{I}^+(I_1^+, I_2^+, I_3^+, I_4^+)$, respectively just before and just after the passive impact with the ground to create a complete cyclic motion.

Now we will consider each sub-phase in more details.

- The swing leg 2 touches the ground just after the end of the ballistic single-support motion on the stance leg 1, and an impact occurs. If the human is equipped with the exoskeleton, then just before contact with the ground of the swing leg 2 (before an impact), in the *first* sub-phase at time-instant $t = T^-$, the knee of the leg 1 is kept locked through an impulsive torque $\Gamma_1^-(t) = I_1^- \delta(t - T^-)$ developed by a brake device mounted in this knee of the exoskeleton. Here $\delta(t - T^-)$ is the Dirac delta-function, which is not zero at the instant $t = T^-$. Impulsive torques $\Gamma_i^-(t) = I_i^- \delta(t - T^-)$ with $i = 2,\ 3,\ 4$ are provided at the same time-instant T^- by the human at the three other inter-link joints. At the same instant T^-, the impulsive ground reaction $\mathbf{r}_1^- = \mathbf{I}_{\mathbf{r}_1}^- \delta(t - T^-)$ is applied in the stance leg tip. Here $\mathbf{I}_{\mathbf{r}_1}^-(I_{\mathbf{r}_{1x}}^-, I_{\mathbf{r}_{1y}}^-)$ is the vector of the magnitudes of the impulsive ground reaction in the stance leg 1. Under the impulsive torques, the velocity vector $\dot{\mathbf{x}}$ of the biped changes instantaneously from the value $\dot{\mathbf{x}}^b$ to some value $\dot{\mathbf{x}}^-$ (unknown). The corresponding equations for the velocities jump can be obtained through the integration of the general equations of motion (1) for the infinitesimal time from T^- to T. The torques provided by the Coriolis and gravity forces have finite values. Thus, they do not influence the velocity jump:

$$\mathbf{A}[\mathbf{x}(T)](\dot{\mathbf{x}}^- - \dot{\mathbf{x}}^b) = \begin{bmatrix}\mathbf{D}_1 & \mathbf{D}_2 & \mathbf{D}_3 & \mathbf{D}_4\end{bmatrix} \begin{bmatrix} I_1^- \\ \mathbf{I}_{3\times1}^- \end{bmatrix} + \mathbf{J}_{\mathbf{r}_1}^{\top} \mathbf{I}_{\mathbf{r}_1}^- . \qquad (11)$$

Here $\mathbf{I}_{3\times1}^-(I_2^-,\ I_3^-,\ I_4^-)$ is the vector-column of the magnitudes of the three impulsive torques applied by human; $\mathbf{x}(T)$ is the configuration of human at the instant of impulsive actions. This configuration $\mathbf{x}(T)$ does not change at the double-support phase i.e. at the instants of the first, second, and third sub-phases.

The velocity of the stance (hind) leg foot remains zero after the first sub-phase. Therefore, the following matrix constraint equation is correct:

$$\mathbf{J}_{\mathbf{r}_1}\dot{\mathbf{x}}^- = \mathbf{0}_{2\times 1} \tag{12}$$

The velocity of the inter-link angle of the stance (hind) leg after first sub-phase remains zero, therefore

$$\mathbf{D}_1^{\top}\dot{\mathbf{x}}^- = 0. \tag{13}$$

Just after first sub-phase the tip of the leg 2 is not on the ground still and the velocity vector of this tip has to be directed downwards to the ground. We have to take into account this condition in our calculations.

- At the *second* sub-phase, mechanically the knee of the leg 1 is unlocked and the knee of the leg 2 is locked. This *second* sub-phase is assumed to be a passive impact, i.e. without torques applied by human in the inter-link joints. We assume this passive impact as absolutely inelastic. The time-instant of this passive impact is $t = T$. Given these conditions, the ground reaction at the instant of an impact and the locking torque provided by the exoskeleton can be considered as impulsive forces and defined by the delta-functions $\mathbf{r}_2 = \mathbf{I}_{\mathbf{r}_2}\delta(t-T)$ and $\Gamma_4(t) = I_4\delta(t-T)$. Here $\mathbf{I}_{\mathbf{r}_2}(I_{\mathbf{r}_{2x}}, I_{\mathbf{r}_{2y}})$ is the vector of the magnitudes of the impulsive ground reaction in leg 2, see [19] and I_4 is the magnitude of the impulsive locking torque in the knee of leg 2 of the exoskeleton. The corresponding equations for the velocities jump can be obtained through the integration of the matrix equation (1) for the infinitesimal time

$$\mathbf{A}\left(\dot{\mathbf{x}}^+ - \dot{\mathbf{x}}^-\right) = \left[\mathbf{D}_1\ \mathbf{D}_2\ \mathbf{D}_3\ \mathbf{D}_4\right]\begin{bmatrix}\mathbf{0}_{3\times 1}\\ I_4\end{bmatrix} + \mathbf{J}_{r_2}^{\top}\mathbf{I}_{\mathbf{r}_2} \tag{14}$$

Here $\dot{\mathbf{x}}^+$ is the velocity vector (unknown) just after an inelastic passive impact. The swing leg 2 after the impact becomes a stance leg. Therefore, its tip velocity becomes zero after the impact,

$$\mathbf{J}_{\mathbf{r}_2}\dot{\mathbf{x}}^+ = \mathbf{0}_{2\times 1} \tag{15}$$

To take into account the locking of the knee of the leg 2, we have to complete equations (14) and (15) with equation:

$$\mathbf{D}_4^{\top}\dot{\mathbf{x}}^+ = 0. \tag{16}$$

The velocity of the stance leg tip 1 before an impact is equal to zero. After the instantaneous passive impact the ground reaction in leg 1 has to be zero and the velocity vector of the leg 1 tip has to be directed upwards - from the ground. We have to take into account this condition in our calculations.

- The swing leg 1 takes off the ground at the *second* sub-phase, which is the passive impact. Then, the next ballistic single-support motion on leg 2 starts. However, before the next ballistic swing motion (just after the take off of the leg 1), in the *third* sub-phase at time-instant $t = T^+$, impulsive torques $\Gamma_i^+(t) = I_i^+\delta(t - T^+)$ are applied by human in the ith ($i = 1, 2$ and 3) inter-link joints to change the velocity vector of the biped instantaneously from the velocity vector just after passive impact $\dot{\mathbf{x}}^+$ to the known velocity vector $\dot{\mathbf{x}}^a$. The locking of the leg 2 knee is kept through the impulsive torque $\Gamma_4^+(t) = I_4^+\delta(t - T^+)$ developed by the brake device mounted in this knee of the exoskeleton. Integrating the differential equations (1) for the infinitesimal time from T to T^+ we come to the following matrix relation:

$$\mathbf{A}\left(\dot{\mathbf{x}}^a - \dot{\mathbf{x}}^+\right) = \begin{bmatrix}\mathbf{D}_1 & \mathbf{D}_2 & \mathbf{D}_3 & \mathbf{D}_4\end{bmatrix}\begin{bmatrix}\mathbf{I}^+_{3\times 1}\\ I_4^+\end{bmatrix} + \mathbf{J}_{\mathbf{r}_2}^{\top}\mathbf{I}_{\mathbf{r}_2}^+ \tag{17}$$

Here $\mathbf{I}^+_{3\times 1} = (I_1^+, I_2^+, I_3^+)^{\top}$.

System (11)–(17) is composed of 27 scalar equations to find 29 unknown variables, which are the components of the vectors and scalars: $\dot{\mathbf{x}}^-(7 \times 1)$, I_1^-, $\mathbf{I}^-_{3\times 1}(I_2^-, I_3^-, I_4^-)^{\top}$, $\mathbf{I}^-_{\mathbf{r}_1}(2 \times 1)$ (for the *first* sub-phase), $\dot{\mathbf{x}}^+(7 \times 1)$, I_4, $\mathbf{I}_{\mathbf{r}_2}(2 \times 1)$ (for the *second* sub-phase), $\mathbf{I}^+_{3\times 1}(I_1^+, I_2^+, I_3^+)^{\top}$, I_4^+ and $\mathbf{I}^+_{\mathbf{r}_2}(2 \times 1)$ (for the *third* sub-phase). Then the problem of impulsive control has an infinite number of solutions. But if the number of equations is less than the number of unknown variables, it is possible to extract a unique solution minimizing some cost functional. The components of the above-mentioned vectors are the subjects of the minimization. Among this set of components, $29 - 27 = 2$ can be defined as parameters to minimize a cost functional.

All equations (11)–(17) to calculate the impulsive torques at the instantaneous double-support phase are correct also for the biped (human) alone—with no exoskeleton. But in this case all torques $\mathbf{\Gamma}_i$ ($i = 1, 2, 3, 4$) are developed by the biped (human). For the biped alone at the first sub-phase, four impulsive torques are applied in all inter-link joints, at the second sub-phase there is no control torques absolutely, and at the third sub-phase again four impulsive torques are applied.

4 Energy Cost of Impulsive Control

The choice of a criterion is difficult and subjective. Furthermore it is not sure if some criterion is optimized during a human walking. Nevertheless for the numerical tests, we consider a criterion, proposed in [29]. This criterion is based on the mechanical energy provided by human. It assumes that the actuated joints are not regenerative (energy cannot be restored in the joints).

In the case of the impulsive torques, the criterion can be expressed as:

$$W = \sum_{i=2}^{4} \int_{T-}^{T} \left| \Gamma_i^-(t)\dot{\theta}_i(t) \right| \mathrm{d}t + \sum_{i=1}^{3} \int_{T}^{T+} \left| \Gamma_i^+(t)\dot{\theta}_i(t) \right| \mathrm{d}t \tag{18}$$

We took into account in expression (18) the torques developed by the human only.

The calculation of the integrals in expression (18) leads to the following formulas, see [19]:

$$W = \sum_{i=2}^{4} W_i^- + \sum_{i=1}^{3} W_i^+ \tag{19}$$

Values W_i^- $(i = 2,\ 3,\ 4)$ are calculated as follows:

$$W_i^- = \left| I_i^- \frac{\dot{\theta}_i^b + \dot{\theta}_i^-}{2} \right| \quad \text{if } \dot{\theta}_i^b \dot{\theta}_i^- \geq 0 \;\; i = 2, 3, \text{ and } 4,$$

$$W_i^- = \left| I_i^- \frac{(\dot{\theta}_i^b)^2 + (\dot{\theta}_i^-)^2}{2\left[\dot{\theta}_i^- - \dot{\theta}_i^b\right]} \right| \quad \text{if } \dot{\theta}_i^b \dot{\theta}_i^- < 0 \;\; i = 2, 3, \text{ and } 4,$$

Values $\dot{\theta}_i^b$ $(i = 2,\ 3,\ 4)$ are the inter-link angular velocities just before the first sub-phase. Values $\dot{\theta}_i^-$ $(i = 2,\ 3,\ 4)$ are the inter-link angular velocities just after the first sub-phase (before the second sub-phase). These velocities are calculated using expressions (3):

$$\begin{aligned} &\dot{\theta}_2^b = \dot{q}_5^b - \dot{q}_2^b, \quad \dot{\theta}_3^b = \dot{q}_5^b - \dot{q}_3^b, \quad \dot{\theta}_4^b = \dot{q}_3^b - \dot{q}_4^b, \\ &\dot{\theta}_2^- = \dot{q}_5^- - \dot{q}_2^-, \quad \dot{\theta}_3^- = \dot{q}_5^- - \dot{q}_3^-, \quad \dot{\theta}_4^- = \dot{q}_3^- - \dot{q}_4^- \end{aligned} \tag{20}$$

Values W_i^+ $(i = 1,\ 2,\ 3)$ are calculated using analogous formulas:

$$W_i^+ = \left| I_i^+ \frac{\dot{\theta}_i^+ + \dot{\theta}_i^a}{2} \right| \quad \text{if } \dot{\theta}_i^+ \dot{\theta}_i^a \geq 0 \;\; i = 1, 2, \text{ and } 3,$$

$$W_i^+ = \left| I_i^+ \frac{(\dot{\theta}_i^+)^2 + (\dot{\theta}_i^a)^2}{2\left[\dot{\theta}_i^a - \dot{\theta}_i^+\right]} \right| \quad \text{if } \dot{\theta}_i^+ \dot{\theta}_i^a < 0 \;\; i = 1, 2, \text{ and } 3.$$

Values $\dot{\theta}_i^+$ $(i = 1,\ 2,\ 3)$ are the inter-link angular velocities just after the second sub-phase. Values $\dot{\theta}_i^a$ $(i = 1,\ 2,\ 3)$ are inter-link angular velocities just after the third sub-phase (at the beginning of the next swing phase). These velocities are calculated using expressions (3):

$$\dot\theta_1^+ = \dot q_2^+ - \dot q_1^+, \quad \dot\theta_2^+ = \dot q_5^+ - \dot q_2^+, \quad \dot\theta_3^+ = \dot q_5^+ - \dot q_3^+,$$
$$\dot\theta_1^a = \dot q_2^a - \dot q_1^a, \quad \dot\theta_2^a = \dot q_5^a - \dot q_2^a, \quad \dot\theta_3^a = \dot q_5^a - \dot q_3^a \tag{21}$$

In simulation, with given time period T and length L of the step, we choose a unique solution of the system (11)–(17) by minimizing the quantity (18) or (19). We take into account the following constraints: $I^-_{r_{1y}} \geq 0$, $I_{r_{2y}} \geq 0$, and $I^+_{r_{2y}} \geq 0$. Furthermore, we ensure that the vector of the linear velocity of the swing leg (leg 2) tip just after the first sub-phase is directed to the ground (downwards). Just after the passive impact the vector of the linear velocity of the leg 1 tip has to be directed from the ground (upwards). Then for the biped with exoskeleton the angular velocities in the knees can not be negative: $\dot\theta_4^- \geq 0$ and $\dot\theta_1^+ \geq 0$. For the biped alone we have to take into account four inequalities: $\dot\theta_1^- \geq 0$, $\dot\theta_4^- \geq 0$, $\dot\theta_1^+ \geq 0$, and $\dot\theta_4^+ \geq 0$. Therefore, our minimization problem is the problem of parametric minimization with constraints. We used the *SQP* method (Sequential Quadratic Programming); see [30, 31] with the *fmincon* function of Matlab ® to solve this problem numerically. This algorithm based on the gradient of the objective with respect to the optimization variables allows to take into account linear and non-linear constraints.

We consider the minimal quantity (18) or (19) corresponding to this solution as the energy cost functional for the biped walking with the given data L and T for several actuation modes of assistance. We will details these modes of assistance in the next section.

5 Simulation Results

The consumption of energy is studied as a function of the velocity of the biped with the exoskeleton and of the biped with no exoskeleton to transport the payload with mass $m_c = 40$ kg. For time T varies from 0.4 s to 0.525 s while the length L is fixed at 0.50 m, see Fig. 4. Then L varies from 0.4 m to 0.525 m while the time T is fixed at 0.45 s, see Fig. 5. When the values of T decrease (with fixed step length L) the biped with the exoskeleton becomes more efficient for the consumption of energy than the biped alone. The same property is observed when the length step L increases (with fixed step time T). It means that the exoskeleton is useful with high velocities of walking.

We see from Figs. 4 and 5 the following property. When the values of T decrease (with fixed step length L) the biped with the exoskeleton becomes more efficient for the consumption of energy than the biped alone. The same property is observed when the length step L increases (with fixed step time T). It means that the exoskeleton is useful with high velocities of walking.

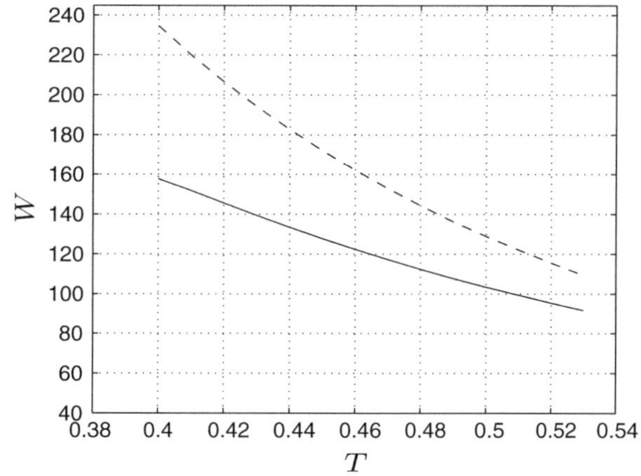

Fig. 4 Energy cost as a function of T for human with the exoskeleton (*solid line*), and for human alone (*dashed line*). The step length is 0.5 m

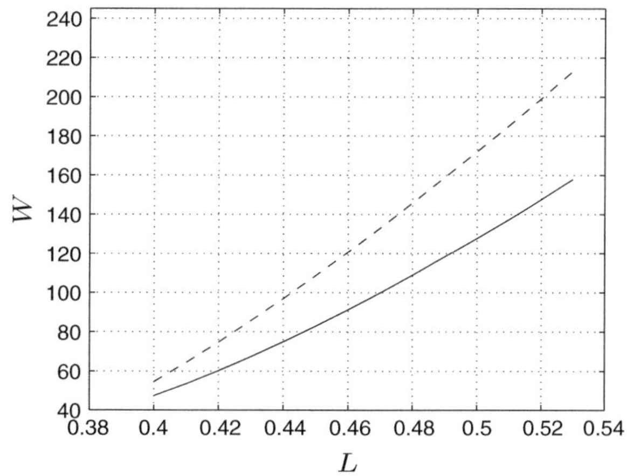

Fig. 5 Energy cost as a function of L for human with the exoskeleton (*solid line*), and for human alone (*dashed line*). The step time is 0.45 s

6 Conclusion

The planar five-link anthropomorphic bipedal mechanism is considered as a mechanical model of a human walking. An exoskeleton to assist human is also considered as a five-link bipedal mechanism (massive) with the same shape and degrees of freedom as mechanical model of a human alone. The links of the exoskeleton are strongly strapped to the corresponding links of the biped. We study passive exoskeleton without any sources of energy and actuators; the knee of the stance leg of our exoskeleton (and as consequence of the human) is locked using mechanical brake device, but the knee of the swing leg is unlocked.

It is shown theoretically the efficiency of mentioned above passive exoskeleton for human carrying a load. The human equipped with the exoskeleton spends less energy than human alone. The study is done in the framework of the ballistic walking problem. Mathematically this problem is reduced to the solving the boundary value problem for the motion equations of the single support and to design the impulsive torques for the instantaneous double support.

Many theoretical problems are still open. Most of the problems are associated with an active exoskeleton equipped with sources of energy and actuators.

Acknowledgments This work is supported by Ministry of Education and Science of Russian Federation, Project No. 7.524.11.4012, and by Région des Pays de la Loire, Project *LMA* and Gérontopôle Autonomie Longévité des Pays de la Loire.

References

1. Dollar, A., Herr, H.: Lower extremity exoskeletons and active orthoses: challenges and state-of-the-art. IEEE Trans. Robot. **24**(1), 144–158 (2008)
2. Zaroodny, S.J.: Bumpusher: A powered aid to locomotion, U.S. Army Ballistic res. Lab., Aberdeen Proving Ground, MD, Technical Note 1524 (1963)
3. Vukobratovic, M., Hristic, D., Stojiljkovic, Z.: Development of active anthropomorphic exoskeletons. Med. Biol. Eng. **12**(1), 66–80 (1974)
4. Main, J.: Exoskeletons for human performance augmentation. In: DARPA Project, 3701 North Fairfax Drive, Arlington (2005)
5. Zoss, A., Kazerooni, H., Chu, H.: On the mechanical design of the berkeley lower extremity exoskeleton (*bleex*). In: Proceedings of IEEE/RSJ International Conference on Intelligent Robots and Systems, pp. 3465–3472. Alberta, Canada (2005)
6. Kazerooni, H., Steger, R.: The berkeley lower extremity exoskeleton. Trans. ASME J. Dyn. Syst. Meas. Control **128**(1), 14–25 (2006)
7. Marcheschi, S., Salsedo, F., Fontana, M., Bergamasco, M.: Body extended: whole body exoskeleton for human power augmentation. In: Proceedings of IEEE International Conference on Robotics and Auomation, pp. 611–616. Shanghai, China (2011)
8. Farris, R.J., Quintero, H.A., Murray, S.A., Ha, K.H., Hartigan, C., Goldfarb, M.: A preliminary assessment of legged mobility provided by a lower limb exoskeleton for persons with paraplegia. IEEE Trans. Neural Syst. Rehabil. Eng. **22**(3), 482–490 (2014)
9. Strausser, K.A., Kazerooni, H.: The development and testing of a human machine interface for a mobile medical exoskeleton. In: IEEE, International Conference on Intelligent Robots and Systems, pp. 4911–4916. San Francisco, USA (2011)
10. Yan, T., Cempini, M., Oddo, C.M., Vitiello, N.: Review of assistive strategies in powered lower-limb orthoses and exoskeletons. Robot. Auton. Syst. **64**, 120–136 (2015). doi:10.1016/j.robot.2014.09.032
11. van den Bogert, A.J.: Exotendons for assistance of human locomotion. Biomed. Eng. Online 2–17 (2003)
12. Walsh, C.J., Pasch, K., Herr, H.: An autonomous, under actuated exoskeleton for load-carrying augmentation. In Proceedings of IEEE/RSJ International Conference on Intelligent Robots and Systems, pp. 1410–1415. Beijing, China (2006)
13. Agrawal, S.K., Banala, S.K., Fattah, A., Scholz, J.P., Krishnamoorthy, V., Hsu, W.L.: A gravity balancing passive exoskeleton for the human leg. In: Robotics: Science and Systems (2006)
14. Agrawal, S.K., Banala, S.K., Fattah, A., Sangwan, V., Krishnamoorthy, V., Scholz, J.P., Hsu, W.L.: Assessment of motion of a swing leg and gait rehabilitation with a gravity balancing exoskeleton. IEEE Trans. Neural Syst. Rehabil. Eng. **15**(3), 410–420 (2007)
15. Dariush, B.: Analysis and simulation of an exoskeleton controller that accommodates static and reactive loads. In: Proceedings of IEEE Conference on Robotics and Automation, pp. 2350–2355. Barcelona, Spain (2005)

16. van Dijk, W., van der Kooij, H., Heckman, E.: A passive exoskeleton with artificial tendons. In: IEEE International Conference on Rehabilitation Robotics, Rehab Week Zurich, ETH Zurich Science City, Switzerland, June 29–July 1, 2011
17. Aoustin, Y.: Walking gait of a biped with a wearable walking assist device. Int. J. Humanoid Robot. **12**(2), 1 550 018–1-11 550 018–20 (2015). doi:10.1142/S0219843615500188
18. Formal'skii, A.M.: Motion of anthropomorphic biped under implusive control. In: Proceedings of Institute of Mechanics, Moscow State Lomonosov University: Some Questions of Robot's Mechanics and Biomechnics, (In Russian), pp. 17–34 (1978)
19. Formalskii, A.M.: Locomotion of Anthropomorphic Mechanisms. [In Russian], Nauka, Moscow, Russia (1982)
20. Formal'skii, A.M.: Ballistic walking design via impulsive control. ASCE, J. Aerosp. Eng. **23**(2), 129–138 (2010)
21. Mochon, S., McMahon, T.: Ballistic walking: an improved model. Math. Bio-sciences **52**, 241–260 (1981)
22. McGeer, T.: Passive dynamic walking. Int. J. Robot. Res. **9**(2), 62–82 (1990)
23. Aoustin, Y., Formalskii, A.M.: 3d walking biped: optimal swing of the arms. Multibody Syst. Dyn. **32**(2013), 55–66 (2013). doi:10.1007/s11044-013-9378-3
24. Wisse, M.: Essentials of dynamic walking, Analysis and design of two legged robots. Ph.D. Thesis (2004). ISBN: 90-77595-82-1
25. Collins, S., Ruina, S., Tedrake, R., Wisse, M.: Efficient bipedal robots based on passive-dynamic walkers. Sci. Mag. **19**, 1082–1085 (2005)
26. Appell, P.: Dynamique des Systèmes - Mécanique Analytique. P. Gauthiers-Villars, Paris (1931)
27. Hurmuzlu, Y., Chang, T.H.: Rigid body collisions of a special class of planar kinematic chains. IEEE Trans. Syst. Man Cybern. **22**(5), 964–971 (1992)
28. Formal'skii, A., Chevallereau, C., Perrin, B.: On ballistic walking locomotion of a quadruped. Int. J. Robot. Res. **19**(8), 743–761 (2000)
29. Beletskii, V.V.: Biped walking. [In Russian], Nauka, Moscow, Russia (1984)
30. Gill, P., Murray, W., Wright, M.: Practical Optimization. Academic Press, London (1981)
31. Powell, M.: Variable Metric Methods for Constrained Optimization. Lecture Notes in Mathematics. Springer, Berlin (1977)

Development of a Robotic Driven Handheld Laparoscopic Instrument for Non-invasive Intraoperative Detection of Small Endoluminal Digestive Tumors

B. Mocan, V.V. Bintintan, S. Brad, C. Ciuce, M. Mocan and M. Murar

Abstract The present paper introduces the development of a sensing laparoscopic instrument based on a framework design for guiding decision-makers towards a superior balance between quality, efficiency and surgical procedure issues in medical instruments development. A prototype of the robotic handheld sensitive laparoscopic instrument for non-invasive intraoperative detection of small endoluminal digestive tumors was designed and developed for validation the instrument. The developed prototype was evaluated by two surgeons in ex vivo experimental conditions by different medical approaches—open and laparoscopic surgery. The surgeons found that the developed prototype is easy to use, satisfactory and useful in precise detection of small endoluminal digestive tumors in 85 % of cases.

Keywords Sensing laparoscopic instrument · Robotic driven handheld laparoscopic instrument · Non-invasive intraoperative detection of small endoluminal digestive tumors · And precise detection of small endoluminal digestive tumors

B. Mocan (✉) · S. Brad · M. Murar
Technical University of Cluj-Napoca, Cluj-Napoca, Romania
e-mail: bogdan.mocan@muri.utcluj.ro

S. Brad
e-mail: stelian.brad@staff.utcluj.ro

M. Murar
e-mail: mircea.murar@muri.utcluj.ro

V.V. Bintintan · C. Ciuce · M. Mocan
University of Medicine and Pharmacy Cluj-Napoca, Cluj-Napoca, Romania
e-mail: vbintintan@gmail.com

C. Ciuce
e-mail: constantinciuce@gmail.com

M. Mocan
e-mail: mihaela.mocan@gmail.com

P. Wenger et al. (eds.), *New Trends in Medical and Service Robots*,
Mechanisms and Machine Science 39, DOI 10.1007/978-3-319-30674-2_15

1 Introduction

1.1 Background and Motivation

Minimally invasive surgery (MIS) is one of the medical procedures that makes small incisions and performs a surgery using the laparoscopic instruments that are inserted through small-diameter trocars placed at the incisions [3, 9, 11]. With the advancement of endoscopic techniques and improvement of patients' addressability to endoscopic evaluations the number of patients with small tumors of the stomach, small intestine, colon and rectum that require surgery has increased significantly in the last years [8, 14, 15, 17].

The MIS has several advantages compared to traditional open surgery, e.g. reduced patient trauma, a fast recovery time, lower health care costs, etc. In addition to the above advantages, the robot manipulator can remove tremor of surgeon's hand and can follow a precise path on a certain angle of the laparoscopic instrument. Industrial robots are still being used today as research and validation tools where immediate clinical use is not contemplated or specialized kinematic design is not essential [9, 15]. Such systems are robust, available, and often have open interfaces suitable for experimentation [12].

In this paper, we introduce a framework design for guiding decision-makers towards a superior balance between quality, cost and surgical procedure issues in medical instruments development and validation of the mechatronic development a laparoscopic sensing instrument for precise localization of the digestive tumors during laparoscopic surgery. Based on the proposed framework we developed a prototype for laparoscopic sensing instrument, that was validated through ex vivo experiments, and which can be used by both the surgeons and by surgeons assisted by a robotic system that handle the instrument, while trying to address the main issues in laparoscopic surgery of small endoluminal digestive tumors such as a precise localisation of the tumors.

1.2 Current Practices and Limitations

When a gastric or colorectal tumor is small in size and doesn't invade the serosa, it is difficult to be identified when approached from the peritoneal surface [8]. Palpation is most of the time helpful, but can be misleading when the tumor is very small or does not have a hard consistency, such as villous adenomas [7].

Laparoscopic surgery has expanded miraculously in the last decades and has become the preferred approach for resection of these small tumors [3]. But laparoscopic identification of a small tumor is even more difficult than in open surgery because the haptic feed-back offered by the laparoscopic instruments cannot match palpation [2].

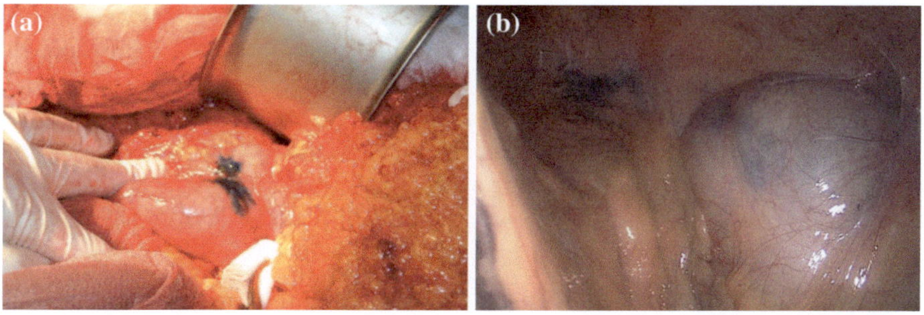

Fig. 1 Methylene-blue dye of a tumor of the ascending colon (Dr. V. Bintintan, 1st Clinic of Surgery, Cluj-Napoca). **a** Methylene-blue dye of a tumor of the ascending colon. **b** Methylene-blue dye has been injected and spilled in the properitoneal space

The location of endoluminal tumors is nowadays marked endoscopically, either before the operation, by endoscopic injection of a dye (Fig. 1a), or intra-operatory a concomitant endoscopic and surgical approach. Preoperative endoscopic injection of a dye, performed in the morning of the day of surgery (for methylene blue) or days before surgery (for India ink or Patent Blue) has the advantage that the endoscopist is not required at the time of surgery, which can be sometimes late in the afternoon, and that the endoscopy is performed in a standardized setting (Endoscopy Department) [21].

However, there are certain disadvantages of this method [9]: (a) a solution is injected in the wall of the colon/rectum using needles that simply cannot be sterile (they are contaminated with the contents of the colon), (b) the dye colours also the neighbouring tissues and the lumen of the colon and modifies chromatically the operative field, a characteristic that can be very distressing for the surgeon and (c) the methylene blue dye vanishes away after a period of 2÷4 h. Also, it was observed, that the patients who used this technique reported the presence of abdominal pain and abdominal guarding signs which suggested a deep injection of the dye directly in the peritoneal cavity or properitoneal space (Fig. 1b). The dye method is not reliable in defining precisely the edges of the tumor and where the line of resection should be.

Other method for identification of endolumenal small tumors of the digestive tract is concomitant endoscopy during surgery [18]. This approach requires the appropriate logistics in the operator-theatre and presence of the endoscopist at the time of the operation. There a few departments in Romania which can afford this set-up and therefore the technique is used quite rarely. Furthermore, insufflation of gas into the lumen of the stomach or colon leads to distention of the bowel which can reduce significantly the working space during laparoscopy [11, 19].

For middle rectal tumors it is often difficult to evaluate by palpation from the pelvis if the abdominal dissection has reached down to the required 2 cm distal to the margin of the tumor [16]. In such instances, a precise tool of identification of the tumor margin is of utmost importance and can improve the radically of resection.

Concomitant endoscopic evaluation can provide accurate measurement from the inferior margin of the tumor to guide adequate resection at least 1–2 cm from the tumor margin but it requires additional set-up of the operator-theatre and specialized personnel, and is therefore seldom used [10]. Unfortunately, due to the limits described in the previous paragraphs and depicted in the Fig. 1b, was not possible when a dye was used for tumor localization [6].

2 Methodology

2.1 *Design Framework for Sensing Laparoscopic Instruments*

Design and development of medical instruments combine engineering principle and techniques with biomedical technology to minimize the unsolved gap between engineering and surgery and apply technical design methodology and engineering problem solving skills to improve medical diagnosis, medical treatment, and surgical operations. The multi-disciplinary team effort from surgeons and engineers, is required to develop efficient and useful medical instruments.

The proposed framework integrates two components, Fig. 2. One of them serves for designing the medical instrument, and the second serves for multi-criteria evaluation of the generated solution. The main objectives of this approach is to direct the creative design process and finally to increase the efficiency and the addressability of the laparoscopic small digestive tumors position identification

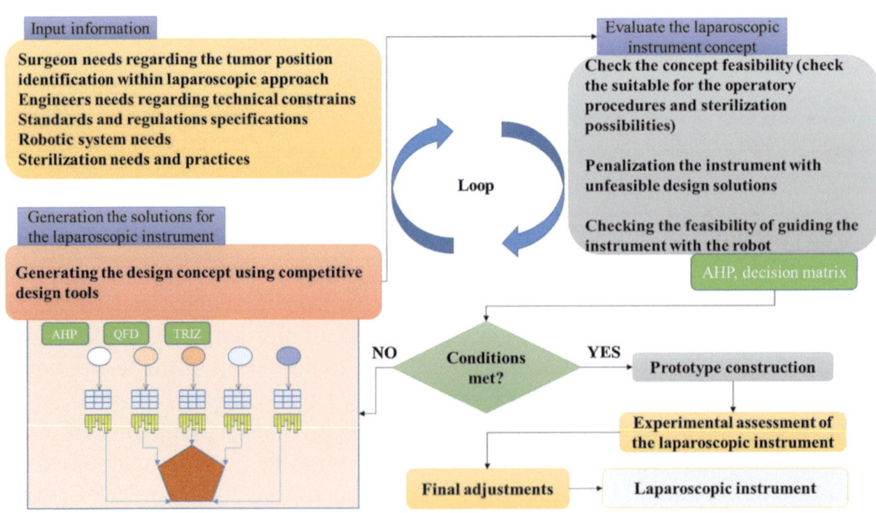

Fig. 2 Graphical representation of the proposed framework

method by developing an instrument for non-invasive intraoperative detection of small endoluminal digestive tumors.

For this during the generation phase a solution is generated by using competitive design algorithms and methods (e.g. AHP [*Analytic hierarchy process*], QFD [*Quality function deployment*], TRIZ [*Theory of Inventive Problem Solving*]) starting from a set of surgeon/medical procedure needs [4, 5]. The steps that have to be followed for generating the design solutions are:

Step 1 Define the specific objectives for laparoscopic instrument functionalities.

Step 2 Define the technical characteristics and target-functions of the laparoscopic instrument (e.g. quality-related).

Step 3 Define a set of specific key requirements and a set of key metrics (value characteristics) for each target-function. For each target-function, locally rank the specific requirements using expert judgements and ranking tools (e.g. AHP). For each target-function, determine the local value weights of the related key metrics by deploying the related specific requirements using a House of Quality frameworks (QFD). For each metric, define adequate targets.

Step 4 For each target-function, transfer all the data from step 2 into a framework for systematic design in order to elaborate local solutions at "mechanism" level. Where conflicting problems occur, call TRIZ (for customer related functions). TRIZ presents a systematic approach for understanding and defining challenging problems: difficult problems require an inventive solution, and TRIZ provides a range of strategies and tools for finding these inventive solutions.

Step 5 Aggregate local solutions into an overall solution. This is a very challenging process as conflicts between the target-functions might occur. In principle, the overall solution should comprise strengths of the local solutions.

Step 6 Highlight the final mechanisms (subsystems) which belong to the overall solution. For each target-function, deploy the key metrics into the final mechanisms. Aggregate local value weights by weighting them with the value weights of the target functions from step 3. Thus, the overall value weights of the final mechanisms of the instrument are determined.

Safety is obviously very important in developing medical instruments and robotic driven medical instruments and must be addressed at all phases of design, manufacture, and application [20, 21, 22]. Having this in mind within the proposed framework we consider several safety basic principles: redundancy in safety-critical systems; avoiding unnecessary speed or power in actuators; rigorous design analysis, documentation, and testing protocols; multiple checkpoint/restart facilities and factored designs allowing not-critical components to be disabled [14].

Also, the proposed framework gives a special importance to the aspects regarding laparoscopic instrument sterilization and/or any part of the robot that could come into contact with the patient or which may contaminate the surgical field. All this stuff must be sterilized or covered with a sterile cover [15].

Finally, the proposed framework has the ability to guide the creative process so that the resulting solution, laparoscopic instrument, can be used manually by the surgeon or by a robot that assist the surgeon. So that, the robot itself is assisting the surgeon in carrying out a surgical procedure that facilitate the position identification of endoluminal digestive tumors.

2.2 Laparoscopic Instrument Design and Development

The proposed framework is applied to develop the laparoscopic instrument for non-invasive intraoperative detection of small endoluminal digestive tumors hereinafter referred to as sensing laparoscopic instrument. The focus within the application example in this section will be on the concurrent planning and design issues, not on detailing each step of the proposed framework.

The surgeons that will use the sensing laparoscopic instrument has formulated the following major surgery procedure-related requirements: (a) allow being sterilized by standard methods (10 %): MR_1; (b) addressing to laparoscopic and classic/open surgery procedures (25 %): MR_2; (c) allowing tumors' position identification extremely accurate (65 %): MR_3. The importance of each requirement, mentioned in brackets, has been formulated by the surgeon department.

Here, five competing target-functions are considered as top inputs in the planning process: high quality (TF_1), affordable costs (TF_2), high efficiency (TF_3), high precision in identification the position of the tumors (TF_4) and easy to handle by the surgeon and by the robot (TF_5). The results of the deployment process according to step 3 of the framework are revealed in Table 1.

Table 1 Planning target-functions

● strong relationship
⊙ medium relationship
O possible relationship
↑ maximization
↓ minimization
++ positive correlation
-- negative correlation

	TF_1					(shaded)
	TF_2				(shaded)	--
	TF_3			(shaded)	++	++
	TF_4		(shaded)	-	++	++
	TF_5	(shaded)	++	++	++	++
	Optimisation trend	↑	↑	↑	↓	↑
Requirements	Importance	TF_5	TF_4	TF_3	TF_2	TF_1
MR_1	10%		⊙		O	O
MR_2	25%	⊙	⊙	O	O	
MR_3	65%	●	●	●		●
	Value weight [%]	24.0	25.9	23.6	8.1	18.4

According to the framework, TRIZ could be applied to overpass the crisis point. The following major conflicts are highlighted: (a) cost minimization versus high quality (material, functions and performances); (b) increasing the efficiency versus increasing the precision of identification the position of the tumors (resolutions performances). In TRIZ-language, the problem is translated as [1]: (a) amount of substance versus convenience of use, accuracy of measurement, reliability and level of automation; (b) energy spent by moving object versus level of automation and accuracy of measurement.

The following key generic inventive principles result for the first case: change the density and the physical state; replace mechanical systems; make immovable parts movable; make use of waste material and energy; arrange objects in advance; use composite materials.

The following key generic inventive principles result for the second case: replace a mechanical means with a sensory (optical, acoustic, taste or smell) means; use electric, magnetic and electromagnetic fields to interact with the object; change from static to movable fields, from unstructured fields to those having structure; use fields in conjunction with field-activated (e.g. ferromagnetic) particles. These principles were further used for the definition of the final solution of the sensing laparoscopic instrument. For example principle "use electric, magnetic and electromagnetic fields to interact with the object" determined us to integrate an inductive proximity sensor within the instrument. The TRIZ innovative principle help designers to identify the possible directions of solving for the current problem based on their knowledge and synthesis capacity.

The final solution is presented in Fig. 3, highlighting all the component function-oriented modules, and the Fig. 4 presents the structural and control scheme for the sensing laparoscopic instrument.

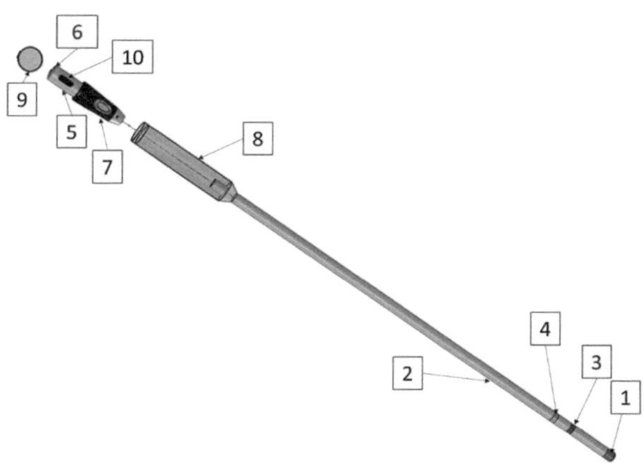

Fig. 3 The designed solution for the sensing laparoscopic instrument. *1* Sensing element, *2* long stalk (36 cm) for use in laparoscopic surgery, *3* visual signal for stand-by position, *4* visual signal when tumor found, *5* command and energy source module, *6* display, *7* ergonomic zone for instrument holding, *8* metallic cover for the command and energy source module, *9* cover, *10* speaker

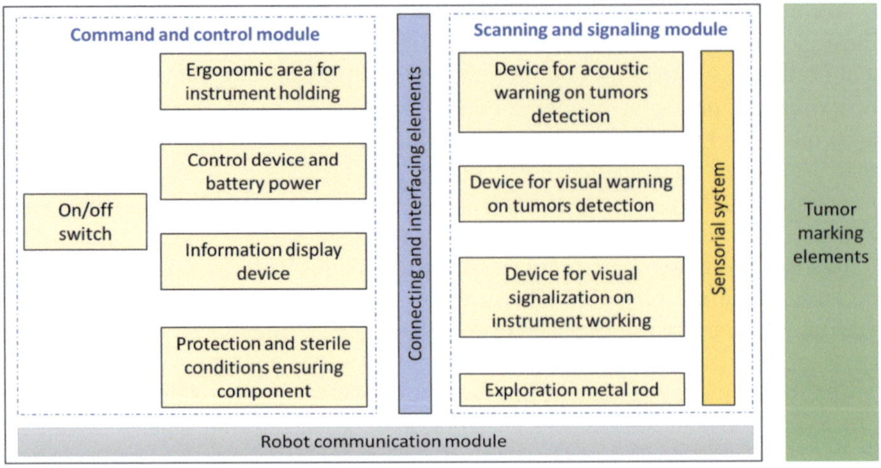

Fig. 4 Structural and control scheme for the sensing laparoscopic instrument

The sensing element that is integrated in laparoscopic instrument is materialized by an inductive proximity sensor. Inductive proximity sensors are used for non-contact detection of metallic objects. Their operating principle is based on a coil and oscillator that creates an electromagnetic field in the close surroundings of the sensing surface. The presence of a metallic object (actuator) in the operating area causes a dampening of the oscillation amplitude [13]. The rise or fall of such oscillation is identified by a threshold circuit that changes the output of the sensor. The operating distance of the sensor depends on the actuator's shape and size and is strictly linked to the nature of the material.

To be able to use the sensing laparoscopic instrument, it requires a preoperative colonoscopy. During this preoperative colonoscopy the upper and lower poles of the tumor on colon tract are market by using metal clips. The metal clips could retain their position in the colon for a period of up to 3 days until surgery is performed. The using method of the instrument exemplified in the Fig. 5 is that the sensing laparoscopic instrument scanning the colon or rectum area where we estimate that the tumor is based on measured distance from the edge of the anus made by the endoscopy specialist in preparatory phase; thus, we accurately identify the location of the upper and lower pole of the tumor already market with the metal clips by the endoscopy specialist.

There are two modalities of using the sensing laparoscopic instrument: one is that in which the instrument is handled by a surgeon (Fig. 6a) and the second way is when the sensing laparoscopic instrument is handled by a robotic system that assist a surgeon (Fig. 6b).

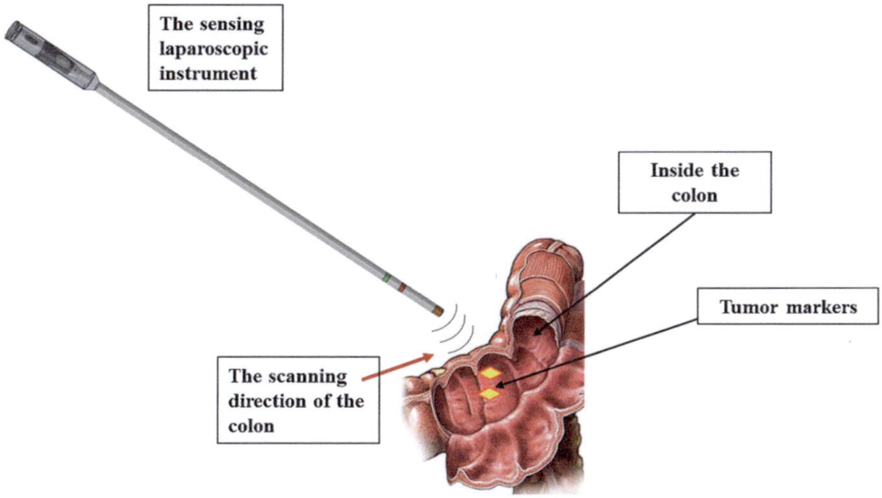

Fig. 5 Method of using the sensing laparoscopic instrument

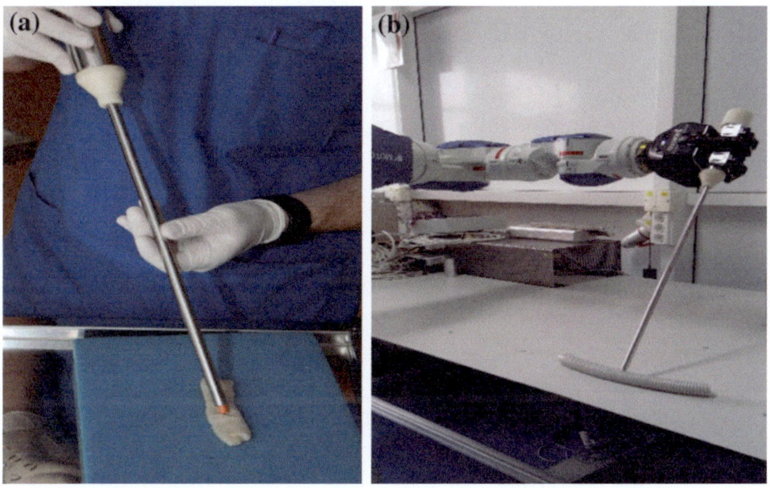

Fig. 6 Modalities of using the sensing laparoscopic instrument. **a** Handled by a surgeon. **b** Handled by a robotic system

The developed prototype of the sensing laparoscopic instrument, based on the designing framework proposed in this paper is highlighted in the Fig. 7. Some of its technical characteristics are: a proximity inductive sensor M8 (sensing distance max. 5 mm); acoustic signaling element; battery unit (2700 mA h; 5 V); electronic command unit; USB communication port, robot communication module.

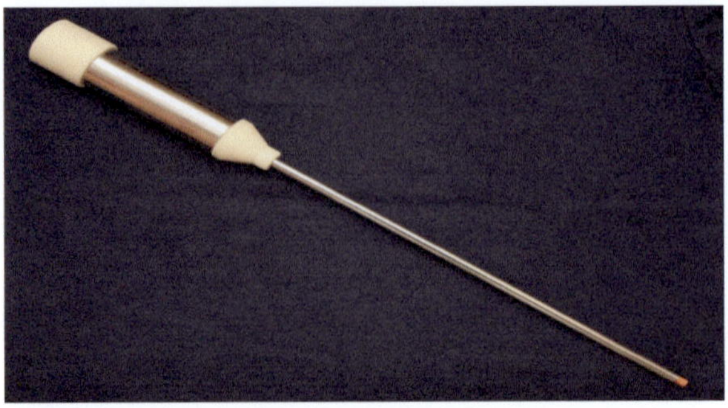

Fig. 7 Prototype of the sensing laparoscopic instrument

3 Experimental Assessment of the Laparoscopic Instrument

3.1 Experimental Setup and Conditions

The sensing laparoscopic instrument (Fig. 9), developed based on the proposed framework, was used to perform a bowel wall scanning for precisely identifying the location of a small tumor previously tagged by the marking elements (various metallic materials).

In all our experiments, the tumor marking elements were mounted inside a small bowel. The marking elements are metal rigid clips that can be applied with the Karl Stroz applier used in laparoscopic surgery. The place where we applied the marking clips was arbitrarily chosen. However, it is hypothetically feasible to place the marking clips to any arbitrary position because in real conditions we have the approximate position of the tumor from the endoscopy and the scanning area decrease. The rationale for extended scanning area in the experiment was to evaluate the efficiency of the sensing instrument, and to evaluate different motion and orientation artifacts that depends on the distance, the motion velocity and the material of the marking elements.

We investigated both static scanning on a fixed position and dynamic motion tracking scanning trajectories. The former was carried out by manual scanning a fixed position of the ex vivo bowel wall while the latter was evaluated based both on manual scanning by the surgeon (Fig. 6a) and also by scanning different trajectories executed by an industrial robot Yaskawa Motoman SDA10D Dual Arm capable to replicate the kinematic constraints associated with minimally invasive procedures, as illustrated in the Fig. 6b.

3.2 Ex Vivo Validation

Validation of the static position analysis was carried out on ex vivo pig small bowel. The medium length of bowel sector was ~20 cm, as illustrated in Fig. 8.

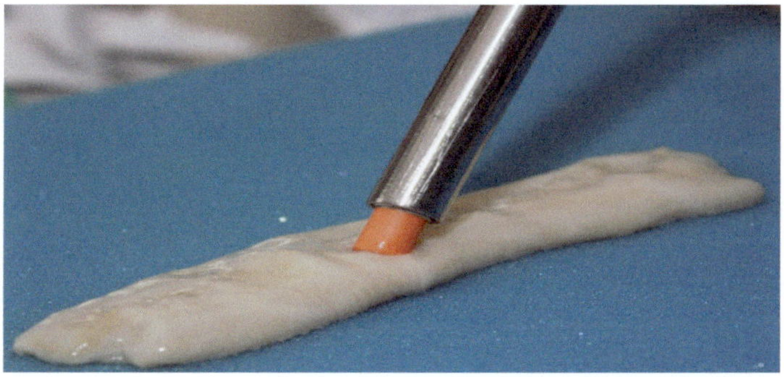

Fig. 8 Detection of the stainless steel clip Ø = 0.5 mm in the small bowel (ex vivo experiment)

Also, it is important to note that the scanning method was not limited to planar scene geometry, and the marking elements were placed sometimes on the upper and sometimes on lower plane of the bowel wall.

Validation of the dynamic motion tracking scanning trajectories was carried out on ex vivo pig small bowel. The medium length of bowel sector was ~20 cm, as illustrated in Fig. 8. First we set some trajectory that have been followed by the surgeon in an attempt to find the tumor marking elements, and allow the surgeon to have also some free hand trajectory. After that the surgeon followed the established trajectories by maintaining the sensing element tip at a certain distance from the bowel wall.

Using the Yaskawa Motoman SDA10D Dual Arm robotic system for handling the sensing laparoscopic instrument we were more confident in maintaining the sensing element tip at a certain distance and in a precise orientation towards the bowel wall.

For marking the tumors area within the pig bowel we have used different custom made clips from different metal material like in Fig. 9.

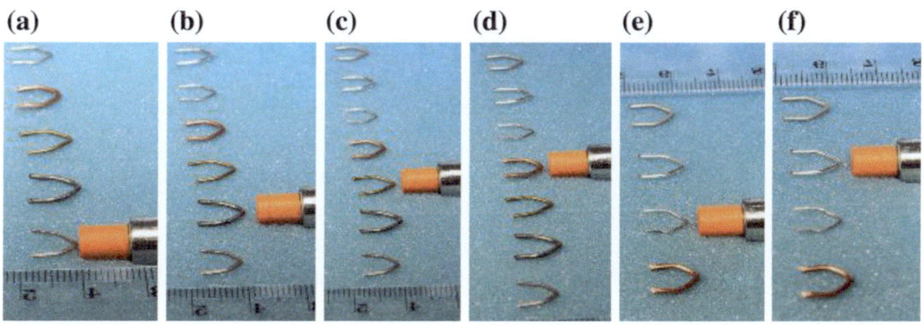

Fig. 9 Comparative detection of different custom made metal clips. **a** titanium, **b** steel Ø = 0.4, **c** cooper Ø = 0.3, **d** cooper Ø = 0.5, **e** stainless steel Ø = 0.2, **f** stainless steel Ø = 0.4

4 Results

4.1 Discussions

A novel method and a new instrument were developed to provide a more precise location identification of the small endoluminal digestive tumors within laparoscopic surgery. The sensing instrument was designed and developed for being used both by the surgeon and also by a robotic system that assist the surgeon in scanning an area of the bowel for identifying the tumor marking elements.

The challenge in conducted ex vivo experiments was to determine the sensing laparoscopic instrument efficiency in identifying tumor marking elements made from different metal materials. The results are shown in Table 2. Based on the presented result we conclude that the efficiency of the sensing laparoscopic instrument highly depend on the type of the material on which the tumor markers elements were made and less on the followed trajectories or on the maintained orientation of the tip of instrument.

We can also say that the freehand trajectory exhibited an error trend that was similar to that of the controlled trajectory when the sensing laparoscopic instrument was handled by the robotic system Yaskawa Motoman SDA10D.

4.2 Limitations and Future Improvements

While the experiments in this study demonstrated feasibility of the proposed design framework for sensing laparoscopic instrument, a more extensive analytical study factoring in the relevant laparoscopic surgery conditions will be conducted in future work for validation its appropriateness for in vivo experimental models.

Regarding the effectiveness of the instrument in identifying the tumor markers it depends on the type of markers material: for example standard endoscopic clips cannot be detected by the sensing laparoscopic instrument; standard titanium laparoscopic clips are detected at a disappointing rate (60 %); clips made of

Table 2 Detection of tumor metallic markers within the bowel

Marking elements material	Detection distance (mm)	Efficiency of detection percentage in bowel wall (%)
Olympus endoscopic clip	5	0
Titanium laparoscopic clip	1.15	60
Steel Ø = 0.4 mm	2.9	85
Cooper Ø = 0.3 mm	2.03	70
Cooper Ø = 0.5 mm	2.4	75
Stainless steel Ø = 0.2 mm	2.5	80
Stainless steel Ø = 0.4 mm	3.5	85

stainless steel are reliably detected with a high rate (85 %). Thus, the present method can be valuable for precise localisation of rectal tumors when custom made, stainless-steel clips are used for marking the margins of the tumor.

Regarding further development, the sensing elements need to be more tested with a robotic system and finally integrated within a medical robot system that could assure a better moving and orientation on a trajectory and finally a better scanning method while the surgeon makes other necessary surgical procedures.

5 Conclusion

A methodology for concurrent planning and design of new products in surgery field considering both multiple medical-functions and other performance functions is introduced in this paper. The effectiveness of the methodology arises from its potential to propose solutions that incorporate a superior balance between the set of considered target-functions. The developed sensing laparoscopic instrument is enough adaptable to be used in both open and laparoscopic surgery and also guided by a robotic system.

The proposed design framework highlights the importance of a structured approach that facilitate systematic introduction of innovation within medical instruments design and its mediating factors in determining efficiency, effectiveness and satisfaction for the final user (surgeons). It also highlights the importance of not considering device design in isolation from the medical procedure or medical regulations and the need to consider the range of stakeholders or users. By taking a systems approach and understanding the complexity of designing, development and utilization of medical instruments, quality, efficiency and satisfaction the surgical needs should be an achievable goal starting from design phase.

Acknowledgments Support within the project Research Grant No. 1495/5/28.01.2014 offered by the University of Medicine and Pharmacy Cluj-Napoca for the study of "Non-invasive intraoperative detection of small endoluminal digestive tumors and their margins using proximity sensors" is acknowledged with gratitude.

References

1. Altshuller, G.: The Innovation Algorithm: TRIZ. Technical Innovation Centre (2000)
2. Beccani, M., Di Natali, C., Sliker, L.J., Schoen, J.A., Rentschler, M.E., Valdastri, P.: Wireless tissue palpation for intraoperative detection of lumps in the soft tissue. IEEE Trans. Biomed. Eng. **61**(2), 353–361 (2014)
3. Bodner, J.C., Zitt, M., Ott, H., Wetscher, G.J., Wykypiel, H., Lucciarini, P., Schmid, T.: Robotic-assisted thoracoscopic surgery (RATS) for benign and malignant esophageal tumors. Ann. Thoracic Surg. **80**, 1202–1206 (2005)

4. Brad, S., Ciupan, C., Pop, L., Mocan, B., Fulea, M.: Manualul de Bază al Managerului de Produs în Ingineria şi Managementul Inovaţiei, Ed. Economică. ISBN: 973-709-265-1/978-973-709-265-6, Bucureşti (2006)
5. Brad, S., Mocan, B., Brad, E., Fulea, M.: Leading Innovation to Improve Complex Process Performances by Systematic Problem Analysis with TRIZ, TFC2014, Global Innovation Convention. EPFL, Lausanne, Procedia CIRP, Elsevier (2014)
6. Brad S., Fulea M., Brad E., Mocan B.: Smart deployment of demonstrators into successful commercial solutions. In: Proceedings of the 24th CIRP Design Conference, Milan, Italy, 14–16 Mar 2014, pp. 165–175 (2014)
7. Cheng, A., Chiu, P., Chan, P., Lam, S.: Endoscopic hemostasis for bleeding gastric strormal tumors by application of hemoclip. J. Laparoendosc. Adv. Surg. Tech. **14**(3), 71–169 (2004)
8. Fuller, J., Scott, W., Ashar, B., and Corrado, J.: Laparoscopic Trocar Injuries: A report from a U. S. Food and Drug Administration (FDA), Center for Devices and Radiological Health (CDRH), Systematic Technology Assessment of Medical Products (STAMP) Committee (2003)
9. Greene, F.L., Kercher, K.W., Nelson, H.: Minimal access cancer management. CA Cancer J. Clin. **57**, 130–146 (2007)
10. Gutt, C.N., Bintintan, V.V., Köninger, J., Müller-Stich, B.P., Reiter, M., Büchler, M.W.: Robotic-assisted transhiatal esophagectomy. Langenbeck's Arch. Surg. **391**(4), 428–434 (2006)
11. Gurusamy, K.S., Aggarwal, R., Palanivelu, L.: Virtual reality training for surgical trainees in laparoscopic surgery. Cochrane Database Syst. Rev. (2009)
12. Hongbin, L., Jichun, L., Xiaojing, S., Seneviratne, L.D., Althoefer, K.: Rolling indentation probe for tissue abnormality identification during minimally invasive surgery. IEEE Trans. Robot. **27**(3), 450–460 (2011)
13. Mocan, B., Fulea, M., Brad, S.: Framework for developing a multimodal programming interface used on industrial robots. Robotica Manage. **19**(2), 29–33 (2014)
14. Mocan, M., Vesa, S., Suciu, S., Blaga, S.N.: Systemic markers of oxidative stress in relation to metabolic syndrome components. Clujul Med. **86**(3) (2013)
15. Mountney, P., Stoyanov, D., Davison, A., Yang, G.Z., Larsen, R., Nielsen, M.: Simultaneous stereoscope localization and soft-tissue mapping for minimal invasive surgery medical image computing and computer-assisted intervention, pp. 347–54. Springer, Berlin/Heidelberg (2006)
16. Müller-Stich, B.P., Reiter, M.A., Wente, M.N., Bintintan, V.V., Köninger, J., Büchler, M.W., Gutt, C.N.: Robot-assisted versus conventional laparoscopic fundoplication: short-term outcome of a pilot randomized controlled trial. Surg. Endosc. **21**(10), 1800–1805 (2007)
17. Nickel, F., Bintintan, V.V., Gehrig, T., Kenngott, H.G., Fischer, L., Gutt, C.N., Müller-Stich, B.P.: Virtual reality does not meet expectations in a pilot study on multimodal laparoscopic surgery training. World J. Surg. **37**(5), 965–973 (2013)
18. Piatt, J., Starly, B., Faerber, E., Sun, W.: Application of computer-aided design methods in craniofacial reconstructive surgery using image-guidance system. J. Neurosurg. **104**, 64–70 (2006)
19. Ruurda, J.P., Draaisma, W.A., van Hillegersberg, R., Borel Rinkes, I.H., Gooszen, H.G., Janssen, L.W., Simmermacher, R.K., Broeders, I.A.: Robot-assisted endoscopic surgery: a four-year single-center experience. Dig. Surg. **22**:313–320 (2005)
20. Ryan, P., McCarthy, S., Kelly, J., Collins, J.K., Dunne, C., Grogan, L., Breathnach, O., Shanahan, F., Carey, P.D., Walsh, T.N., O'Sullivan, G.C.: Prevalence of bone marrow micrometastases in esophagogastric cancer patients with and without neoadjuvant chemora-diotherapy. J. Surg. Res. **117**, 121–126 (2004)
21. Starly, B., Fang, Z., Sun, W., Regli, W.: Three-dimensional reconstruction for medical-CAD modeling. J. Comput.-Aided Des. Appl. **2**(1–4), 431–438 (2005)
22. Schostek, S., Ho, C.-N., Kalanovic, D., Schurr, M.O.: Artificial tactile sensing in minimally invasive surgery—a new technical approach. Minim. Invasive Ther. Allied Technol. **15**(5), 296–304 (2006)

Modeling and Dynamic Identification of Medical Devices: Theory, Issues and Example

A. Jubien and M. Gautier

Abstract This paper deals with the dynamic identification of medical devices. The majority of medical devices are like serial robots. On robotic, the usual identification method is based on the Inverse Dynamic Identification Model and the Least Squares estimation (*IDIM-LS* method). This method was validated on industrial robots and several prototypes. However, the safety constraints applied on medical devices add some issues. Both typical examples are the use irreversible gearbox and the use of brakes during constant position level unlike conventional robot. This paper presents the theory of identification and how to apply it on medical devices. A simple example of modeling and experimental identification of medical device is presented.

Keywords Dynamic · Identification · Parameters · Medical · Medicine · Robot

1 Introduction

Accurate dynamic system models are needed to control and simulate their motions with precision and reliability. The medical devices are like serial robot with bodies, reducers, motors and drive chains. So the robotic identification methods can be used for medical devices.

The modeling and the identification of robots has been widely investigated in the last decades [1]. The usual identification process is based on the Inverse Dynamic Model and Least Squares estimation (*IDIM-LS* method). This method has been

A. Jubien (✉) · M. Gautier
IRCCyN (Institut de Recherche en Communication et Cybernétique de Nantes),
University of Nantes, Nantes, France
e-mail: anthony.jubien@univ-nantes.fr

M. Gautier
e-mail: maxime.gautier@irccyn.ec-nantes.fr

P. Wenger et al. (eds.), *New Trends in Medical and Service Robots*,
Mechanisms and Machine Science 39, DOI 10.1007/978-3-319-30674-2_16

performed on several prototypes and industrial robots with accurate results. The identified parameters are more accurate than those from CAD, furthermore the offset and frictions parameters are identified.

However, the medical devices add some issues over conventional and industrial robots, particularly medical safety constraints.

The safety constraints are for patients' protection in case of power failure. In addition of electromagnetic power-off brakes, each gearbox is quasi-irreversible or irreversible for redundant safety. Therefore, it is necessary to extend the *IDIM-LS* method to this issue.

The usual *IDIM-LS* method requires the measurement of motor currents/torques and the measurements of motor positions. It has several advantages:

- the inverse dynamic identification model is done automatically with software,
- no initial conditions on parameters and positions are necessary,
- the time computation is low (no simulation of direct dynamic model),
- the base parameters (only the identifiable parameters) are computed automatically.

However, the velocities and accelerations must be computed for inverse dynamic identification model. This requires a well-tuned filtering.

In this paper, we explain how to extend this identification method to medical devices with medical issues.

This paper is divided into 6 sections. Section 2 describes the robot modeling. Section 3 presents the usual method for dynamic identification of robots, the *IDIM-LS* method. Section 4 presents the extension of *IDIM-LS* method to medical devices. Section 5 is devoted to a very simple modeling example of medical device and his experimental identification. Section 6 is the conclusion.

2 Modeling

2.1 Modified Denavit and Hartenberg Notation

The kinematics of serial robots is defined using the Modified Denavit and Hartenberg (*MDH*) notation [2]. In this notation, the link j fixed frame is defined such that: the axis z_j is taken along joint j axis; the x_j axis is along the common normal between zj and z_{j+1}; α_j and d_j parameterize the angle and distance between z_{j-1} and z_j along x_{j-1}, respectively; θ_j and r_j parameterize the angle and distance between x_{j-1} and x_j along z_j, respectively.

2.2 Inverse Dynamic Model

The inverse dynamic model of a robot calculates the torques τ_{idm} as a function the joint positions, velocities and accelerations. It can be obtained from the Newton-Euler or the Lagrangian Eq. [2]. It is given by the following relation:

$$\begin{aligned} \boldsymbol{\tau}_{\mathrm{idm}} &= \mathbf{Ia}\ddot{\mathbf{q}} + \boldsymbol{\tau}_{\mathrm{L}} + \boldsymbol{\tau}_{\mathrm{f}} \\ \boldsymbol{\tau}_{\mathrm{L}} &= \mathbf{M}(\mathbf{q})\ddot{\mathbf{q}} + \mathbf{C}(\mathbf{q},\dot{\mathbf{q}})\dot{\mathbf{q}} + \mathbf{Q}(\mathbf{q}) \\ \boldsymbol{\tau}_{\mathrm{f}} &= \mathbf{Fv}\dot{\mathbf{q}} + \mathbf{Fc}\,\mathrm{sign}(\dot{\mathbf{q}}) \end{aligned} \tag{1}$$

where $\mathbf{q}$, $\dot{\mathbf{q}}$ and $\ddot{\mathbf{q}}$ are respectively the (nx1) vectors of joint positions, velocities and accelerations; $\mathbf{M}(\mathbf{q})$ is the (nxn) robot inertia matrix; $\mathbf{C}(\mathbf{q},\dot{\mathbf{q}})\dot{\mathbf{q}}$ is the (nx1) vector of centrifugal forces/torques; $\mathbf{Q}(\mathbf{q})$ is the (nx1) vector of gravity forces/torques; $\mathbf{Fv}$ is the diagonal matrix of viscous frictions and $\mathbf{Fc}$ is the diagonal matrix of Coulomb friction. n is the number of moving links. In practice, the joint positions, velocities and acceleration are equal to motor positions, velocities and accelerations expressed on joint side and the torques $\boldsymbol{\tau}$ are equal to motor torques expressed on joint side for rigid robots.

The choice of the modified Denavit and Hartenberg frames attached to each link allows a dynamic model that is linear in relation to a set of standard dynamic parameters $\boldsymbol{\chi}_{\mathrm{st}}$ [3]:

$$\begin{aligned} &\boldsymbol{\tau}_{\mathrm{idm}} = \mathbf{IDM}_{\mathrm{st}}(\mathbf{q},\dot{\mathbf{q}},\ddot{\mathbf{q}})\chi_{\mathrm{st}} \\ &\text{with } \boldsymbol{\chi}_{\mathrm{st}} = \begin{bmatrix} \boldsymbol{\chi}_{\mathrm{st1}}^{\mathrm{T}} & \boldsymbol{\chi}_{\mathrm{st2}}^{\mathrm{T}} & \cdots & \boldsymbol{\chi}_{\mathrm{stn}}^{\mathrm{T}} \end{bmatrix}^{\mathrm{T}} \end{aligned} \tag{2}$$

where $\mathbf{IDM}_{\mathrm{st}}(\mathbf{q},\dot{\mathbf{q}},\ddot{\mathbf{q}})$ is (nxNs) the Jacobian matrix of $\boldsymbol{\tau}_{\mathrm{idm}}$, with respect to the (Nsx1) vector $\boldsymbol{\chi}_{\mathrm{st}}$ of the standard parameters. $\boldsymbol{\chi}_{\mathrm{stj}}$ is composed of standard dynamic parameters of axis j:

$$\begin{aligned} \boldsymbol{\chi}_{\mathrm{stj}} = [\mathrm{XX_j} \quad & \mathrm{XY_j} \quad \mathrm{XZ_j} \quad \mathrm{YY_j} \quad \mathrm{YZ_j} \quad \mathrm{ZZ_j} \\ & \mathrm{MX_j} \quad \mathrm{MY_j} \quad \mathrm{MZ_j} \quad \mathrm{M_j} \quad \mathrm{Ia_j} \quad \mathrm{Fv_j} \quad \mathrm{Fc_j}]^{\mathrm{T}} \end{aligned} \tag{3}$$

where:

- XX_j, XY_j, XZ_j, YY_j, YZ_j, ZZ_j are the six components of the robot inertia matrix of link,
- MX_j, MY_j, MZ_j are the components of the first moments of link j,
- M_j is the mass of link j,
- Ia_j is a total inertia moment for rotor and gears of actuator of link j,
- Fv_j and Fc_j are the viscous and Coulomb friction parameters of joint j,
- Ns is the number of standard parameters.

3 Inverse Dynamic Identification Model with Least Squares Method

Because of perturbations due to noise measurement and modeling errors, the actual torque $\boldsymbol{\tau}$ differs from $\boldsymbol{\tau}_{\mathrm{idm}}$ by an error e, such that:

$$\boldsymbol{\tau} = \mathbf{IDM}(\mathbf{q}, \dot{\mathbf{q}}, \ddot{\mathbf{q}})\boldsymbol{\chi} + \mathbf{e} \tag{4}$$

The vector $\boldsymbol{\chi}$ is the least squares (LS) solution of an over determined system built from the sampling of (4), while the robot is tracking exciting trajectories [4]:

$$\mathbf{Y} = \mathbf{W}\boldsymbol{\chi} + \boldsymbol{\rho} \tag{5}$$

where: $\mathbf{Y}$ is the measurement vector, $\mathbf{W}$ the observation matrix, and $\boldsymbol{\rho}$ is the vector of errors. The vector $\boldsymbol{\chi}$ is composed of the b base parameters [3, 5]. Standard deviations $\hat{\sigma}_{\hat{\chi}_i}$, are estimated assuming that $\mathbf{W}$ is a deterministic matrix and $\boldsymbol{\rho}$, is a zero-mean additive independent Gaussian noise, with a covariance matrix [6]:

$$\mathbf{C}_{\rho\rho} = \mathrm{E}(\boldsymbol{\rho}\boldsymbol{\rho}^{\mathbf{T}}) = \sigma_{\mathrm{p}}^{2}\mathbf{I}_{\mathrm{r}} \tag{6}$$

where E is the expectation operator and $\mathbf{I}$r, the (rxr) identity matrix. An unbiased estimation of the standard deviation σ_{p} is the following:

$$\hat{\sigma}_{\rho}^{2} = \frac{\|\mathbf{Y} - \mathbf{W}\hat{\boldsymbol{\chi}}\|^{2}}{(\mathrm{r} - \mathrm{b})} \tag{7}$$

The covariance matrix of the estimation error is given by:

$$\mathbf{C}_{\chi\chi} = \hat{\sigma}_{\rho}^{2}\left(\mathbf{W}^{\mathrm{T}}\mathbf{W}\right)^{-1} \tag{8}$$

The relative standard deviation $\%\sigma_{\hat{\chi}_{\mathrm{ri}}}$ is given by:

$$\%\hat{\sigma}_{\hat{\chi}_{\mathrm{ri}}} = 100\frac{\hat{\sigma}_{\hat{\chi}_{\mathrm{i}}}}{|\hat{\chi}_{\mathrm{i}}|} \text{ for } |\hat{\chi}_{\mathrm{i}}| \neq 0 \tag{9}$$

where $\sigma_{\hat{\chi}i}^{2} = C_{\chi\chi}(i, i)$ is the ith diagonal coefficient of $\mathbf{C}_{\chi\chi}$. Calculating the LS solution of (5) from perturbed data in $\mathbf{W}$ and $\mathbf{Y}$ may lead to bias if $\mathbf{W}$ is correlated to error terms. Then, it is essential to filter data in $\mathbf{Y}$ and $\mathbf{W}$ before computing the LS solution. Velocities and accelerations are estimated by means of a band-pass filtering of the positions (Butterworth filter). To eliminate high frequency noises and torque ripples, a parallel decimation is performed on $\mathbf{Y}$ and on each column of $\mathbf{W}$ (Decimate filter). More details about data filtering can be found in [6, 7].

We recall the advantages of *IDIM-LS* method:

- no necessary initial conditions,
- the time computation is low,
- the base parameters are computed automatically.

However, the computation of velocities and accelerations requires a well-tuned filtering.

4 Issue of Medical Devices

In majority of rigid robotic case, the motor can be in operation in four quadrants [8, 9] (see Fig. 1):

- Quadrant 1 : $P_{Lj} > 0,\ \dot{q}_j > 0,\ \tau_{Lj} > 0$
- Quadrant 2 : $P_{Lj} < 0,\ \dot{q}_j < 0,\ \tau_{Lj} > 0$
- Quadrant 3 : $P_{Lj} > 0,\ \dot{q}_j < 0,\ \tau_{Lj} < 0$
- Quadrant 4 : $P_{Lj} < 0,\ \dot{q}_j > 0,\ \tau_{Lj} < 0$

where $P_{Lj} = \dot{q}_j \tau_{Lj}$ is the transmitted power of joint j (joint power).

In medical robotic case, the first issue is the using of quasi-irreversible or irreversible gearbox [10, 11] (see Fig. 2).

In this case, the transmission efficiency is not the same between quadrants 1 and 3 ('motor quadrants') and quadrants 2 and 4 ('generator quadrants'). The inverse dynamic model (1) become the following [10]:

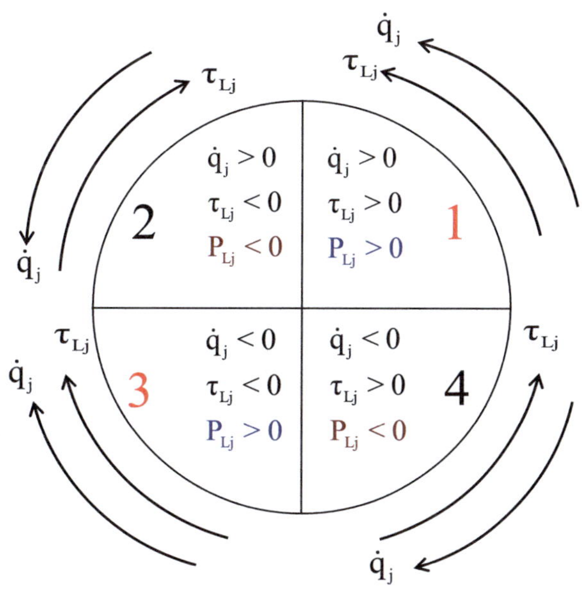

Fig. 1 Schematic of four quadrants

Fig. 2 An irreversible gearbox: parts and schematic

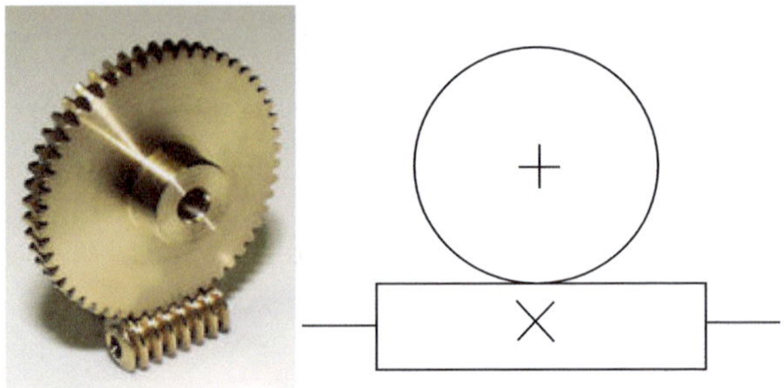

$$\boldsymbol{\tau}_{idm\_m} = \mathbf{Ia}\ddot{\mathbf{q}} + \mathbf{R}\boldsymbol{\tau}_L + \boldsymbol{\tau}_{fmp} + \boldsymbol{\tau}_{fmn}$$

$$\text{with} \begin{cases} R_{jj} = fp\left(\tau_{Lj}\dot{q}_j\right)R_{pj} + fn\left(\tau_{Lj}\dot{q}_j\right)R_{nj} \\ \tau_{fmp\,j} = fp\left(\dot{q}_j\right)\left(Fc_{p\,j} + Fv_{p\,j}\dot{q}_j\right) \\ \tau_{fmn\,j} = fn\left(\dot{q}_j\right)\left(Fc_{n\,j} + Fv_{n\,j}\dot{q}_j\right) \\ fp(u) = (1 + \mathrm{sign}(u))/2 \\ fn(u) = (1 - \mathrm{sign}(u))/2 \end{cases} \tag{10}$$

where R_{pj} and R_{nj} are the transmission efficiency coefficients in motor and generator quadrants of joint j respectively. The frictions terms are not the same for these two cases (X_{pj} for motor quadrants and X_{nj} for generator quadrants).

The second issue of medical devices is the use of electromagnetic power-off brakes during constant position level. All samples of Eq. (4) with $\dot{q}_j = 0$ must be deleted.

5 Modeling and Experimental Identification of Medical Device

5.1 Modeling

In this section, we propose to modeling a simple medical device: the Discovery IGS 730 of General Electric Healthcare (see Fig. 3).

It is C-arms architecture used for capture X-ray 3D image with mobile platform. Consequently, the patient can be immobile for interventional procedure. It is a very simple serial structure with one rotational joint. Its kinematics is defined using the MDH notation described in Sect. 2.2 (see Fig. 4). The geometric parameters defining the robot frames are given in Table 1.

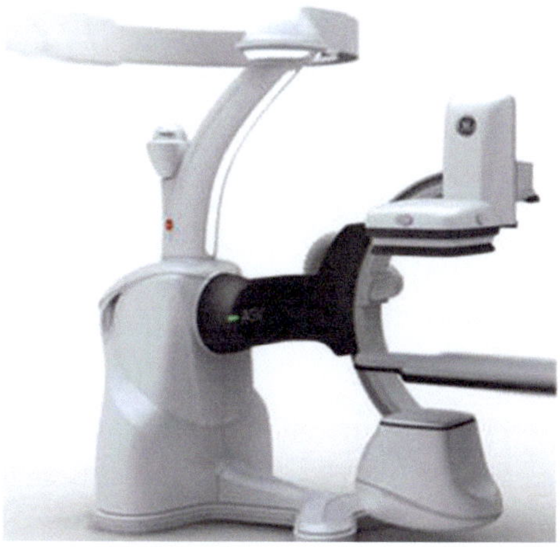

Fig. 3 The Discovery IFS 730 by General Electric Healthcare

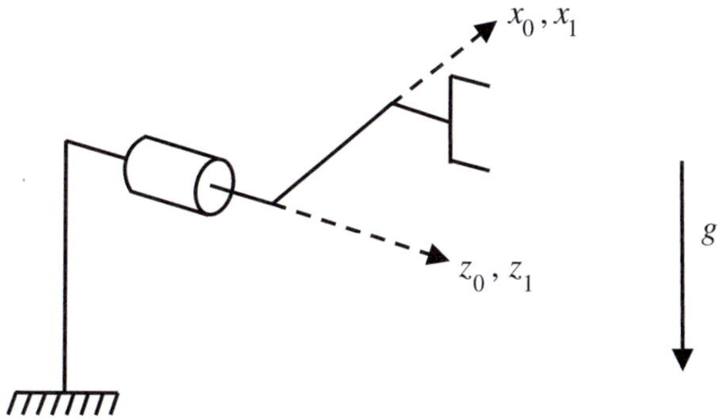

Fig. 4 Link frame of rigid model of the Discovery IFS 730 (g is the gravity vector)

Table 1 MDH parameters of rigid model of the Discovery IFS 730

j	μ_j	σ_j	α_j	d_j	θ_j	r_j
1	1	0	0	0	q_1	0

All mechanical variables are given in SI unit in joint side. The classic dynamic inverse model of rigid robot is the following:

$$\begin{aligned}\tau_{idm\_m1} = {} & (Ia_1 + ZZ_1)\ddot{q}_1 - MX_1 g\cos(q_1)\ldots \\ & + MY_1 g\sin(q_1) + Fv_1\dot{q}_1 + Fc_1\mathrm{sign}(\dot{q}_1)\end{aligned} \tag{11}$$

Due to the use of quasi-irreversible or irreversible gearbox, the inverse dynamic model (11) becomes the following from (10):

$$\begin{aligned} \tau_{idm\_m1} = & fp(\dot{q}_1)\left(Fc_{p1} + Fv_{p1}\dot{q}_1\right) + fn(\dot{q}_1)(Fc_{n1} + Fv_{n1}\dot{q}_1) + Ia_1\ddot{q}_1 \ldots \\ & + fp(\tau_{L1}\dot{q}_1)R_{p1}(ZZ_1\ddot{q}_1 + MY_1 g\sin(q_1) - MX_1 g\cos(q_1)) \ldots \\ & + fn(\tau_{L1}\dot{q}_1)R_{n1}(ZZ_1\ddot{q}_1 + MY_1 g\sin(q_1) - MX_1 g\cos(q_1)) \end{aligned} \quad (12)$$

Consequently, the inverse dynamic identification model is written as follow:

$$\boldsymbol{\tau} = \mathbf{IDM}(\mathbf{q}, \dot{\mathbf{q}}, \ddot{\mathbf{q}})\boldsymbol{\chi} + \mathbf{e}$$

with

$$\begin{cases} \boldsymbol{\tau} = \tau_{m1} \\ \mathbf{IDM} = \left[\ddot{q}_1 \quad fp(\tau_{L1}\dot{q}_1)\,\ddot{q}_1 \quad fn(\tau_{L1}\dot{q}_1)\,\ddot{q}_1 \quad -fp(\tau_{L1}\dot{q}_1)g\cos(q_1) \quad \ldots \right. \\ -fn(\tau_{L1}\dot{q}_1)g\cos(q_1) \quad fp(\tau_{L1}\dot{q}_1)g\sin(q_1) \quad fn(\tau_{L1}\dot{q}_1)g\sin(q_1) \quad \ldots \\ \left. fp(\dot{q}_1)\dot{q}_1 \quad fn(\dot{q}_1) \quad fp(\dot{q}_1)\dot{q}_1 \quad fn(\dot{q}_1)\right] \\ \boldsymbol{\chi} = [\,Ia_1 \quad ZZ_1R_{p1} \quad ZZ_1R_{n1} \quad MX_1R_{p1} \quad MX_1R_{n1} \quad \ldots \\ MY_1R_{p1} \quad MY_1R_{n1} \quad Fv_{p1} \quad Fv_{n1} \quad Fc_{p1} \quad Fc_{n1}\,]^T \end{cases} \quad (13)$$

5.2 *Experimental Identification*

The sign of power depends of joint torque and can be approximated with a priori parameters (X^{ap}):

$$\begin{aligned} \mathrm{sign}(\tau_{L1}\dot{q}_1) &= \mathrm{sign}((ZZ_1\,\ddot{q}_1 + MY_1 g\sin(q_1) - MX_1 g\cos(q_1))\dot{q}_1) \\ &\approx \mathrm{sign}\left((ZZ_1^{ap}\,\ddot{q}_1 + MY_1^{ap} g\sin(q_1) - MX_1^{ap} g\cos(q_1))\dot{q}_1\right) \end{aligned} \quad (14)$$

The inertia ZZ_1 is a positive value (physical constraint). Due to the use of C-arm architecture, the gravity terms MX_1 and MY_1 are close to zero:

$$\begin{aligned} ZZ_1^{ap} &> 0 \\ MX_1^{ap} &= 0 \\ MY_1^{ap} &= 0 \end{aligned} \quad (15)$$

So the sign of power can be approximated with this relation:

$$\mathrm{sign}(\tau_{L1}\dot{q}_1) \approx \mathrm{sign}(\ddot{q}_1\,\dot{q}_1) \quad (16)$$

The motor position is measured by the motor encoder. The motor torque τ_{m1} depends of motor current I_1 (measured by the controller):

Table 2 Identified parameters of rigid model

Par.	$\hat{\chi}$	$2\%\sigma_{\hat{\chi}_r}$
$g_{\tau 1}ZZ_1R_{p1}$	3.40	1.6
$g_{\tau 1}ZZ_1R_{n1}$	1.35	3.2
$g_{\tau 1}Fc_{p1}$	1.50	3.0
$g_{\tau 1}Fc_{n1}$	1.39	3.6

$$\tau_{m1} = g_{\tau 1} I_1 \tag{17}$$

where $g_{\tau 1}$ is the gain of joint drive chain of joint j. In practice, his value is not given by the manufacturer, so all parameters are identified with this term.

IDIM-LS method is performed with the inverse dynamic model (13). The cut-off frequency of the Butterworth filter and decimate filter are tuned at 30 (Hz) and 5 (Hz) respectively. The sample acquisition frequency is 1 (kHz). The exciting trajectories consist of short movement of C-arm at different velocities with several position levels. The identification results are given in Table 2.

The identified parameters have very low standard relative deviations so the identification is relevant. The relative error between measured torque and reconstructed torque is $\|\mathbf{W}\boldsymbol{\chi}\text{-}\mathbf{Y}\|/\|\mathbf{Y}\| = 9.4\ \%$. The gear efficiency is 2.5 times better quadrants 1 and 3 than quadrants 2 and 4.

6 Conclusion

In this paper, we expose the dynamic identification issues of medical devices. The usual identification method based on the Inverse Dynamic Identification Model and the Least Squares estimation can be used for dynamic identification of medical devices. However, some constraints must be taken into account: the use irreversible gearbox and the use of brakes during constant position level. The extension of *IDIM-LS* method with these constraints is presented and allows to simply apply this identification method to medical devices.

References

1. Hollerbach, J., Khalil, W., Gautier, M.: Model identification. In: Springer Handbook of Robotics. Springer (2008)
2. Khalil, W., Dombre, E.: Modeling, Identification and Control of Robots, 3rd edn. Taylor and Francis Group, New York (2002)
3. Gautier, M., Khalil, W.: Direct calculation of minimum set of inertial parameters of serial robots. IEEE Trans. Robot. Autom. 368–373 (1990)
4. Gautier, M., Khalil, W.: Exciting trajectories for the identification of base inertial parameters of robots. In: IEEE Conference on Decision and Control, pp. 494–499 (1995)

5. Mayeda, H., Yoshida, K., Osuka, K.: Base parameters of manipulator dynamic models. IEEE Trans. Robot. Autom. 312–321 (1990)
6. Gautier, M.: Dynamic identification of robots with power model. In: IEEE International Conference on Robotics and Automation, vol. 3, pp. 1922–1927 (1997)
7. Pham, M.T., Gautier, M., Poignet, P.: Identification of joint stiffness with bandpass filtering.In: IEEE International Conference on Robotics and Automation, vol. 3, pp. 2867–2872 (2001)
8. Jubien, A., Gautier, M.: Global identification of spring balancer, dynamic parameters and drive gains of heavy industrial robots. In: IEEE/RSH International Conference on Intelligent Robots and Systems (IROS), pp. 1355–1360 (2013)
9. Jubien, A., Gautier, M., Janot, A.: Dynamic identification of the Kuka LWR robot using motor torques and joint torque sensors data. In: World Congress of the International Federation of Automatic Control (IFAC), pp. 8391–8396 (2014)
10. Abba, G., Chaillet, N.: Robot dynamic modelling using a power flow approach with application to biped locomotion. Auton. Robots **6**, 39–52 (1999)
11. Al Assad, O.: Etude d'une méthodologie de modélisation et de commande d'un robot multiaxe pour une application en radiologie médicale. Université de Paris-Sud 11 (2009)

A Legged Robotic System for Remote Monitoring

F. Tedeschi and G. Carbone

Abstract The paper outlines the evolution of the robotics series named "Cassino Hexapod", highlighting main design issues and operational features. The Cassino Hexapod is an hybrid robot, equipped with legs and wheels, characterized by design solutions having low-cost and user-friendly features. Main task is aimed at monitoring and analysis of historical or archaeological sites.

Keywords Hexapod · Walking robot · Leg-wheel · Low-cost design

1 Introduction

In recent past, at LARM, various research activities have been carried out, aiming at developing Hexapod Walking Robots (HWR) [2, 11]. The key features of the design proposals have been focused on the use of architectures and mechanisms having low-cost and user friendly features [1, 4]. The research activities that have been carried out at LARM, led the development of the so-called "Cassino Hexapod" series.

The Cassino Hexapod is an hybrid HWR, that is equipped with legs and wheels, whose main task is monitoring and analysis of historical or archaeological sites [5]. The proposed robot can be easily operated, even by non-expert users, and it is able to move in a non-invasive way within archaeological or historical sites, performing operations such as inspection, detection or monitoring [13]. More generally, the robot is able to operate in environments not accessible or dangerous to human operators. This application of robotic systems is considered of great interest

F. Tedeschi · G. Carbone (✉)
LARM; DICEM, University of Cassino and Southern Latium, Cassino, Italy
e-mail: carbone@unicas.it

F. Tedeschi
e-mail: franco.tedeschi@unicas.it

P. Wenger et al. (eds.), *New Trends in Medical and Service Robots*,
Mechanisms and Machine Science 39, DOI 10.1007/978-3-319-30674-2_17

by Architects and operators working on cultural heritage goods, aiming to overcome the common problems in their investigations with the help of user-friendly devices.

2 The Attached Problem

At present time, survey and preservation of historical sites, have been attracting more and more attention from the media. Many sites such as Pompei, for example, seem to require significant efforts to ensure their proper conservation. There are many problems associated with the analysis, preservation and conservation of historical sites, such as described, for example in [9]. The modern survey processes consist of interconnected activities such as measurements, survey, control and comparison of the data collected, as shown in [7].

HWR, have particular features that make them suitable for the inspection and architectural survey. For example, they can overcome obstacles that are comparable with the size of their legs, they can have a low impact on the ground and they can have a high mobility in natural environments or uneven terrains [6]. This latter aspect is of fundamental importance when it is essential preserve the soil from damages [7]. There are many design solution for an HWR. For example, an hexapod robot can be based on biologically inspired legs or non-zoomorphic legs. Biologically inspired legs can be slower and more difficult to design and operate as compared with non-zoomorphic legs. As a compromise solution one can choose a design with legs and wheels at the same time. This type of walking machines may range from wheeled devices to true walking machines with a set of legs to overcome particularly difficult obstacles, or wheels to enhance the speed when moving on flat terrains. Hexapod robots are also able to easily maintain a static balance and they can move with various kinds of gaits in order to comply with different speeds or loads. Hexapod robots can be equipped with various sensors including 3D laser scanning systems [8]. This innovative technology allows to create models of large and complex objects with significant level of definition.

Service robotics has a strong potential to solve the many problems associated with cultural heritage monitoring and maintenance. A challenge can be the use of hexapod robots that perform complex tasks, aimed at the analysis in scenarios such as proposed in Fig. 1.

At first stage, design requirements and operation characteristics have been investigated. Since the variety of irregular terrain is very large, it is has been difficult to cover all the different cases of operation. In order to study this problem the real features have been simplified into standard geometric features. Figure 2 shows the geometric features and related parameters that have been considered in term of crests, ditches and vertical steps. In the Figure, W stand for the Width and H stand for Height of the obstacle. Typical values have been identified, by referring to previous experiences at Montecassino Abbey, as

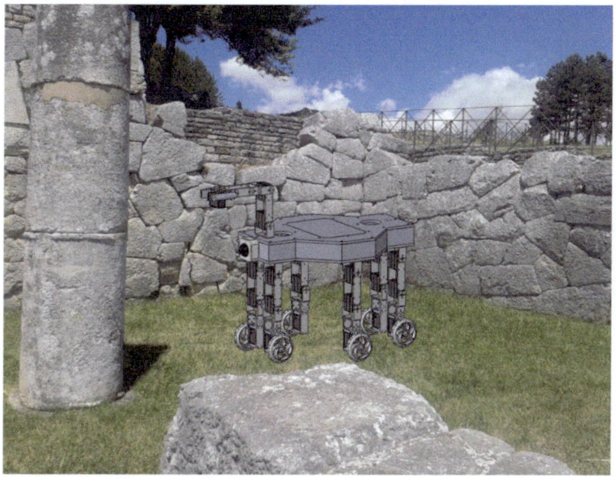

Fig. 1 3D simulation of a survey activity by hexapod walking robot

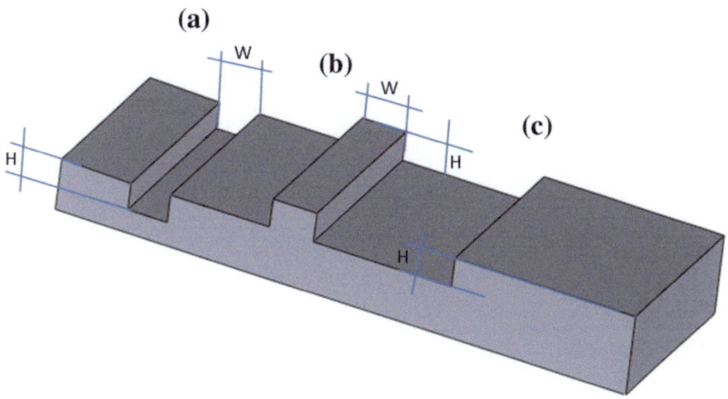

Fig. 2 Basic obstacle that have been considered with main sizes

- Ditch (Fig. 2a): W_{Max} = 60 mm; H_{Max} = 80 mm;
- Crest (Fig. 2b): $W_{Max=}$ 60 mm; H_{Max} = 50 mm;
- Vetical Step (Fig. 2c): H_{Max} = 50 mm;

3 Design Evolution of Cassino Hexapod

The first prototype of the series, shown in Fig. 3a, was developed in 2006 with the name of Cassino Hexapod I [2]. The control architecture was implemented by using an on board commercial PLC. An external DC power supply was used to provide

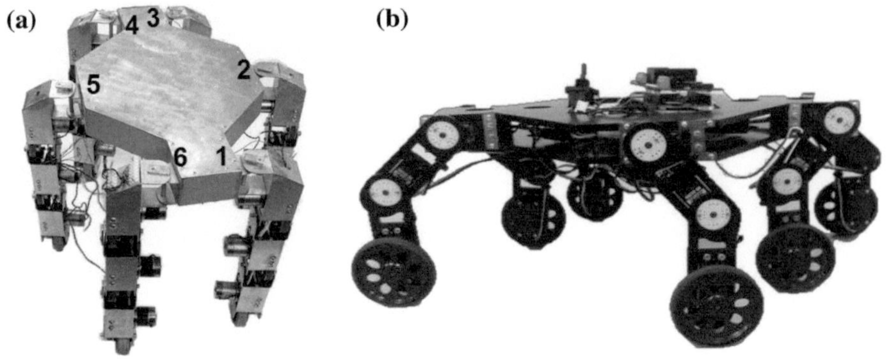

Fig. 3 Robotics series Cassino Hexapod. a Hexapod I. b Hexapod II

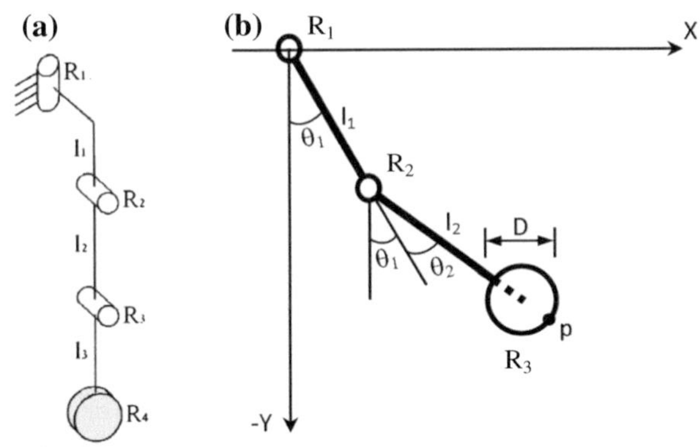

Fig. 4 Architecture of locomotion. a Kinematic scheme of Cassino Hexapod I. b Kinematic scheme of Cassino Hexapod II

power to the hexapod. The size of the external shape of the robot was 0.6 × 0.6 × 0.5 m. The overall weight of the robot was 21.6 kg. The main disadvantage of Cassino Hexapod I was represented by the high weight and the high power consumption, which prevented the use of any on board energy storage, making it necessary to use an umbilical cable for power supply. High weight and high power consumption in the first prototype, originate mainly from the high number of DC motors adopted in order to actuate the hexapod.

A new design was proposed in 2012 with the name of Cassino Hexapod II (Fig. 3b). Figure 4 report the kinematic scheme of Cassino Hexapod I and Cassino Hexapod II in order to much better explain the difference between the two prototypes. Basically the Cassino Hexapod II was inspired to the mechanical simplicity by using low cost architectures.

The Cassino Hexapod II has been built by using commercial thermoplastic alloy (Delrin), the kinematic architecture has been described in [12]. The maximum size of the robot was 0.36 × 0.27 × 0.2 m. The prototype was powered by 18 RC servomotors, 12 of which were used to give mobility to the legs, while the other six were used to drive the wheels. The control system was based on a commercial, low cost platform Arduino Mega 2560. A customized software has been developed to allow the operation of the whole hexapod. The remote control interface has been developed by means a Wi-Fi Arduino shield. The high-level control, implemented on PC, has been developed in a Java environment and allows the task planning through Wi-Fi network. A Li-Po battery, 7.4 V–2200 mAh provides power to the control board and the actuators [4].

A novel solution is currently under patenting [3] with the aim to improve the performance of Cassino Hexapod II in terms of walking speed, load capacity, stiffness, survey activity. This novel solution has been proposed with the name of Cassino Hexapod III as shown in Fig. 5. This prototype has been equipped with omni-wheels in order to improve the strategy for turning left and right. Each omni-wheel has a diameter of 60 mm and it is driven by an independent continuous rotation servo. A suitable control strategy of omni-wheels allows the robot steering. The legs operation has been carried out by means 12 digital servomotors with a output torque of 1.5 Nm. The new design can also include a robotic arm placed on the upper base of the body hexapod, to carry out measurements using laser scanners or grasping operations. Further details on the design process and operation of Cassino Hexapod III are reported in [12, 15, 16].

SolidWorks and MSC.ADAMS environments have been used for kinematic, static, dynamic analysis of the operation, in order to verify its performance in various operating modes. Details, can be found in [14, 15].

Table 1 summarizes the main features of the robotics series Cassino Hexapod in order to allows a numerical comparison between the three prototypes.

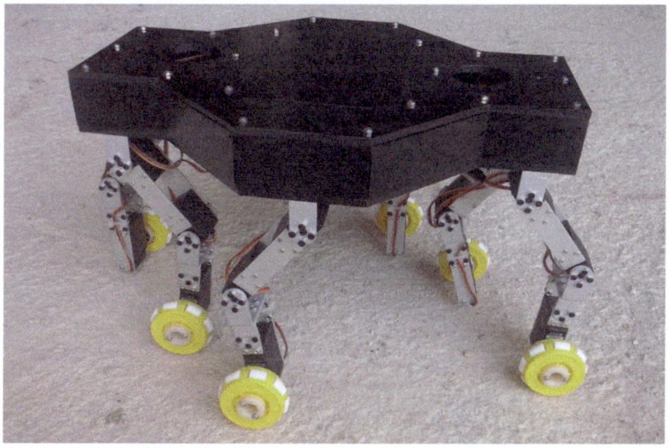

Fig. 5 A built prototype of Hexapod III

Table 1 Main features of Cassino Hexapod series

Main features	Hexapod I	Hexapod II	Hexapod III
Sizes (m)	0. 6 × 0.6 × 0.5	0.36 × 0.27 × 0.2	0 .4 × 0.3 × 0.3
Weight (kg)	21.6	3.9	3.1
Walking speed (m/s)	0.05	0.06	0.08
Wheeled speed (m/s)	0.1	0.15	0.17
Control architecture	PLC simatic S7-200	Mega 2560	Mega 2560
Power supply	12 V DC	7.4 V DC	7.4 V DC
Actuators	18 DC motor	18 Servo RC	18 Digital servo

4 Sensing Architecture of Cassino Hexapod III

Cassino Hexapod III can be remotely operate by PC or smartphone through Wi-Fi network, according to the scheme of Fig. 6.

A low-cost, commercial card Arduino Mega 2560 has been selected as suitable on board control, in order to manage the servomotors. A specific shield has been adopted as power interface. An Arduino Yun platform allows the communication link and wireless operation. The Cassino Hexapod III can be equipped with various kind of sensors, such as the wireless Inertial Measurements Unit LPMS-B [10], an high resolution camera, a vision system or 3D laser scanner.

Figure 7a shows a robotic arm for Cassino Hexapod III, equipped with a low-cost solution for 3D laser scanning [8] that can be attached on the main body of the robot. Figure 7b shows a set-up example for 3D shape acquisition; Fig. 7c shows a result of acquisition. In particular, Fig. 7c is a result of a laser scanning test aiming to produce a very large cloud of points for 3D image reconstruction.

5 Operation Strategy

Attention has been addressed to operation features in terms of basic operation strategies for survey operation such as walking and obstacle overpassing. Walking strategies in tripod gaits has been simulated in virtual environments.

Tripod gait, such as shown in Fig. 8, is a regular, periodic gait, where the front and back legs on one side lift at same time with the contralateral middle leg, forming alternating tripods. For each tripod, the legs are lifted, lowered, and moved forwards and backwards at same time.

Figure 9 show a tripod gait with main step frames of a simulated walking for the first tripod (0 ÷ T/2). Similarly Fig. 10, by referring to the second tripod (T/2 ÷ T). They also include plots of the joints angle values as function of time in the form of cyclogram, where L_1 and R_1 stand for first leg left and right, respectively. Similarly ϑ_1 and ϑ_2 stand for waist and knee joints respectively.

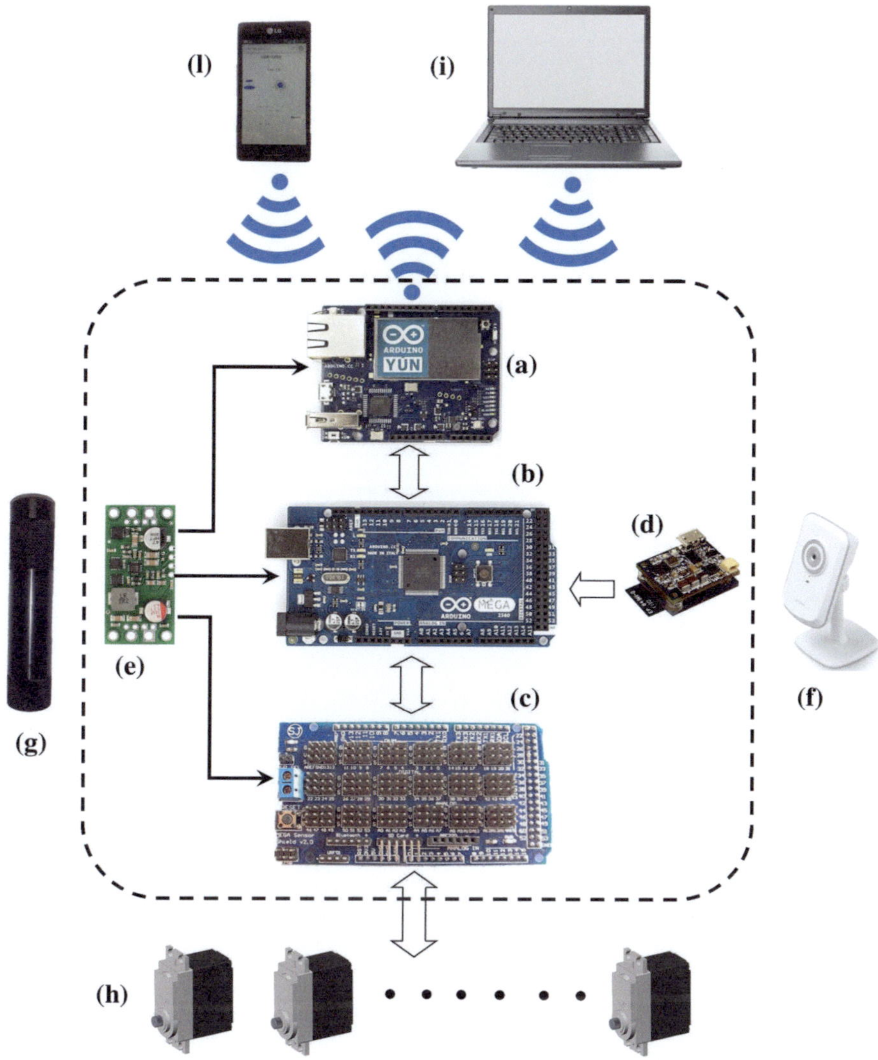

Fig. 6 Control and sensing architecture of Cassino Hexapod III: **a** Arduino Yun; **b** Arduino Mega 2560; **c** Power shield; **d** IMU sensor; **e** Power regulator; **f** Camera; **g** Laser scanner; **h** Servomotors; **i** PC; **j** Smartphone

The key characteristics emphasized in the new design of the robot have been oriented on the ability to move within the area to be analyzed, carrying the equipment for the acquisition of the data and to perform the operations of survey as also detailed in [3].

The actuated Mecanum-wheels, placed at the extremity of the legs allow the robot to move fast on flat surfaces. Additionally, Mecanum-wheels are

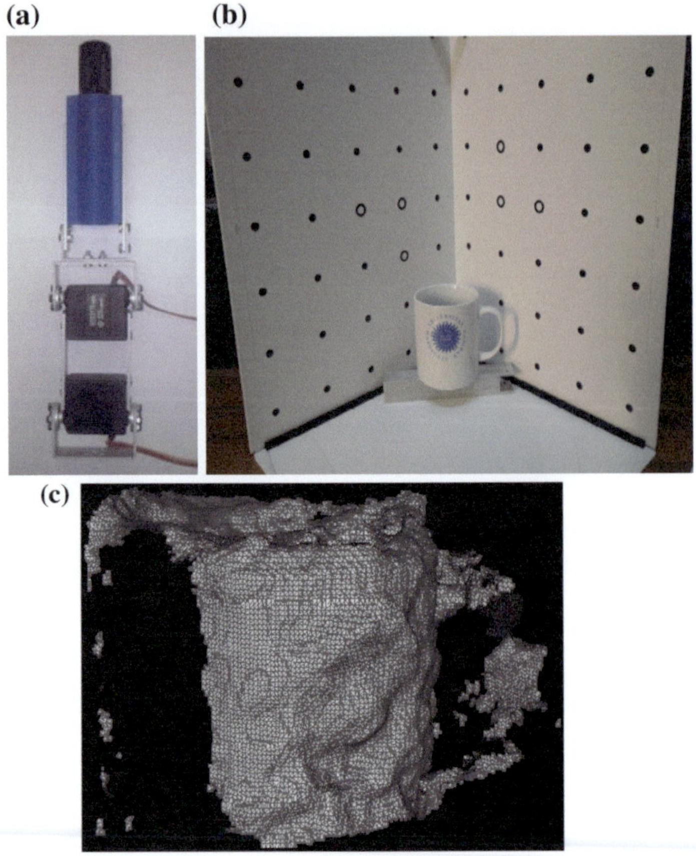

Fig. 7 Remote sensing sensor of Cassino Hexapod III. **a** Robotic arm equipped with 3D Laser scanner. **b** Example of set-up for 3D acquisition. **c** Results of acquisition process

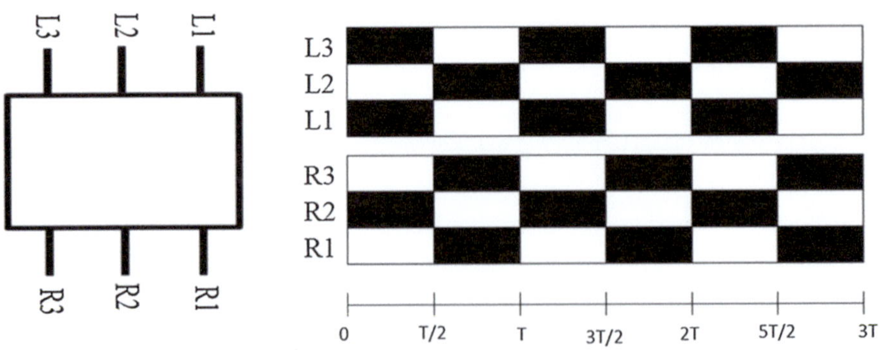

Fig. 8 Walking strategy of Cassino Hexapod III: tripod gait. *Black color* indicates that the foot is in ground contact and the *white color* otherwise, T(s) is the gait period

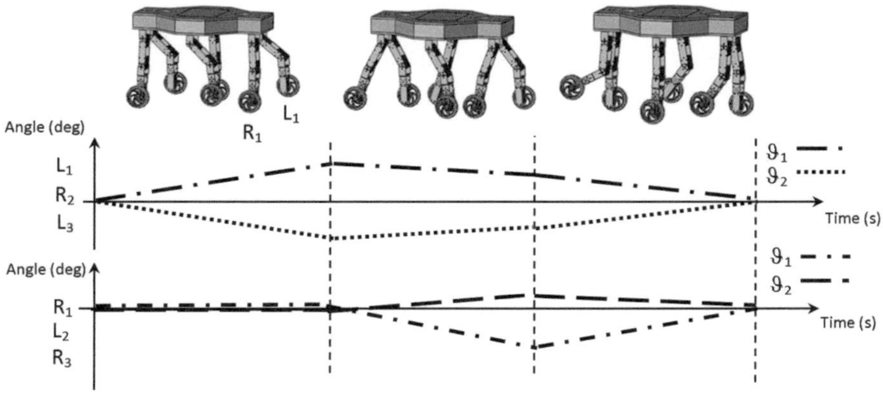

Fig. 9 Walking strategy of Cassino Hexapod III: first tripod

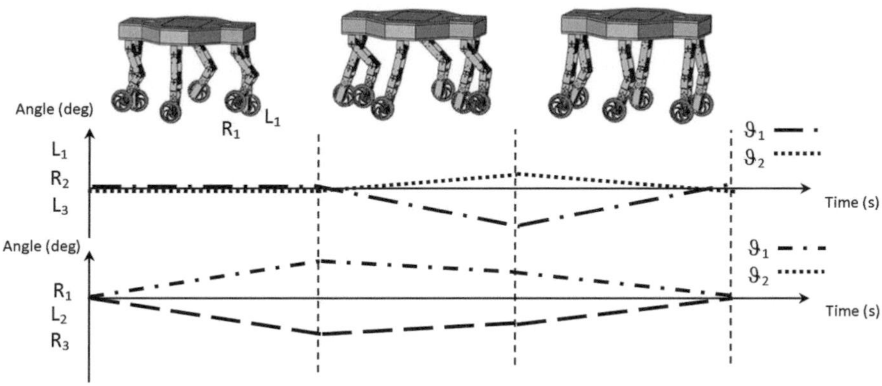

Fig. 10 Walking strategy of Cassino Hexapod III: second tripod

omni-directional wheels having 45° inclined rolling discs around their circumference. The effect is that the wheel can roll, but can also slide laterally. Accordingly, Mecanum-wheels allow the robotic platform to easily perform lateral changes of direction.

Figure 11 shows some frames that have been taken during an experimental crest overcoming test. In particular, Fig. 11a shows the robot that approaches the obstacle; Fig. 11b shows the robot that raises the front leg aside to match the height of the obstacle and then it goes forward by using the wheels; Fig. 11c shows the robot that lean the front leg on the ground; Fig. 11d shows the robot that lean the front legs on the ground and then it overcomes the obstacle. Additional details on the design and operation of Cassino Hexapod III are given in [15, 16]..

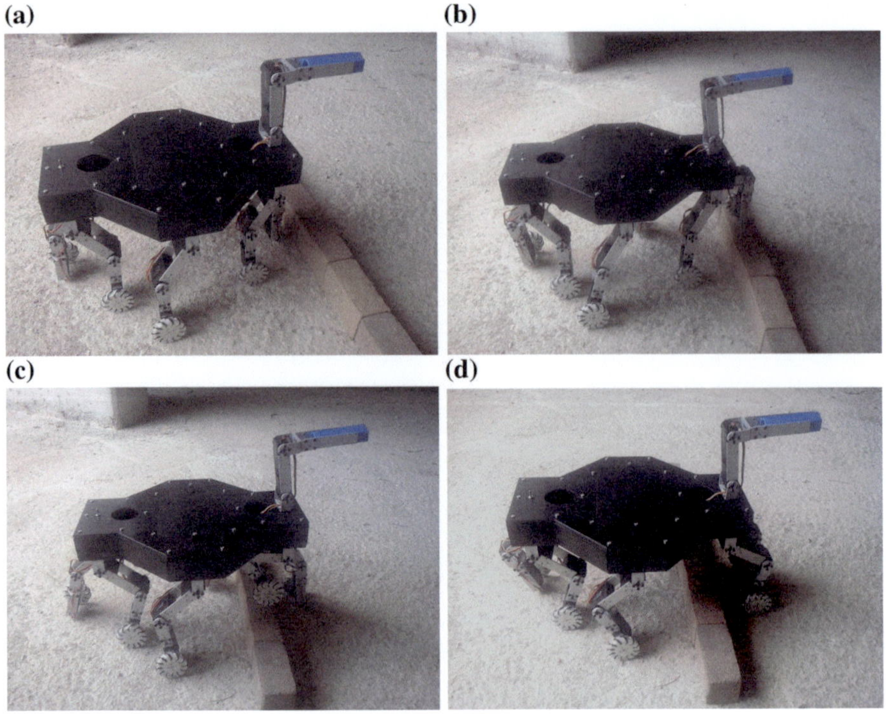

Fig. 11 Main frames related to the obstacle overcome strategy of Cassino Hexapod III

6 Conclusions

This paper outlines the evolution of the robotics series “Cassino Hexapod”, specifically dedicated to inspection/survey of cultural heritage goods. Several design and prototypes have been described with design considerations, simulations and experimental results. The results confirm the possibility of using the system for robotic operations in the architectural survey and monitoring of sites of historical interest. The most recent design solution is currently under patenting.

References

1. Carbone, G., Ceccarelli, M.: A mechanical design of a low-cost easy-operation anthropomorphic wheeled leg for walking machines. Int. J. Robot. Manager **9**(2), 3–8 (2004)
2. Carbone, G., et al.: Operation strategy for a low-cost easy-operation Cassino Hexapod. Appl. Bion. Biomech. **4**(4), 149–156 (2007)
3. Carbone, G., Tedeschi, F.: A legged robotic system for remote sensing, Patent Application N. IS 2014A1 (2014)

4. Carbone, G., Tedeschi F.: A low cost control architecture for Cassino Hexapod II. Int. J. Mech. Control, vol. 14 N° 01 2013 pp. 19–24 (2013)
5. Carbone, G., Tedeschi, F., Cigola M.: The challenge of analysis, survey and conservation of historical sites for service robotics. In: Proceedings of International Advanced Robotics Program, Frascati, Roma, pp. 1–6 (2014)
6. Carbone, G., Ceccarelli, M.: Legged Robotic Systems, Cutting Edge Robotics, pp. 553–576. ARS Scientific Book, Wien (2005)
7. Cigola, M.: Architectural survey and robotics: new frontiers in study, preservation and restoration of historical sites. In: Proceedings of International Conference on Innovative Methods in Product Design, Padova, paper 147 (2011)
8. David Homepage. http://www.david-3d.com/en. Accessed 14 Jan 2015
9. Docci, M., Maestri, D.: Handbook of Architectural and Urban Survey. Roma (1996)
10. Life Performance Research homepage. http://www.lp-research.com/. Accessed 14 Jan 2014
11. Nava Rodríguez, N.E. et al.: A new design of Cassino Hexapod robot. In: Proceedings of the 10th Biennial ASME Conference on Engineering Systems Design and Analysis ESDA2010, Istanbul, Turkey, 12–14 July 2010
12. Tedeschi, F. et al.: Design and operation of Cassino Hexapod. Int. J. Mech. Control, vol. 15 N° 01 pp. 19–25 (2014) ISSN 1590-8844
13. Tedeschi, F., Carbone, G.: Design of Hexapod Walking Robots: Background and challenges in Handbook of Research on Advancements in Robotics and Mechatronics IGI Global. Hershey, USA (2014)
14. Tedeschi F., Carbone G.: Design issues for hexapod walking robots. Robotics **3**(2), 181–206. ISSN 2218-6581. doi:10.3390/robotics3020181 (2014)
15. Tedeschi, F, Carbone, G.: Toward the design of a wheel-leg walking robot. In: 10th IEEE/ASME International Conference on Mechatronics and Embedded Systems and Applications. 10–12 Sep 2014, Senigallia Italy (2014)
16. Tedeschi, F., Carbone, G.: Hexapod walking robots locomotion in motion and operation planning of robotics system. Mech. Mach. Sci. **29**. Springer International Publishing Switzerland (2015)

Development of Human-Centered Social Robot with Embedded Personality for Elderly Care

Aleksandar Rodić, Milica Vujović, Ilija Stevanović and Miloš Jovanović

Abstract The paper regards to research and development of a human-centric, social, care-robot for elderly people and persons with reduced ability to improve quality of their life and to create conditions for more independent living at their homes. Paper presents new mechanical design of personal robot assistant operating in an informational structured environment arranged in the form of a smart house. The paper suggests mechanical structure of the robot that meets ergonomic standards adapted to the low mobile or immobile patients. Fine ergonomic characteristics of robot allow better support for low mobile patients while walking and relatively easy to use services offered by the robot such as: adding of items, medications, personal belongings, serving drinks and meals, connecting and use of the Internet or social networks, phone calls to family members or friends, use Skype services, etc. The robot has a built-in security features such as emergency for medical services, emergency call to family members, etc. Proposed care-robot includes artificial intelligence additionally enhanced by the emotional intelligence interface that enables better adaptability to different personality profiles. In the paper, the care-robot is put in the context of a cloud system that enables enhanced sensing, fast communication between agents as well as real-time decision making and operation. The way of personality embodiment with care-robot is described in

A. Rodić (✉) · M. Vujović · I. Stevanović · M. Jovanović
Mihajlo Pupin Institute, University of Belgrade, Volgina 15, Belgrade, Serbia
e-mail: aleksdandar.rodic@pupin.rs

M. Vujović
e-mail: milica.vujovic@pupin.rs

I. Stevanović
e-mail: ilija.stevanovic@pupin.rs

M. Jovanović
e-mail: milos.jovanovic@pupin.rs

P. Wenger et al. (eds.), *New Trends in Medical and Service Robots*,
Mechanisms and Machine Science 39, DOI 10.1007/978-3-319-30674-2_18

the paper and the methodology proposed was explained by an example—the use case entitled "broken glass". In the conclusion, main novelties and research objectives are stressed out as well as the future work is proposed.

Keywords Human-centric robots · Care-robots · Assistive-living technologies · Embedded personality

1 Introduction

Estimates from the United Nations suggest the population over 65 worldwide will increase 181 % between 2010 and 2050, compared to a 33 % increase in people aged 15–65. That shift will create a large incentive to automate at least some assistive work. Because over the next 20 years the ratio of people over the age of 65 to the number of people under 65 is going to change rather dramatically. As robots become safer, smarter, and more capable, robotics companies are eyeing elder care as a huge potential market. A rapidly expanding elderly population could also necessitate other new forms of home-assistance i.e. assistive-living technology.

Personal assisted, human-centered, care and social robots could play an important role with respect to the health and psychological well-being of the elderly. Objectives of assistive social robots are believed to be useful in eldercare for two reasons, a functional one and an affective one. Such robots are developed to function as an interface for the elderly with digital technology, and to help increase the quality of life of the elderly by providing companionship. The use of these mechatronic devices in particular is justified in the attendance of elderly and people with limited physical and mental abilities in order to support their more independent lifestyle, and a better and safer life in his home. The growing of elderly population enlarges need for larger number of caregivers, cost of medical and social care and life insurance. Also, some scientific research in America and Europe have shown that most of elderly people feel happier and more comfortable if they are attended in their own homes rather than in shelters or elderly dormitories for the care of the elderly. In that sense, the level of care, attention, mental communication, emotional contact with these persons is of special interest. Is it possible by robots, as advanced intelligent devices, to respond to those psycho-physical, socio-economic and cultural challenges, is the question laid in front of the experts from both the humanitarian and the technical and technological sciences. The fact is that the global IT industry follows the needs and requirements of modern mankind and tries to offer right solutions in this sense.

The paper is organized as follows. State-of-the-art in the field is given in Sect. 2. The overview of the prototype structure as a whole is given in the Sect. 3. Problem setting in the context of an ambient-assisted living is done in Sect. 4. Development of the cognitive features of the system is considered in Sect. 5 through building of the embedded personality. The closing section contains a conclusion and future research.

2 State-of-the-Art

Companies are developing elder care robots with the hope of making people more independent in their life. Researchers and robotics companies worldwide are designing prototypes to provide automated assistance to the elderly at home, targeting a market that promises to grow as people live longer. In the past ten years a lot has been done in developing the so-called personal robots for care of the elderly, children, the sick and the handicapped. There are plenty of attempts making such service robots that have been developed for laboratory research. Truly speaking, the examples which are in commercial use are rare because there are still significant technological constraints and lacking knowledge of how to transfer human emotional intelligence to the robots.

One of the most successful help and care robot assistants for household is *Care-O bot 4* designed at the IPA Fraunhofer [1], Fig. 1a. The fourth edition of the Care-O bot range of caring and socially interacting robots has a more adaptable personality than any of its predecessors from this family of robots. It has a visual display which can depict various atmospheres, and the entire model has a more caring and personal feel about it. The Care-O bot 4 is incredibly adaptable, and can be used in various scenarios, including as a drinks waiter and a mobile information point. One of the main positive features of Care-O bit 4 is the attempt to decrease construction costs.

The Robosoft care-robot called *Kompaï* [2] resembles a plastic kiosk on training wheels, Fig. 1b. This robot features a touch-screen display on an easel and a bowling ball–size white head with a "face". The vision for Kompaï is as follows: Family members would call the robot via Skype. The robot would then use ultrasonic sensors to detect the location of the person being called and navigate to that person, who answers the Skype videoconference call via Kompaï's multitouch tablet PC and Webcam. Kompaï could likewise be used as an interface to *Facebook*, *MySpace* or some other social network. Interactive speech recognition would be available to help elderly or otherwise dependent people access the Internet using a simple graphic and tactile interface. Kompaï could also store a person's daily schedule and shopping lists, and access online calendars or weather. Robosoft also was looking for partnership with companies that make wireless physiological sensors worn by a robot's user that could communicate blood pressure, pulse, body temperature and other data via Bluetooth to the robot, which would then relay that information to the personal doctor.

The Robosoft company also developed a prototype of the RobuWalker [3], a human-assisted robot to help humans walking. This robot is only available in its research version (Fig. 1c). The RobuWalker is automated version of the passive walker device.

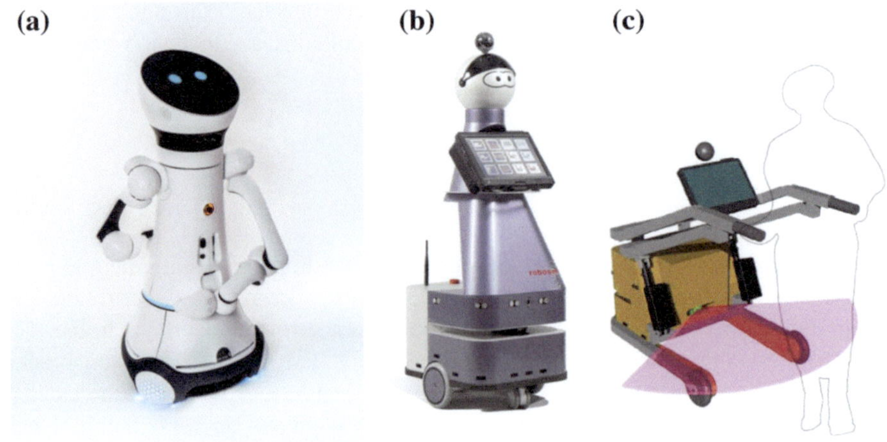

Fig. 1 **a** Care-O bot 4 human-assisted indoor robot, **b** The care-robot *Kompaï,* **c** The Robosoft RobuWalker

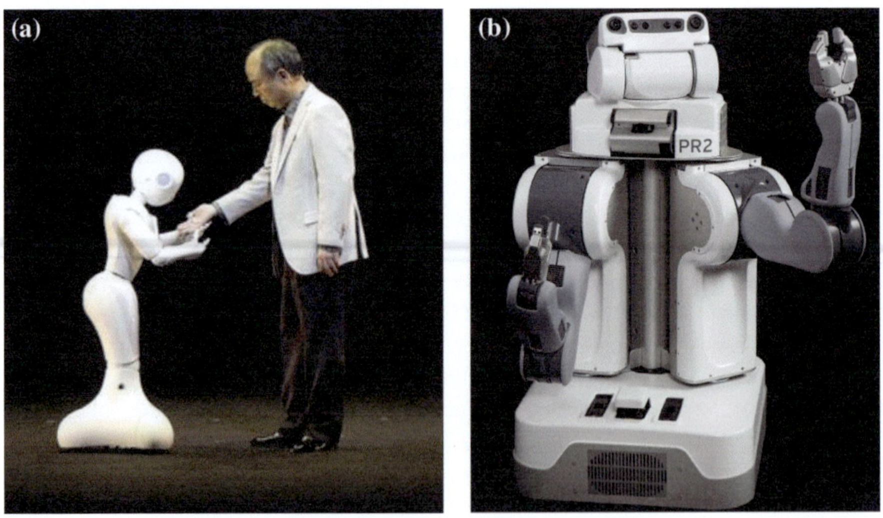

Fig. 2 **a** The SoftBank care-robot Pepper, **b** The Willow Garage personal robot PR-2

The Japanese *Pepper* robot (Fig. 2a) [4] uses a cloud-based AI system so that units learn from one another. Japanese technology giant SoftBank has unveiled a robot they claim is capable of understanding human emotions using an "emotional engine" and cloud-based AI. Standing roughly a meter tall with a tablet computer fixed to its chest, *Pepper* is expected to be used in a range of roles from caring from the elderly to baby-sitting. Pepper reportedly learns from human interactions, with each experience helping to teach a cloud-based AI shared by all units. It has fully articulated arms and hands but moves about on wheels hidden under a curved plastic skirt.

One of the most popular robots in the country is *Paro* [5], a furry, seal-like bot programmed to bond with its owners and show emotions such as happiness and surprise. Paro is an advanced interactive robot developed by AIST, a leading Japanese industrial automation pioneer. It allows the documented benefits of animal therapy to be administered to patients in environments such as hospitals and extended care facilities where live animals present treatment or logistical difficulties.

Willow Garage's first major robot is called *PR2* (Fig. 2b) [6]. It is of a size similar to a human. PR2 is designed as a common hardware and software platform for robot researchers. *PR2* is a robotics platform being developed at Stanford University. *PR* stands for "personal robot".

In parallel with development personal robots scientists focus their interest in developing robots with attributes of human personality to increase their cognitive capabilities. New generation of robots will not be a cold machine but ones that perceive emotion of others and are able to manage their own affective and social behavior. Recently Google has patented customizable robot personalities [7]. Newly-patented system would allow users to download the personality of one to a robot. Google has been granted a patent that would allow the company to develop downloadable personalities for robots drawn from the cloud. Robots that mimic humans are still very much in their infancy, and truthfully there's no telling where this technology can go—especially when backed by giants like Google. And while there's no guarantee that this patent will ever come to fruition, it may very well be the next step in making human-robot relationship a reality. This paper is contribution in that direction. The researches described in this paper refers to the progress in the following directions: (i) more attention was devoted to ergonomic design and better support for mobility of elderly, and (ii) better emotional and social adaptability of robot to the patients through embodiment of personality.

3 Mechanical Design

The body of the robot represents a monolithic entity with amorphous shape. Its form is intended to make the robot aesthetically attractive and ergonomic for humans (Fig. 3). Robot body carries the robot head placed on the collar (neck) that is basically continuation of the body and two 6 DOF robot arms with graspers.

Robot body doesn't have the ability to turn around its axis, but robot arms that have 6 DOF, collar and robot head that turns around vertical axis allow its mobility and operability in various positions. Robot body is equipped with ultrasonic sensors placed around lower part of the body, speaker and led light in the chest zone. Collar contains three cameras and it can rotate independently of the body and the head. Shape of the robot body is designed in a way that the lower part is wider and upper part is narrower so that the overall dimension would not exceed anthropometric

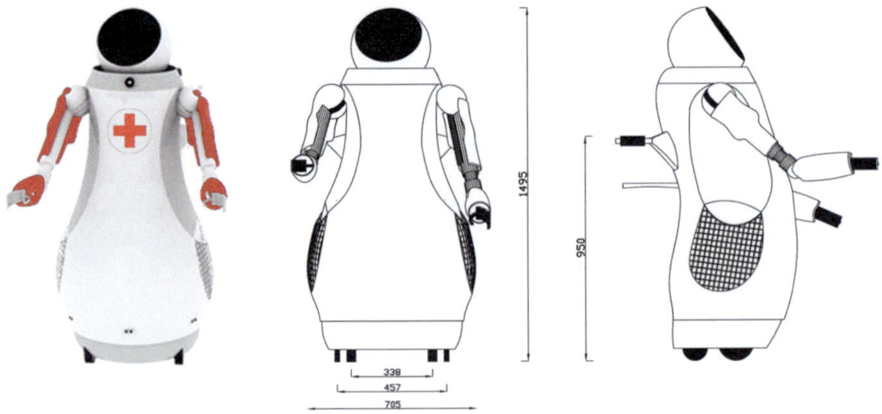

Fig. 3 CAD model of the human-centered care-robot of ergonomic characteristics

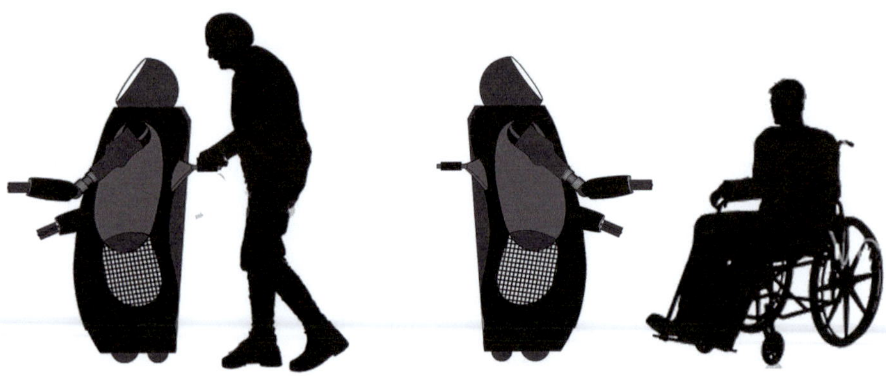

Fig. 4 Care-robot applications—supported mobility (*left*), human assistance (*right*)

limits when add robot arms. Following shape's design, two side pockets are added which serve as baskets for transporting lightweight objects or food. They are made of elastic net in order to provide ventilation for fresh fruit or vegetables that are carried in it. The bi-manual manipulation system consists of two lightweight robot arms of industrial quality. Arms are equipped with grippers. Two-arm manipulation system, combined with ability of turning head, provides good manipulation properties of the overall system and fine functionality (Fig. 4).

The robot head contains: (i) kinematic mechanism with 1 DOF, (ii) touch screen for command input and display information, (iii) three microphones with increased sensitivity, and (iv) optional visual depth sensor placed on the crown of the head. The head has good kinematic abilities of rotation around vertical axes. Based on fine visual and audio capabilities, the robot head can be rotated in direction of the source of the light and/or sound.

4 Ambient-Assisted Living

Advanced approach to support daily life activities of elderly people consists of creating a living environment supported by different technologies including wireless sensor networks and service robot(s). The elderly and people with disabilities tend to have difficulty in performing basic daily activities. Adjusting the physical environment (ambient) to make space more comfortable and ergonomic is not enough. It is necessary to set up an informational structured environment to enhance benefits of different technologies to be applied. Such systems represent adaptive systems, where the context is customizable, and adjustment is done by integrating circuitry in an intelligent system. In other words, living or working space for people turns into an intelligent environment—the smart house [8].

The robot is actually just part of the system (Fig. 5), which includes a kind of smart home aspect to it, with environmental sensors around the house feeding back information about the inhabitant's movements, movement objects, and physiological sensors to track their health. Motion sensors track if someone is in a certain room, while pressure sensors under beds and sofas can tell if someone is sitting down. There are also sensors that are activated when certain appliances are plugged in, and sensors that monitor when doors and windows are open or closed, temperature and humidity trackers, etc. Also, there are wearable body devices (Fig. 5) that measure

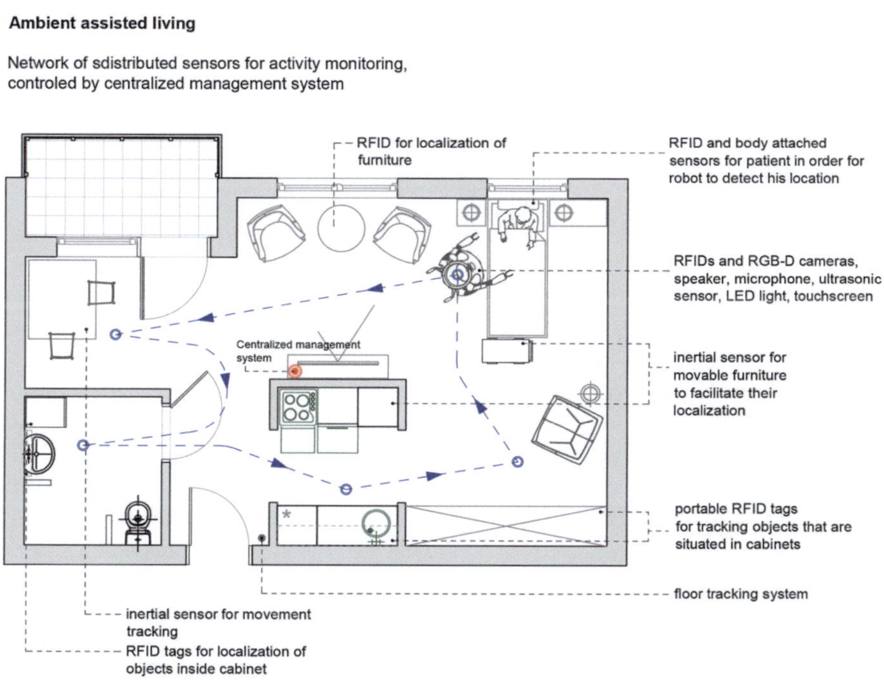

Fig. 5 The context of ambient-assisted living with care-robot of elderly

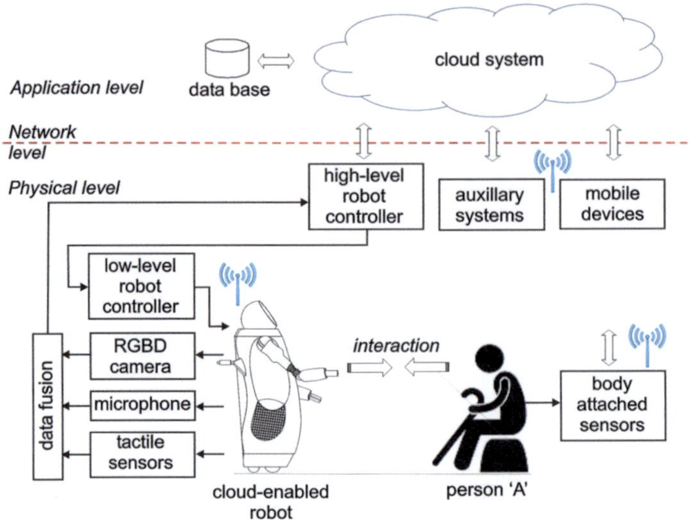

Fig. 6 High level system description—cloud-enabled care-robot operation

blood pressure, heart pulse, motion acceleration and so on. All of the data from the sensors is stored in the database. Based on this information we can extract some activities, like if the person is sleeping or the person got up during the night, the person is watching television or cooking, the person is anxious or calm, etc. The care robot, which is not autonomous, complements these tasks by allowing virtual visits from friends, family, and healthcare professionals. It's basically the equivalent of Skype on wheels. The user calls the robot and is able to direct it around the home to check in on the inhabitant. It's intended to make visits easier for those who aren't immediately at hand. Care robot on command is able to find and bring own objects required by patient(s), bring medicaments, meal or drinks. Based on RGB-D camera robot observes elderly gestures (body gestures as well face mime) and deliver information acquired to the cloud system [9, 10] (Fig. 6). The robot, devices and sensors put and used together create a 24 h monitoring system that demonstrates quite how machines can outperform us in roles that are traditionally considered inherently human, like looking after loved ones. Then there's the issue of collecting and fusion all that data into the cloud system developing a suitable interface for interpreting the constant stream of data over physical and social environment. By respecting privacy, only authorized persons (members of family or medical team) have access to the information, and they're able to see either a weekly or monthly report based on the data collected. The efficiency of the system depends on capacity of the cloud system (Fig. 6) that should enable fast and reliable communication amongst the system agents (robot(s), sensors, objects, human), processing and storing information. Overall system comprises three basic levels: (i) physical level that includes humans, robots, objects, sensors, etc., (ii) network level that enables reliable wireless communication between agents, and (iii) application level that collects, processes and store information about specific application including information about patient physical and psychological condition. The care-robot performs different caregiver service tasks such as assistance, nursing, monitoring, amusing, communicating and so on at the physical level but logistics for that (instructions how to do that, where, etc.) it receives from the application level.

Each activity of the robot requires certain activities of the environment. This activity of the environment is primarily there to help the robot and relieve him of additional sensors and complex algorithms.

5 Embedded Personality

Personality psychology is a branch of psychology that studies personality and its individual differences [11]. According to the theory, "personality" is a dynamic and organized set of characteristics possessed by a person that uniquely influences individual cognitions, emotions, motivations, and behaviors in various situations. Personality also refers to the pattern of thoughts, feelings, social adjustments, and behaviors consistently exhibited over time that strongly influences one's expectations, self-perceptions, values, and attitudes. It also predicts human reactions to other people, problems, and stress [12, 13]. This scientific discipline uses the Myers-Briggs Type Indicator (MBTI) assessment as a psychometric questionnaire designed to measure psychological preferences in how people perceive the world and make decisions [14]. The MBTI sorts psychological differences into four opposite pairs, i.e. dichotomies (*Extravert-Introvert*, *Sensing-intuitive*, *Feeling-Thinking* and *Perceiving-Judging*). That results in 16 possible psychological types. None of these types are better or worse. However, Briggs and Myers theorized that individuals naturally prefer one overall combination of type differences [15]. In the same way that writing with the left hand is hard work for a right-hander, so people tend to find using their opposite psychological preferences more difficult, even if they can become more proficient (and therefore behaviorally flexible) with practice and development. The 16 personality types are typically referred to by an abbreviation of four letters, e.g. ESTJ, INTJ, ISTP, etc. They can be acquired by filling out the on-line questionnaire available at [16]. The characteristics of all particular personality traits according to theory of Meyers and Briggs are presented in [15]. Here in Table 1 is listed only for the pair E-I with aim to explain the procedure of modeling human psychological behavior.

According to the Diagnostic and Statistical Manual of the American Psychiatric Association, personality traits are "enduring patterns of perceiving, relating to, and thinking about the environment and oneself that are exhibited in a wide range of social and personal contexts." Theorists generally assume that: (a) traits are relatively stable over time, (b) traits differ among individuals, and (c) traits influence behavior. They consistently are used in order to help define people as a whole. Traits are relatively constant; they do not usually change. Traits are also bipolar; they vary along a continuum between one extreme and the other (e.g. friendly vs. unfriendly).

Table 1 Personality traits of the dichotomy pair (E)-(I)

Extraverted versus Introverted (E)-(I)	
Talkative and sociable	Private
Expressive	Reserved
Would rather speak than listen	Would rather listen than speak
Comfortable around people	Tire quickly in social settings
Dislike being alone	Comfortable being alone
Get energized by communicating with other people	Get energized by being alone
Think while speaking	Think before speaking

Table 2 Overview of type temperaments and corresponding behavior attributes

Temperament	Behavior attributes
Sanguine (Sg)	Fast and short emotional reactions
	Variable mood
	Cheerful and optimistic person
Choleric (Ch)	Powerful emotions
	Impulsive and irascible person
	Affective
Phlegmatic (Ph)	Weal emotions and rare reactions
	Quite and poised
	Without abrupt change in emotional experience and reactions
Melancholic (Ml)	Rare but intensive and long-lasting reactions
	Long lasting mood under the influence of emotions
	Prone to the negative emotions, sadness and worry

Under the notion "temperament" it is assumed in psychology the individual kinds of the psyche traits that determine dynamics of human psychological activity [17]. The temperament traits are expressed in an even manner in any activity nevertheless to its' content, goals and motives, remaining invariant in the later years and which, in their interconnections, characterize the type of temperament. The temperaments are: *sanguine* (pleasure-seeking and sociable), *choleric* (ambitious and leader-like), *melancholic* (introverted and thoughtful), and *phlegmatic* (relaxed and quiet). The characteristics of different temperament types are summarized in Table 2 [17, 18]. A temperament type can be determined by filling corresponding questionnaires (tests) available at the Internet [19].

The embodiment of personality in robots can be achieved by implementing model of psychological behavior (i.e. the model of human affective and social behavior) with the attributes of personality and temperament [20, 21]. The model parameters are determined based on experience and experimental results obtained by processing of adequate filled out on-line questionnaire with human examinees (for detecting the type of personality [16], temperament [19] and the degree of affective reactions induced by particular excitation events). To do this, 237 patients of different gender and age have been treated. In determining the type of personality the Myers-Briggs type indicator was used which is based on the theory known in personality psychology [11, 14]. The mentioned theory emerged as the elaboration of Jung's (Carl Gustav Jung) theory of personality types [22]. When developing psychological (affective and social) personality model, research started from the original assumption that human behavior depends on several factors [18, 20] some of which are acquired by birth while others have evolved in the course of an individual's life as a result of the influence of physical and social environment on personality development.

According to this assumption, the factors that determine our behavior are: (i) the excitation event—called "trigger", (ii) type of personality, (iii) temperament, (iv) interior stimuli, and (v) external factors. The above listed factors cause changes in the emotional state of human, resulting in appropriate social-affective reactions (gestures, verbal, and/or physiological reactions). Excitation event or excitation case (trigger) is an event or circumstance in the environment that cause changes of human's emotional state and cause an appropriate response to developments in the surroundings. The interior stimuli are related to the physical and mental state of a person such as for example: fatigue, depression, illness, excitement, love, etc. External factors that influence behavior in humans are largely sociological factors like for example family upbringing, education, wealth, society influence, belonging to a community (religious and cultural), etc. It's difficult to say which of the above factors are more or less dominant upon behavior and there is no agreement among experts on this issue.

The dominance of the influence depends significantly on the tradition and culture of the nation to which an individual belongs. However, psychologists are of the opinion that the type of personality and temperament are dominant factors profiled by the man's emotional and social behavior. These factors are mainly acquired at birth, but in the course of life they somewhat vary depending on the living conditions and circumstances. Adopted psychological model of personality is presented on the block scheme in Fig. 7. The model was implemented as a three stage fuzzy

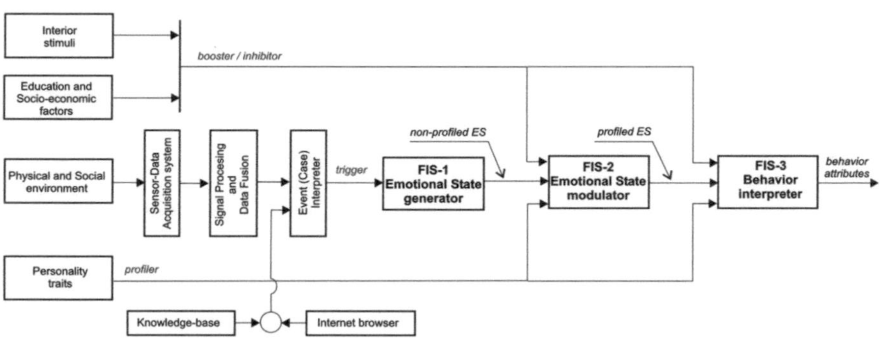

Fig. 7 Structure of the three-stage emotion-driven behavior model with the following fuzzy blocks: emotionally state generator, emotionally state modulator and behavior interpreter

logic, multi input—multi output (MIMO) system. Man as a biological being represents a multivariable dynamic MIMO system. The man behaves in a fuzzy way, often using incomplete or symbolic information. Input and output variables of behavior model are linguistic values as the example big-small, far-near, sad-happy, strong-moderate-low, etc. Fuzzy logic problem formulation allows it to translate the situation described by the symbolic or incomplete way into the determined numerical domain which can be implemented/processed in/by the microprocessor or in the robot controller [21].

The proposed model (affective machine or generator of affective behavior) has three stages of generating emotional state and behavior. At the output of the first stage (FIS-1 block) is obtained the so-called "non-profiled" emotional intermediary state (impersonal emotional state induced by trigger event), at the output of the second stage the profiled state is obtained (characteristic of a particular personality profile), and at the third output represents the emotion-driven behavior is obtained that characterizes the behavior of an exactly one person with corresponding type of personality and temperament. According to the model shown in Fig. 7 interior stimuli and external factors act as boosters or inhibitors of affective behavior. The model shown in Fig. 7 therefore represents a model of emotional intelligence and basis for building EI-controller [21].

Role of the robot EI-controller is to enable robot to acquire, to perceive (understand) and manage emotions (affects) of others and oneself. Having EI-controller robot achieves better social inclusion into the living environments and better adaptability to other persons. Core of the EI-controller represents a knowledge-based model presented in Fig. 7 [18]. The membership functions of the fuzzy blocks FIS-1 to FIS-3 are tuned based on experimental data obtained from the experiments with human examinees (using on-line questionnaires).

In the following paragraph we will describe how to implement the proposed model of psychological behavior in the robot controller. We discuss how to embody the personality traits within machines (robots). In order to achieve that, it is necessary to use appropriate sensorial system and communication equipment installed to the robot together with use advantages of cloud computing. Methodology will be explained by a simple example (use case) of a robot application. Let's call this use-case "broken glass".

Demo use case: Robot is required to bring a glass of water and medication to the patient. It is done in a way that the cloud forwards the information on a particular command to the system. Cloud takes the information about where the cup/glass is from the database, and where the water can be found. In the smart home, there are many sensors and many objects marked by the RFID markers. Also, the shelves are equipped with sensors that detect whether all the objects are in place or are relocated. This information is available for cloud system that sends the necessary information (notifies) to other agents in the room, according to their request for information. So, the robot moves to a location to take the cup, then to a place where it can fill up a glass of water. Path planning can also be dislocated outside of the robot controller on the cloud systems in order to relieve the robot controller of planning movement. It is done at the cloud application level (Fig. 6). Upon execution of this part of the task the robot is sent back to the user—patient. The robot approaches the patient and gives him voice information that it brings him water and medicine. Box with the medications robot carries in the side nets for disposal of objects (see Fig. 3). Robot lets know to the patient that the medication is in the side net and he/she can take it over if capable of doing manipulation. If not, the robot puts a glass of water and drug pill on a tray and carries complete tray to the service user. While approaching the patient robot provides him with information that it brought him water and medicine. The patient, who expected service, moves his hand to grab a glass but it seems weak and physically clumsy. Glass gets out of the hands, falls down to the floor and breaks. Consequently the water spills on the floor. The patient responds affectively (physically and mentally) in accordance with the feelings that are mixed: surprised, frightened and frustrated. Depending on personality traits and temperament his/her affective reactions can be very expressive, moderate or weak which can be appropriately defined in accordance with fuzzy logic forms. On the other hand, the robot carefully "observes" what happened. Based on the video stream from the stereo camera, sensor information from sensors attached to the patient (on the change of pulse, blood pressure and acceleration due to e.g. re-jerk reflex) robot finds out what happened (enabled by the cloud) and understands the context in which the event occurred. On the basis of the information made known in advance about the patient (personality type, temperament, medical indicators that preceded the event) the robot is expected to act in accordance with medical, social and ethical principles in a way that is desirable and beneficial for the older person.

In certain situations it is desirable that the robot has a complementary personality to the patient's personality profile of whom takes care of, to be tolerant, kind, devoted, full of understanding (supporting) for others, etc. In psychology, complementary personality types and temperaments which mutually agree are well known. In this sense, the robot was awarded traits that are desirable in a given situation. Cloud system as a global structure supports adaptive approach to building personality with robots. How to concretely embody (implement) certain attributes of personality in the robot will be shown through the following semantic table. Table links incentive event, personality type and temperament with output affective states. The meaning of symbols in the table is as follows: '+' increases the level of experience, '−' decreases, '++' and '−−' significantly increases/significantly decreases.

Based on semantic table given in Table 3 fuzzy rules of the model of affective behavior can now be applied for instance considering the case "broken glass".

Table 3 Semantic table—trigger versus affective state

Trigger event	E	I	Sg	Ch	Ph	Ml	Affective state
"Broken glass"	+	−	+	+	−−	+	Suprised
	+	−	+	+	−	++	Frightened
	+	−	+	++	−	+	Frustrated

If you introduce a degree of gradation among attributes of behaviors (e.g., et al., slightly, moderately, significantly, extremely) and introduce the membership functions in the form of Gaussian curves and then apply semantic rules defined in Table 3, the following fuzzy rules can be written. Derived scheme for writing rules also applies to other event that causes the same feelings of surprise, fear and anger with people. Derived rules have for example the form where 'PT' stands for personality type, 'TE' for temperament, and 'AS' for affective state:

Rule 1: if (PT = slightly 'E') .and. (TE = slightly 'Sg' .or. TE = slightly 'Ml') then (AS = slightly 'Surprised')
Rule 2: if (TE = moderately 'Ch') then (AS = extremely 'Frustrated')
Rule 3: if (TE = moderately 'Ph') then (AS = slightly 'Surprised') …

In the considered case the personality profile determines the intensity of affective behavior. Semantic tables and fuzzy rules are determined based on experience or on the basis of experiments performed on a number of subjects. The quality of tests performed (sincerity of respondents fully understanding the point of the matter) depends on the accuracy of derivative fuzzy model and it can be successively upgraded and further improve. The number of cases processed (in the field of application) in the database depends on the generality of the cloud model and its applicability to a broader set of tasks within the application. As shown emotional states in humans and robots can be numerically already estimated and expressed in percentages. It provides many other features not only application in robotics but also in medical diagnostics, therapy, stimulating the patient's motivation, etc. In a similar way the rule-base can be updated and completed to cover application.

6 Conclusion and Future Work

The paper presents results of research conducted with a goal to develop emotionally intelligent, social, service robot for care of elderly. The main novelties in this paper regards to:(i) original mechanical design of robot that allows better mobility of patients and meets ergonomic design standards, (ii) application-oriented cloud robotic system architecture, and (iii) development of robot EI-controller that enable personality embodiment and a better understanding of emotional and social behavior of patients. It ensures better social acceptability of new technologies.

The laboratory prototype shown in Figs. 6 and 7 will be built, tested and evaluated in typical household tasks, which should open up the possibilities for its commercial applications. Future work will be done with aim of improving technical performances: sensory-motor skill as well as extensive cognitive capabilities. Also, one of the most important tasks to be fulfilled in the future is to complete the data-base at the application level to give system more applicative freedom.

Acknowledgment The work is supported by the Serbian Ministry of Education, Science and Technology Development within the project no. TR-35003 entitled "Research and Development of Ambient Intelligent Service Robots of Anthropomorphic Characteristics". The research is partially supported by the Alexander von Humboldt Foundation (Germany), under the title "Building attributes of artificial emotional intelligence aimed to make robots feel and sociable as humans (Emotionally Intelligent Robots—EI*robots*)", contract no. 3.4-IP-DEU/112623.

References

1. Care-O bot 4: http://www.care-o-bot.de/en/care-o-bot-4.html. Accessed 16 July 2015
2. Kompai robot: http://www.robosoft.com/robotic-solutions/healthcare/kompai/index.html. Accessed 18 June 2015
3. RobuWalker: http://www.robosoft.com/robotic-solutions/healthcare/robuwalker/index.html. Accessed 16 July 2015
4. Pepper robot: http://www.independent.co.uk/life-style/gadgets-and-tech/japanese-robot-with-a-heart-will-care-for-the-elderly-and-children-9491819.html. Accessed 16 July 2015
5. Paro robot seal: http://www.parorobots.com/. Accessed 16 July 2015
6. Personal robot: http://wiki.ros.org/Robots/PR2. Accessed 16 July 2015
7. Google patent: http://spectrum.ieee.org/automaton/robotics/robotics-software/why-googles-robot-personality-patent-is-not-good-for-robotics. Accessed 16 July 2015
8. Smart home: http://www.cedia.org/blog/what-is-a-smart-home-the-basics-of-home-automation. Accessed 16 July 2015
9. Cloud robotics-1: http://servicerobotics.dei.unipd.it/. Accessed 16 July 2015
10. Cloud robotics-2: http://roboearth.org/. Accessed 16 July 2015
11. Personality psychology: http://en.wikipedia.org/wiki/Personality_psychology. Accessed 16 July 2015
12. Myers, D.G.: Psychology, 9th edn. Worth Publishers, New York (2010)
13. Winnie, J.F., Gittinger, J.W.: An introduction to the personality assessment system. J. Clin. Psychol. Monograph Supplement, 38, 1–68 (1973)
14. MBTI: http://en.wikipedia.org/wiki/Myers-Briggs-Type-Indicator. Accessed 16 July 2015
15. Myers-Briggs theory: http://www.myersbriggs.org/my-mbti-personality-type/mbti-basics/. Accessed 17 July 2015
16. On-line personality test: http://www.16personalities.com/free-personality-test. Accessed 16 July 2015
17. Temperament types: http://en.wikipedia.org/wiki/Four_temperaments. Accessed 16 July 2015
18. Rodić, A., Addi, K.: Mathematical modeling of human affective behavior aimed to design of robot EI-controller. In: Rodic, A., Pisla, D., Bleuler, H. (eds.) New Trends in Medical and Service Robots. Challenges and Solutions. Mechanisms and Machine Science, vol. 20, 384 p, pp. 141–163. Springer Publishing House (2014). ISSN: 2211-0984. doi:10.1007/978-3-319-05431-5
19. On-line temperament test: http://neoxenos.org/wp-content/blogs.dir/1/files/temperaments/temperament_test.htm. Accessed 16 July 2015
20. Rodić, A., Jovanović, M.: How to make robots feel and social as humans. In: The 6th IARIA International Conference on Advanced Cognitive Technologies and Applications (COGNITIVE 2014), pp. 133–139. 25–29 May 2014, Venice, Italy. ISSN: 2308-4197. ISBN: 978-1-61208-340-7
21. Rodić, A., Jovanović, M., Stevanović, I., Karan, B., Potkonjak, V.: Building technology platform aimed to development service robots with embedded personality and enhanced communication with social environment. Digital Commun. Netw. **1**(2), 112–124 (2015). ISSN: 2352–8648. doi:10.1016/j.dcan.2015.03.002
22. McLeod, S.A.: Carl Jung. www.simplypsychology.org/carl-jung.html (2014)

Morphological Optimization of Prosthesis' Finger for Precision Grasping

J.L. Ramírez, A. Rubiano, N. Jouandeau, L. Gallimard and O. Polit

Abstract In this paper, we present the morphological optimization of our tendon driven under-actuated robotic hand prosthesis' finger, to improve precision grasping. The optimization process is performed with a black box optimizer that considers simultaneously kinematic and dynamic constraints. The kinematic is computed with the Denhavit-Hartenberg parameterization modified by Khalil and Kleinfinger and the dynamic is computed from the virtual displacements and the virtual works. All these constraints are considered as a fitness function to evaluate the best morphological configuration of the finger. This approach gives a way to introduce and improve soft and flexible considerations for the grasping robots such as hands and grippers. Theoretical and experimental results show that flexible links combined with morphological optimization, lead in more precise grasping. The results of the optimization, show us an important improvement related to size, torque and consequently energy consumption.

Keywords Morphological optimization · Mechanisms prehension · Precision grasping · Soft robotic

J.L. Ramírez (✉) · A. Rubiano · L. Gallimard · O. Polit
LEME Université Paris Ouest Nanterre La Défense, Paris, France
e-mail: jl.ramirez_arias@u-paris10.fr

A. Rubiano
e-mail: astrid.rubiano@unimilitar.edu.co

N. Jouandeau
LIASD Université Paris 8, Paris, France
e-mail: n@ai.univ-paris8.fr

A. Rubiano
Universidad Militar Nueva Granada, Bogotá, Colombia

P. Wenger et al. (eds.), *New Trends in Medical and Service Robots*,
Mechanisms and Machine Science 39, DOI 10.1007/978-3-319-30674-2_19

1 Introduction

Frequently, robots are designed as rigid structures, but recently some works have shown that the use of flexible bodies, actuators, and sensors could improve considerably the performance of the robots to interact with the environment, this kind of robots is known as soft robots. Soft robotic [1] systems could be able to improve grasping and manipulation, because they use: (i) elastic and deformable bodies, (ii) unconventional materials (like smart materials, shape memory alloy [2], i.a.) and (iii) high number of degrees of freedom.

In this context, the University of Bologna developed the UB-HAND IV, also called DEXMART Hand [3]. The hand is based on an endoskeletal structure articulated via pin joints, the actuators are located remotely with tendon-based transmissions, it has a soft cover and the mechanical structure of the hand was manufactured using additive technologies [4].

With the aim of building a robust and safe hand the University of Pisa and the Advanced Robotics Department of the Italian Institute of Technology in Genoa proposed the Pisa-IIT Soft Hand. This hand incorporated traditional and rolling contact joints with elastic ligaments. The rolling contact joints ensure a correct motion while the hand is actuated. In case of impacts, these joints provide an easy disengage and allow deformations. The hand has a single tendon, passing through all the joints simultaneously. The tendon produces flexion-extension and adduction-abduction of the fingers during the actuation [5].

Consequently, an important tool named Mooveit! [6] incorporates the latest advances in motion planning, manipulation, control and navigation of arms, grippers and hands i.a. Even if the tool is designed for rigid robots it constitutes an interesting approach.

The consideration of a tendon driven under-actuated mechanisms, flexible links and soft articulations in kinematics chains, introduces the necessity of optimal analysis of the morphological parameters. In this domain, one important development is presented by Jouandeau [7], which is related to "Enhancing Humanoids Walking Skills through Morphogenesis Evolution Method", in that work the optimization was performed using confident local optimization for noisy black-box parameter tuning (CLOP) [8].

Based on our first prototype, we observe that an optimization of the finger lengths is wide important to increase the precision and reduce the torque requirements. Consequently, considering that the target of our robotic hand is the precision grasping, we begin the design process with the optimization of the finger that is the key element of the robotic hand.

Therefore, in this paper we propose the application of CLOP to improve the performance of our tendon driven finger, during the precision grasping. Our approach is to use the mathematical model of the kinematic (based on the Denhavit-Hartenberg parameterization modified by Khalil and Kleinfinger) and dynamics (based on the virtual displacements and virtual works) as the fitness function to evaluate the best morphological configuration of the finger. This approach gives a way to introduce and improve soft and flexible considerations for the grasping robots such as hands and grippers.

2 Kinematic and Dynamic Modelling of the Robotic Hand Prosthesis' Finger

2.1 Description of the Robotic Hand Prosthesis' Finger

Our approach is a bio-inspired tendon-driven finger composed of three joints, the metacarpophalangeal (MP), the proximal interphalangeal (PIP) and the distal interphalangeal (DIP). The MP joint has two degrees of freedom (DoF); one rotation (to perform flexion-extension), and one passive translation that allows the vertical alignment of the joint with the motor axis. The PIP and DIP joints have one DoF to perform flexion and extension.

The finger is under-actuated, so it is controlled by only one servo motor. The drive mechanism uses two tendons for transmitting motion to the finger, one tendon flex the finger and the other extend the finger. Considering that the tendons are attached to the motor pulley and the fingertip, as shown in Fig. 1, the clockwise rotation of the servo motor causes a flexion, and the anticlockwise rotation produce an extension. Due to the under actuation the rotation angles of the PIP (θ_{35}) and DIP (θ_{36}) joints are linked with the rotation angle of MP (θ_{33}) joint. The relation between angle is given as $\theta_{35} = 0.23\theta_{33}$ and $\theta_{36} = 0.72\theta_{33}$, where θ_{33} is the MP joint angle, θ_{35} is the PIP joint angle and θ_{36} is the DIP joint angle.

The kinematic and the dynamic modeling are presented in the following subsections. For the kinematics, the Denhavit-Hartenberg parameterization modified by Khalil and Kleinfinger (DHKK) is used and for the dynamics we use the virtual

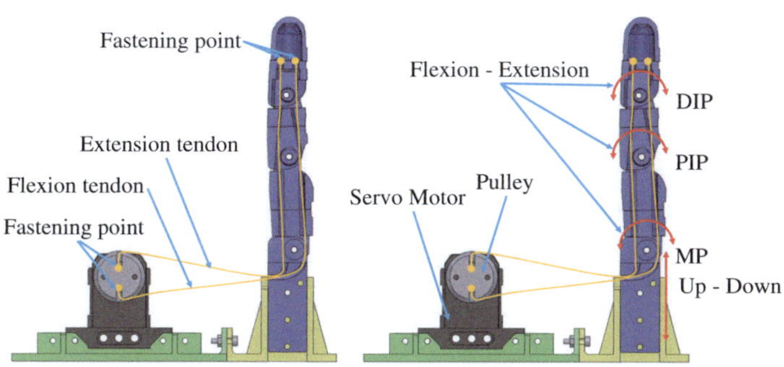

Fig. 1 Section view of the finger mechanism

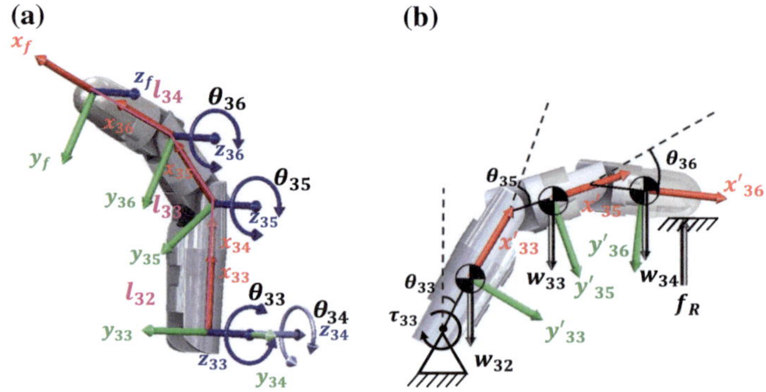

Fig. 2 Equivalent models of the finger. **a** Kinematic model. **b** Dynamic model

displacements and virtual works approach. The equivalent mechanical model of the finger is shown in Fig. 2a for the kinematic and in Fig. 2b for the dynamic.

In Fig. 2a, the parameters l_{32}, l_{33} and l_{34} are the lengths of the proximal, medial and distal phalanges respectively. The angles θ_{33}, θ_{34}, θ_{35} and θ_{36} correspond to MP, PIP and DIP joints rotations. The frameworks (x_{33}, y_{33}, z_{33}) and (x_{34}, y_{34}, z_{34}) are associated to the MP joint. The framework (x_{35}, y_{35}, z_{35}) is associated to the PIP joint and the framework (x_{36}, y_{36}, z_{36}) associated to the DIP joint. The framework (x_f, y_f, z_f) corresponds to the fingertip position. In the same way, in Fig. 2b, w_{32}, w_{33} and w_{34} are the weights of the proximal, medial and distal phalanges respectively, and are placed in the points (x'_{33}, y'_{33}), (x'_{35}, y'_{35}) and (x'_{36}, y'_{36}). F_r is the applied force that is equivalent to the reaction force.

2.2 *Kinematic Model of the Robotic Hand Prosthesis' Finger*

To propose a method to model the kinematic of our robotic hand prosthesis' finger, we use the DHKK. This convention, allows the representation of open-loop and close-loop kinematic chains, and presents a convenient definition of:

- The rotation axis $\mathbf{z}_i$ of each ith joint
- The angle of rotation θ_i around $\mathbf{z}_i$
- The rotation α_i around $\mathbf{x}_{i-1}$
- The distance a_i along of $\mathbf{x}_{i-1}$
- The distance d_i along of $\mathbf{z}_i$

These parameters θ_i, α_i, a_i and d_i are known as DHKK parameters, and are calculated for each joint M_i with coordinates (x_i, y_i, z_i), in Fig. 3 a graphical representation of these DHKK parameters is presented. The rotations are performed using the transformation matrix shown in Eq. (1) [9].

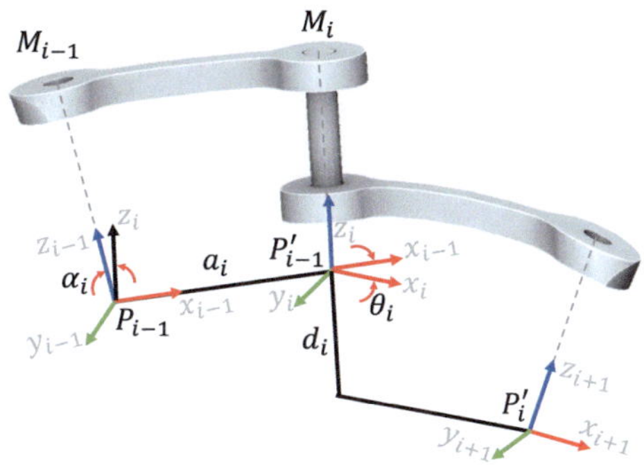

Fig. 3 Graphical representation of DHKK parameters

$$^{i-1}T_i = \begin{bmatrix} \cos\theta_i & \sin\theta_i & 0 & a_i \\ \sin\theta_i\cos\alpha_i & \cos\theta_i\cos\alpha_i & \sin\alpha_i & \sin\alpha_i d_i \\ \sin\theta_i\sin\alpha_i & \cos\theta_i\sin\alpha_i & \cos\alpha_i & \cos\alpha_i d_i \\ 0 & 0 & 0 & 1 \end{bmatrix} \tag{1}$$

Consequently, the kinematics of a robot composed of n joints is the matrix ^0T_n, which is a composition of the 3×3 orientation matrix ^0_nR, and the position vector $[^0P^x_n, ^0P^y_n, ^0P^z_n]^T$, as shown in the following expression:

$$^0T_n = \prod_{i=1}^{n} {}^{i-1}T_i = \left[\begin{array}{ccc|c} & ^0_nR & & ^0P_n \\ \hline 0 & 0 & 0 & 1 \end{array}\right] \tag{2}$$

Usually, the formulation of DHKK parameters is difficult, because is performed manually, and is more difficult when there are multiple kinematic chains. Even that, a method to automatically generate these parameters is presented in [10], and is the adopted methodology to parameterize in the present work. The DHKK parameter for our finger are shown in Table 1, using the configuration shown in Fig. 2a.

Operating the Eq. (1) with the DHKK parameters of the robotic hand prosthesis' finger, shown in Table 1, we get a set of five matrices $^0T_{33}$, $^{33}T_{34}$, $^{34}T_{35}$, $^{35}T_{36}$ and $^{36}T_f$, that describe the transformation between the links of the kinematic chain. Applying the Eq. (2) with the calculated $^{i-1}T_i$ matrices, we get the position $[^0P^x_n, ^0P^y_n, ^0P^z_n]^T$ and orientation ^0_nR of the joints.

Table 1 DHKK parameters of the robotic hand prosthesis' finger

Link	α_i	a_i	d_i	θ_i
33	$-\pi/2$	0	0	θ_{33}
34	$\pi/2$	0	0	θ_{34}
35	$-\pi/2$	l_{32}	0	θ_{35}
36	0	l_{33}	0	θ_{36}
f	0	l_{34}	0	0

Considering that the frameworks M_{33} and M_{34} are in the same position of the reference framework, the position vectors of ${}^0T_{33}$ and ${}^0T_{34}$ are zero (see Eq. (3), and Eq. (4)). From Eq. (3) to Eq. (7) we use the abbreviations $C_i := \cos(\theta_i)$ and $S_i := \sin(\theta_i)$.

$$
{}^0T_{33} = \left[\begin{array}{ccc|c} C_{33} & -S_{33} & 0 & 0 \\ 0 & 0 & 1 & 0 \\ -S_{33} & -C_{33} & 0 & 0 \\ \hline 0 & 0 & 0 & 1 \end{array}\right] \tag{3}
$$

$$
{}^0T_{34} = \left[\begin{array}{ccc|c} C_{33}C_{34} & -C_{33}S_{34} & S_{33} & 0 \\ S_{34} & C_{34} & 0 & 0 \\ -C_{34}S_{33} & S_{33}S_{34} & C_{33} & 0 \\ \hline 0 & 0 & 0 & 1 \end{array}\right] \tag{4}
$$

The following equation corresponds to the position $[{}^0P^x_{35}, {}^0P^y_{35}, {}^0P^z_{35}]^T$ and orientation ${}^{0}_{35}R$ of the joint M_{35}.

$$
{}^0T_{35} = \left[\begin{array}{ccc|c} C_{33}C_{34}C_{35} - S_{33}S_{35} & -C_{35}S_{33} - C_{33}C_{34}S_{35} & -C_{33}S_{34} & l_{32}C_{33}C_{34} \\ C_{35}S_{34} & -S_{34}S_{35} & C_{34} & l_{32}S_{34} \\ -C_{33}S_{35} - C_{34}C_{35}S_{33} & C_{34}S_{33}S_{35} - C_{33}C_{35} & S_{33}S_{34} & -l_{32}C_{34}S_{33} \\ \hline 0 & 0 & 0 & 1 \end{array}\right] \tag{5}
$$

The following equation corresponds to the position $[{}^0P^x_{36}, {}^0P^y_{36}, {}^0P^z_{36}]^T$ and orientation ${}^{0}_{36}R$ of the joint M_{36}.

$$
{}^0T_{36} = \left[\begin{array}{ccc|c} {}^{0}_{36}r_{11} & {}^{0}_{36}r_{12} & C_{33}S_{34} & {}^0P^x_{36} \\ S_{34}(-S_{36}S_{35} + C_{36}C_{35}) & -S_{34}(S_{36}C_{35} + C_{36}S_{35}) & -C_{34} & {}^0P^y_{36} \\ {}^{0}_{36}r_{31} & {}^{0}_{36}r_{32} & -S_{33}S_{34} & {}^0P^y_{36} \\ \hline 0 & 0 & 0 & 1 \end{array}\right] \tag{6}
$$

where
$$
\begin{aligned}
{}^{0}_{36}r_{11} &= C_{34}(-S_{36}S_{35} + C_{36}C_{35})C_{33} - S_{33}(S_{36}C_{35} + C_{36}S_{35}) \\
{}^{0}_{36}r_{12} &= -C_{34}(S_{36}C_{35} + C_{36}S_{35})C_{33} - S_{33}(-S_{36}S_{35} + C_{36}C_{35}) \\
{}^{0}_{36}r_{31} &= (-S_{36}C_{35} - C_{36}S_{35})C_{33} - C_{34}S_{33}(-S_{36}S_{35} + C_{36}C_{35}) \\
{}^{0}_{36}r_{32} &= (S_{36}S_{35} - C_{36}C_{35})C_{33} + C_{34}S_{33}(S_{36}C_{35} + C_{36}S_{35}) \\
{}^0P^x_{36} &= C_{34}(l_{32} + l_{33}C_{35})C_{33} - l_{33}S_{33}S_{35} \\
{}^0P^y_{36} &= S_{34}(l_{32} + l_{33}C_{35}) \\
{}^0P^z_{36} &= -S_{33}(l_{32} + l_{33}C_{35})C_{34} - l_{33}C_{33}S_{35}
\end{aligned}
$$

The following equation corresponds to the position $[{}^0P_f^x, {}^0P_f^y, {}^0P_f^z]^T$ and orientation ${}^0_fR$ of the fingertip.

$$
{}^0T_f = \left[\begin{array}{ccc|c}
{}^0_fr_{11} & {}^0_fr_{12} & -C_{33}S_{34} & {}^0P_f^x \\
S_{34}S_{35}S_{36} & -S_{34}(S_{36}C_{35} + C_{36}S_{35}) & C_{34} & {}^0P_f^y \\
{}^0_fr_{31} & {}^0_fr_{32} & S_{33}S_{34} & {}^0P_f^z \\
\hline
0 & 0 & 0 & 1
\end{array}\right] \tag{7}
$$

where
$$
\begin{aligned}
{}^0_fr_{11} &= C_{34}(-S_{36}S_{35} + C_{36}C_{35})C_{33} - S_{33}(S_{36}C_{35} + C_{36}S_{35}) \\
{}^0_fr_{12} &= -C_{34}(S_{36}C_{35} + C_{36}S_{35})C_{33} - S_{33}(-S_{36}S_{35} + C_{36}C_{35}) \\
{}^0_fr_{31} &= (-S_{36}C_{35} - C_{36}S_{35})C_{33} - C_{34}S_{33}(-S_{36}S_{35} + C_{36}C_{35}) \\
{}^0_fr_{32} &= (S_{36}S_{35} - C_{36}C_{35})C_{33} + C_{34}S_{33}(S_{36}C_{35} + C_{36}S_{35}) \\
{}^0P_f^x &= ((l_{33} + l_{34}C_{36})C_{35} + l_{32} - l_{34}S_{36}S_{35})C_{34}C_{33} \\
&\quad - (C_{35}S_{36}l_{34} + S_{35}(l_{33} + l_{34}C_{36}))S_{33} \\
{}^0P_f^y &= ((l_{33} + l_{34}C_{36})C_{35} + l_{32} - l_{34}S_{36}S_{35})S_{34} \\
{}^0P_f^z &= -((l_{33} + l_{34}C_{36})C_{35} + l_{32} - l_{34}S_{36}S_{35})S_{33}C_{34} \\
&\quad - C_{33}(C_{35}S_{36}l_{34} + S_{35}(l_{33} + l_{34}C_{36}))
\end{aligned}
$$

2.3 *Dynamic Model of the Robotic Hand Prosthesis' Finger*

The proposed dynamic model uses the principle of the virtual displacements and virtual works [11]. We use the dynamic equilibrium to define a model of the input torque as function of the applied force. The virtual work δW is calculated for the external forces (e.g. weight, applied force and input torque) in Eq. (8) and the inertial forces (e.g. centrifugal forces) in Eq. (9).

$$\delta W_e = Q_e^T \delta r_e \tag{8}$$

where Q_e^T is the external forces vector and δr_e is the virtual displacement vector of the forces application points.

$$\delta W_i = M\ddot{q}^T \delta r_i \tag{9}$$

where M is the diagonal mass matrix composed of the masses m_i and inertias J_i, $\ddot{q}^T$ is the acceleration vector and δr_i is the virtual displacement vector of the inertial frameworks.

The dynamic equilibrium is given by Eq. (10), but as in our model the rigid bodies have movements restrictions, the displacements in the points where forces are applied aren't independent, so to solve the equilibrium equation it is necessary separate the coordinates into dependent and independent coordinates.

$$\delta q^T [M\ddot{q} - Q_e] = 0 \tag{10}$$

In order to separate coordinates, the transformation shown in Eq. (11) is proposed, as result we have the equilibrium equation proposed in Eq. (12), which is separable.

$$\delta q = B \delta q_{ii}, B = \begin{bmatrix} -C_{qd}^{-1} C_{qi} \\ I \end{bmatrix} \tag{11}$$

where C_{qd} is the jacobian of dependent coordinates, C_{qi} is the jacobian of independent coordinates and I is the identity matrix.

$$\delta q_{ii}^T B^T [M\ddot{q} - Q_e] = 0 \tag{12}$$

Solving the Eq. (12), we obtain the dynamic function which give us the input torque τ_{33} as function of the force Fr and the kinematics $q, \dot{q}, \ddot{q}$. The resulting expression is shown in Eq. (13), where we use the abbreviations $C_i := \cos(\theta_i)$ and $S_i := \sin(\theta_i)$.

$$\tau_{33}(Fr, q, \dot{q}, \ddot{q}) = \frac{H_0 - 4\, l_{32}\, H_{12} + H_{13}\left(l_{33}\, S_{35} - 4\right)}{8\, l_{33}\, S_{35} - 32} \tag{13}$$

where $H_0 = 2\, {l_{32}}^2 \ddot{\theta}_{33} \left(l_{33} \left(m_{33} + m_{32}\right) S_{35} - 6\, m_{33} - 4\, m_{32}\right) \left(S_{33}\right)^2$

$$H_1 = \left(\left(3\, \ddot{\theta}_{35} + \ddot{x}_{33}\right) m_{33} + 2\, \ddot{\theta}_{35} m_{34} + \left(m_{34} + 2\, m_{33} + m_{32}\right) g - 2\, Fr\right) l_{33}\, S_{35}$$
$$H_2 = \left(\left(m_{33} + 2\, m_{34}\right) {l_{33}}^2 + 4\, m_{34}\, l_{33}\, l_{34} + 2\, m_{34}\, {l_{34}}^2\right)$$
$$H_3 = \left(\left(1/2\, m_{33}\, \ddot{y}_{33} + m_{34}\, \ddot{y}_{35}\right) l_{33} + l_{34}\, \ddot{y}_{35}\, m_{34}\right) C_{35}$$
$$H_4 = 2\, \ddot{\theta}_{36} S_{36} l_{34}\, m_{34} - 6\, \ddot{x}_{33}\, m_{33} + 2\, J_{33}\, \ddot{\theta}_{35} - 4\, \ddot{x}_{35}\, m_{34}$$
$$H_5 = \left(-6\, m_{33} - 4\, m_{32} - 4\, m_{34}\right) g$$
$$H_6 = 1/4\, {l_{32}}^2 \ddot{\theta}_{33} \left(3/2\, m_{33} + m_{32}\right) \left(C_{33}\right)^2$$
$$H_7 = \left(\left(m_{33} + 2/3\, m_{34}\right) l_{33} + 2/3\, l_{34}\, m_{34}\right) \ddot{\theta}_{35} C_{35}$$
$$H_{11} = 1/4\, m_{33}\, l_{33}\, C_3 5 l_{32}\, C_3 3 \ddot{\theta}_{33} + 1/4\, \ddot{\theta}_{35} H_2 {C_{35}}^2$$
$$H_{12} = \left(-1/2\, m_{33}\, {l_{33}}^2 {S_{35}}^2 \ddot{\theta}_{35} + H_1 + H_{11} + H_3 + H_4 + H_5 + 8\, Fr\right) S_{33}$$
$$H_{13} = 8\, \left(H_6 + 3/8\, l_{32}\, \left(H_7 + 2\, m_{33}\, \ddot{y}_{33} + 4/3\, m_{34}\, \ddot{y}_{35}\right) C_3 3 + J_{32}\, \ddot{\theta}_{33}\right)$$

3 Finger Prototype Test Platform Set-Up

With the aim of test the drive mechanism, we design a platform to carry out several experiments, the experiments seek to measure the kinematics of the finger and fingertip force using several servo motors. The platform permits to adjust the position of the MP joint with respect to the actuator axis, which guarantees that the actuator torque is transmitted to the tendons in the same condition. The CAD model of the test platform is shown in Fig. 4.

3.1 *Materials and Methods*

The experiments are performed using two standard servo motors HS-422 and Traxxas 2065 with torques of 0.324 nm and 0.225 nm respectively, and three serial servo motors Dynamixel XL-320, AX-12a and MX-106R with torques of 0.390 nm, 1.50 nm and 10.0 nm respectively. To measure the force, we use a resistive-based force sensor Flexiforce®, that measure up to 5 N, connected to a circuit that uses an inverting operational amplifier arrangement to produce an analog output based on the sensor resistance, the output voltage is registered with a digital oscilloscope. The sensor is calibrated in the range 0.6 N–4.8 N. The sensor is placed in a support (platform) which is located in the trajectory of the fingertip.

Considering that the finger performs flexion and extension in 2D, the kinematic is measured using a high-performance 4 megapixel CCD camera Prosilica GE-2040, to track black markers placed on the finger joints and the fingertip.

3.2 *Kinematic Tracking and Force Measure*

As result of the test, shown in Fig. 5, which corresponds to the measure of the position of each M_i joint (using the Traxxas 2065 servo motor), it is possible to identify several peaks, i.e. the ${}^0P_f^x$ value shows a perturbation after contact. These overshoots are produced by different phenomena as friction forces and other external causes. The

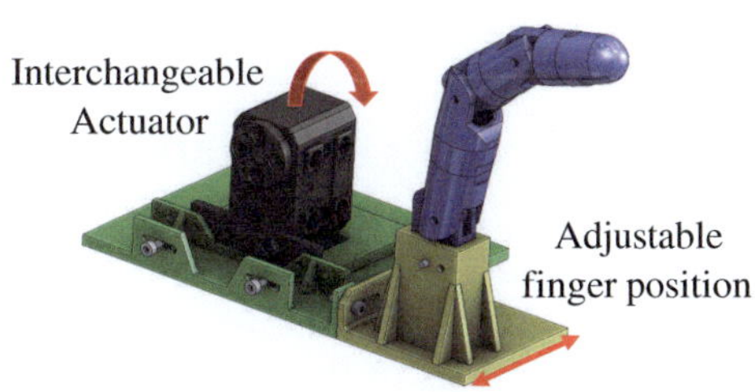

Fig. 4 CAD Model of the test platforms

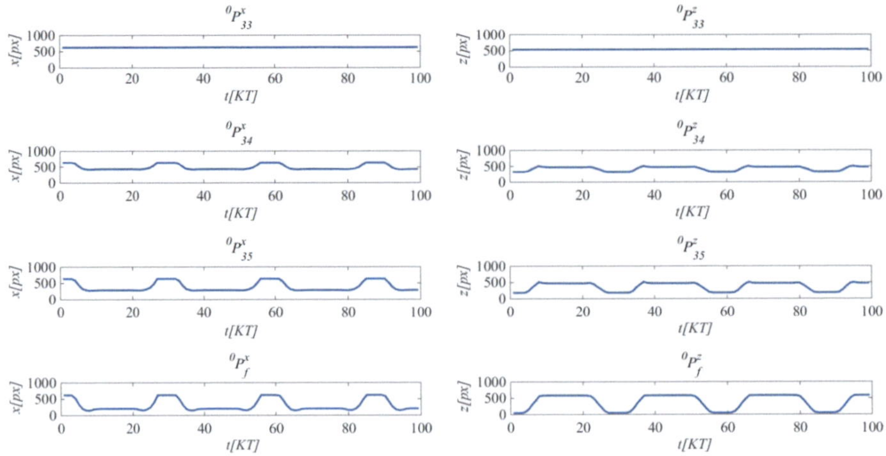

Fig. 5 Results of the position tracking using the Traxxas 2065 servo motor

Fig. 6 Results of the fingertip force using the Traxxas 2065 servo motor

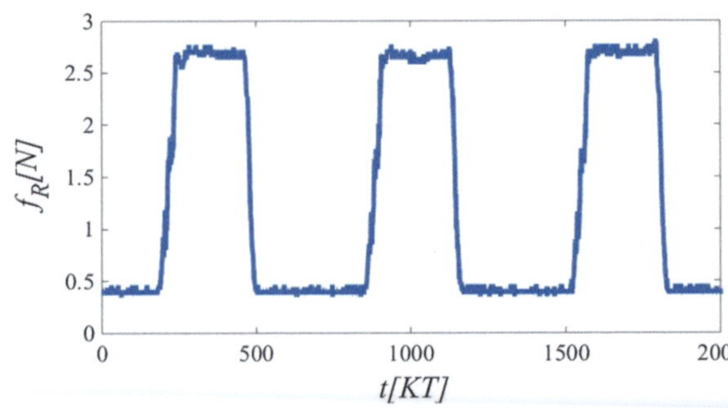

maximal force value is 2.82 N, (using the Traxxas 2065 servo motor) Fig. 6 shows the fingertip force f_r during three repetitions of flexion and extension.

Although we cannot control external conditions, we identify that the performance of the finger is affected by the phalanges lengths. The lengths of the finger could increase the amount of torque needed to apply the same force over an object, and also may impact the precision of the grasping. So that, we propose a morphological optimization of the lengths of the finger phalanges, which is presented in Sect. 4.

4 Morphology Optimization

This section introduces the proposed optimization process, which improves the movement of the finger during the precision grasping. This process seeks to find the optimal lengths of the finger phalanges, to reduce the position error during a grasping movement and also to reduce the torque τ_{33} to apply a force of 5 N.

The used method is confident local optimization (CLOP) for noisy black-box parameter tuning, which was developed to tune parameters in artificial intelligence for games. In our case, we follow the methodology proposed in [7] for enhancing the humanoids walking skills through morphogenesis evolution so that CLOP is implemented in two stages: evolution and evaluation.

4.1 Evolution Process

The evolution process (based on an heuristic evaluation) uses as parameters the set $\mathscr{H}$ (which contains Motors, Torques $< M, T >$ and $lengths_{new}$ parameters, and their maximum and minimum values) and the eval function to calculate the fitness of the results. For each iteration, a new set of lengths is calculated and evaluated, the best result is updated when the founded solution is better than the stored one. The evolution process is presented in Algorithm 1.

Algorithm 1 `evolution` $< M, T >(n, \mathscr{H},$ `eval`$)$

$(\mathscr{H}, \mathscr{L}) \leftarrow (\emptyset, \emptyset)$;
for $i = 0$ to n **do**
    $lengths_{new} \leftarrow$ `newParam` $< M, T >(\mathscr{H})$;
    $(d, m) \leftarrow$ `move` $(lengths_{new}, q_{initial}, q_{obj}, U, dt)$;
    $score \leftarrow$ `eval` (d, m);
    if $score == ACCEPT$ **then**
        `insert` $((lengths_{new}, score), \mathscr{L})$;
    end if
    `insert` $((lengths_{new}, score), \mathscr{H})$;
end for
return `best` $(\mathscr{L})$;

4.2 Evaluation Process

The evaluation, use the results of the kinematic and the dynamic simulation to evaluate the fitness. The eval function determines two Euclidian distances: (i) distance d between the fingertip and the objective position (positioning error), and (ii) distance d_{best} between the best position founded and the objective position. Both distances are compared and the best result is updated only if d is lower than d_{best}. In the same way, the function analyses if the input torque m (which corresponds to τ_{33}) is lower than the best to modify the result. The eval function is presented in Algorithm 2

Algorithm 2 `eval` (d, m)

if $d < d_{best}$ **then**
    $(d_{best}, m_{best}) \leftarrow (d, m)$;
    return *ACCEPT*;
else if $m \geq 0$ **then**
    if $m < m_{best}$ **then**
        $(d_{best}, m_{best}) \leftarrow (d, m)$;
        return *ACCEPT*;
    end if
end if
return *REJECT*;

4.3 Experiment Setting and Application

To perform the experiment, two functions are defined, $f(lengths, q, u, dt)$ to describe the movement before the contact with the object to grasp and $g(lengths, x, u, dt)$ to describe the movement after the contact with the object.

Before contact, the parameter u is a speed control law defined as a ramp, which handle the engine speed to a maximal value with a constant slope. After contact u is a

Algorithm 3 `kinematicMove` $(lengths_{new}, q_{initial}, q_{obj}, U, dt)$

$q \leftarrow q_{initial}$;
$t \leftarrow 0$;
while `contact` $(q) == false$ **do**
    $(u, t) \leftarrow$ `next` (U, t, dt);
    $q \leftarrow$ `f` $(lengths_{new}, q, u, dt)$;
end while
return (`dist` $(q, q_{obj}), -1)$;

Algorithm 4 `DynamicMove` $(lengths_{new}, x_{initial}, q_{obj}, Fr, U, dt)$

$q \leftarrow$ `position` $(x_{initial})$;
$x \leftarrow x_{initial}$;
$t \leftarrow 0$;
while `contact` $(q) == false$ **do**
    $(u, t) \leftarrow$ `next` (U, t, dt);
    $x \leftarrow$ `g` $(lengths_{new}, x, u, dt)$;
    $q \leftarrow$ `position` (x);
end while
while `torque` $(x) < Fr$ **do**
    $(u, t) \leftarrow$ `next` (U, t, dt);
    $x \leftarrow$ `g` $(lengths_{new}, x, u, dt)$;
end while
return (`dist` $(q, q_{obj}), u)$;

force control law that handles the applied force to a maximal value *Fr* with a constant slope. The algorithms to implement both functions are presented in Algorithms 3 and 4.

5 Results

The experiment, which was executed 150 times, search to minimize the position error and the torque τ_{33}. The evaluation process generates iteratively solutions, from the first (where l_{32} is 22.1 mm and τ_{33} is 46 Nmm) to the last (where l_{32} is 22.2 mm and τ_{33} is 50.7 Nmm). Each solution is equivalent or better than the previous. By applying the morphological optimization on l_{32}, l_{33}, l_{34} and τ_{33} parameters that produce f_R, we change parameters from (36.6, 24, 25 mm, 225 Nmm) to (22.2, 9.2, 10 mm, 50.7 Nmm) that improves f_R by a factor of 2 with a single finger experiment. Such gain over output force on each finger will be more important with a prosthetic hand with multiple fingers.

The complete experiment, corresponding to the last row of Table 2, is shown in Fig. 7a, where is possible to follow the evolution of the phalanges lengths and the trajectory described from the initial position to the objective position. Consequently,

Table 2 Seven best results of the CLOP experiments

l_{32} (mm)	l_{33} (mm)	l_{34} (mm)	τ_{33} (Nmm)
22.1	19.6	16	46
26.5	15.3	13.3	58.6
26.2	10	18.9	55.1
23.1	12.9	10.6	52.3
22.9	12.8	10.3	51.8
18.9	9.9	13.1	40.3
22.2	9.2	10	50.7

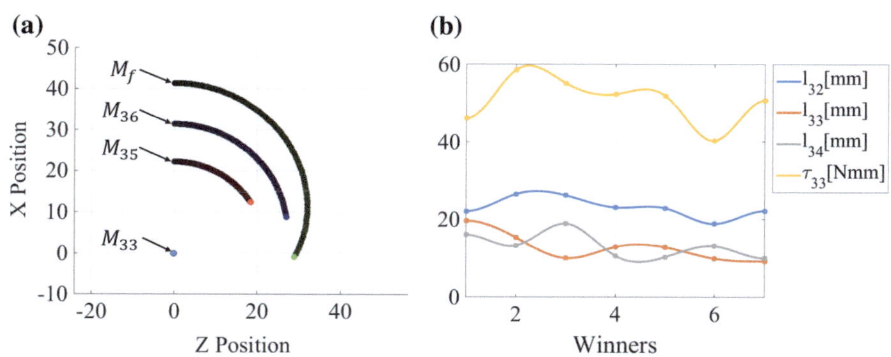

Fig. 7 Equivalent models of the finger. **a** Kinematic model. **b** Dynamic model

the result shows a direct relationship between the length of the phalange l_{32} and the torque τ_{33}, and as can be shown in the Fig. 7b, the values are converging around a mean value.

6 Perspectives

The consideration of a tendon driven under-actuated mechanisms, introduces the necessity of torque control after the contact with the object to grasp, which in our case is the result of the optimal analysis of the morphological parameters. The morphological optimization performed, leads us to envisage a new finger, which should involve soft and flexible considerations for the design of the links and articulations, in order to achieve the grasping task in a more appropriate way. The results of the optimization, show us an important improvement related to size, torque and consequently energy consumption. Therefore, the next stage will be the integration of the optimal finger. Further investigations should also be tested to improve usability of robotic hand prosthesis with soft and flexible components.

7 Conclusions

The CLOP optimizer is a performant method that deals automatically with non-negative Hessians, which is the case of the proposed dynamic method. Consequently, the morphological optimal values allow to propose an evolution of our robotic finger. The obtained results show a smooth trajectory that is important for precision grasping. A similar optimization process could be applied to create an adaptive torque control grasping system.

The results of the performed torque optimization, give us an energetic performance, which render the robotic finger ideal to be used in our hand prosthesis. This energetic performance also lets the robotic hand prosthesis be more convenient to the patient according to the fact that we reduce the weight and increase the autonomy of the robot.

Acknowledgments Through this acknowledgement, we express our sincere gratitude to the Université Paris Lumières UPL for the financial support through the project PROMAIN This work has been partly supported by Université Paris Lumières UPL and by a Short Term Scientific Mission funding from LEME-UPO-EA4416/LIASD-UP8-EA4383. We also acknowledge Colciencias—Colombia and the Universidad Militar Nueva Granada for the financial support of the Ph.D. students.

References

1. Nurzaman, S., Iida, F., Laschi, C., Ishiguro, A., Wood, R.: Soft robotics [tc spotlight]. Robot. Autom. Mag. IEEE **20**(3), 24–95 (2013)
2. Andrianesis, K., Tzes, A.: Design of an innovative prosthetic hand with compact shape memory alloy actuators. In: 21st Mediterranean Conference on Control Automation (MED), pp. 697–702 (2013)
3. Palli, G., Scarcia, U., Melchiorri, C., Vassura, G.: Development of robotic hands: the UB hand evolution. In: IEEE/RSJ International Conference on Intelligent Robots and Systems (IROS), pp. 5456–5457 (2012)
4. Ficuciello, F., Palli, G., Melchiorri, C., Siciliano, B.: Postural synergies of the UB hand IV for human-like grasping. Robot. Auton. Syst. **62**(4), 515–527 (2014)
5. Ajoudani, A., Godfrey, S., Catalano, M., Grioli, G., Tsagarakis, N., Bicchi, A.: Teleimpedance control of a synergy-driven anthropomorphic hand. In: IEEE/RSJ International Conference on Intelligent Robots and Systems (IROS), pp. 1985–1991 (2013)
6. Chitta, S., Sucan, I., Cousins, S.: Moveit! [ros topics]. IEEE Robot. Autom. Mag. **19**(1), 18–19 (2012)
7. Jouandeau, N., Hugel, V.: Enhancing humanoids walking skills through morphogenesis evolution method. In: Brugali, D., Broenink, J., Kroeger, T., MacDonald, B. (eds.) Simulation, Modeling, and Programming for Autonomous Robots. Lecture Notes in Computer Science, vol. 8810, pp. 412–423. Springer International Publishing (2014)
8. Coulom, R.: Clop: confident local optimization for noisyblack-box parameter tuning. In: van den Herik, H., Plaat, A. (eds.) Advances in Computer Games. Lecture Notes in Computer Science, vol. 7168, pp. 146–157. Springer, Berlin Heidelberg (2012)
9. Harada, K., Anzai, T.: Multiple sweeping using quaternion operations. Comput. Aided Des. **34**(11), 815–822 (2002)
10. Hugel, V., Jouandeau, N.: Automatic generation of humanoids geometric model parameters. In: RoboCup 2013: Robot World Cup XVII, pp. 408–419. Springer (2014)
11. Yamane, K., Nakamura, Y.: O(n) forward dynamics computation of open kinematic chains based on the principle of virtual work. IEEE Int. Conf. Robot. Autom. ICRA **3**, 2824–2831 (2001)

Correction Method for Spine Flexion Tracking with Markers

S. Butnariu and C. Antonya

Abstract The aim of the present paper is to accomplish a virtual model for testing the properties of the outer layers of the human body (skin, adipose tissue, muscle) in order to estimate and calculate the displacements of certain points on the skin surface in relation to the bones (which are considered fixed points). The proposed correction method will be used in the development of a device for tracking the human body postures and the spine movement by using different types of sensors for establishing a preliminary diagnosis of it. There is a major problem identified in this case of tracking the spine with markers: the skin sliding in connection with the bones. In order to obtain a precise calculus, it requires great knowledge of this phenomenon and the ability to establish a clear relationship between the position of bones and the position of the corresponding points on the skin, taking into account the different characteristics of material and measurement conditions.

Keywords Lumped mass model · Skin behavior · Multi-point system · Spine tracking

1 Introduction, Description of Problem

The position of the spine can be estimated by tracking the posture of the human body. This can be done by optical tracking using reflective markers bonded on the human body, so the data obtained can be used to set up a human body posture (Fig. 1). In our studies, the question arises whether at a certain time in the process of the movement of the subject, the position of one point on the surface of the human

S. Butnariu (✉) · C. Antonya
Transilvania University of Brasov, Braşov, Romania
e-mail: butnariu@unitbv.ro

C. Antonya
e-mail: antonya@unitbv.ro

P. Wenger et al. (eds.), *New Trends in Medical and Service Robots*,
Mechanisms and Machine Science 39, DOI 10.1007/978-3-319-30674-2_20

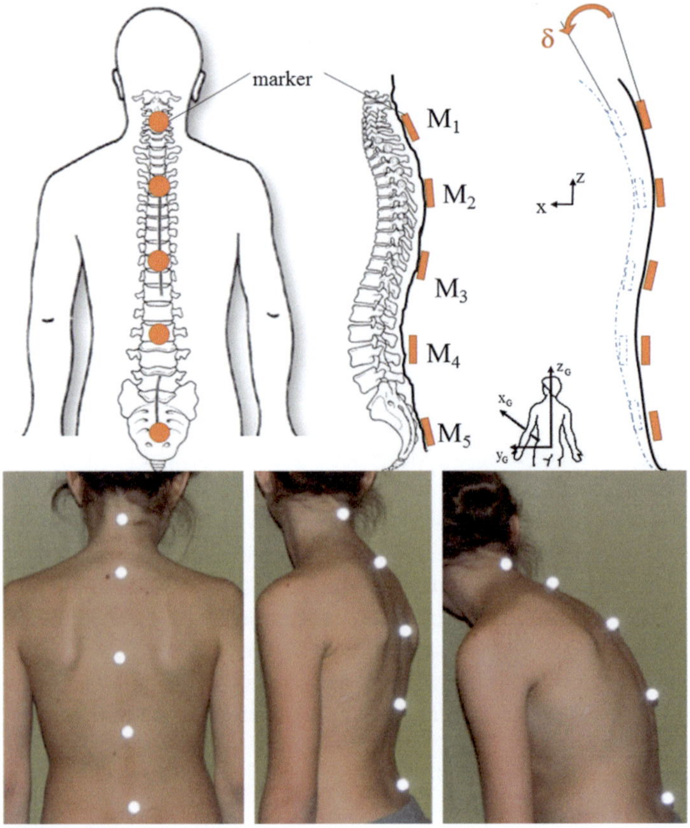

Fig. 1 Measured human posture using reflective markers

body (tracked by the marker) corresponds to its the initial position measured in a fixed reference frame attached to a point on the spine (on the spine vertebra).

Specifically, we consider that during normal movement of the body, due to the elastic properties of the skin, for a point situated on the human body surface, characterized by an initial position on a fixed reference frame, its position will change depending on various factors. We assume that these factors are controlled by the intrinsic characteristics of the tissue, but also the amplitude of the body movement.

The question is: the values of outer tissue deformation can be used to estimate the spine flexion and extension? If this is possible, then we can calculate a correction factor to be taken into account when it will be reconstructed the spine posture based on human body tracking.

Because the markers are glued directly on the skin, and taking into account the skin deformation during movement, we cannot consider a rigid approach for involved bodies and surfaces. The skin has a relative motion to the bone, which is called skin artifacts [2, 9, 15]. This property is the main source of the errors in human motion analysis using reflective markers.

2 Human Body Modeling

Due to significant developments in computer sciences in the last 20–30 years, particularly in hardware and software technology, we have finally passed on to a new level of testing on virtual models in a lot of fields which used until recently traditional and analogical research methods, of determining how the human body works and what are its characteristics. In this way, research costs and test duration have been reduced and at the same time the test' versatility has increased, also bringing significant financial savings.

During the last years, analysis models and software for various human activities have been developed, such as reconstruction of accidents, human body biomechanics, applications in ergonomics, medicine, sports and arts. However, the testing of various applications on virtual models involves a laborious work in developing models and validating them.

The applications that use virtual models can be classified into:

- deterministic applications (results of an action on the model may be predicted using estimated parameters representing some features of the human body and the environment with which it interacts, according to the laws of physics);
- statistical applications (used to assess the proper relationship between loading conditions and results obtained).

Creating the models used for human body testing relies on various principles: the lumped mass models (consists of rigid bodies with masses connected by spring and dampers, 1D or 2D), the multi-body models (MBS, elements connected by various joint types through which the number of degrees of freedom between the elements can be constrained, 2D or 3D) and finite element models (the body is divided into a number of finite volumes, 3D). Note: the lumped model may be considered as a particular case of the multi-body model.

The multi-body model is a very effective method for complex kinematic connections, such are those in the human body. The finite element method can describe the local structural deformations and stress distribution, but it is not very attractive for optimization studies involving many designing parameters. However, an option combining the two methods is considered optimal.

There are several approaches to human body modeling in the literature. Thus, there are different identifiable models of the human body or of certain parts of it.

Human body modeling as a whole is done in order to analyze its kinematics. There are neuromuscular pathologies that lead to motor system dysfunctions. An important challenge for professionals is to identify muscular problems by analyzing the walking kinematics and/or patient's movement. In this case, the model is carried out using the MBS, being a general method.

The same method is also used to shape parts of the human body, usually comprising some kinematic and couplings (spine, limbs, hands etc.). The tracking can be conducted using with or without markers through various methods and concentrating specially on the position and movement of rigid elements of the human body (bones) [11, 14, 15].

3 Working Methodology

Regarding the skin sliding over the spine, we have two main issues to be considered: skin artifacts and 6D relative movement of the spine joints. In the present work we opted for a very small segment analysis, taken from the dorsal surface of the human body, in the region of thoracic vertebrae $T_1 \dots T_4$. At the same time, we tried to simplify the analysis model, eliminating a number of possible movements of the vertebrae, one from the other. Thus, for this study, we considered a single rotation between two adjacent vertebrae (Fig. 2), in sagittal plane (XZ plane, see Fig. 1). We analyzed only clockwise rotation between vertebrae (Fig. 4b), which causes skin stretching.

Unlike other applications, where skin artifacts can get extremely large values (such as knee) [8, 9], in spine case study we will consider a linear model.

The skin properties will be modeled using a multi-point system with springs and dampers (Fig. 3), which will be set in motion due to the connections to the vertebrae.

The skin deformation is modeled with a collection of inter-constrained mass points, using the multi-particle system (MPS) formulation [12]. The multi-particle

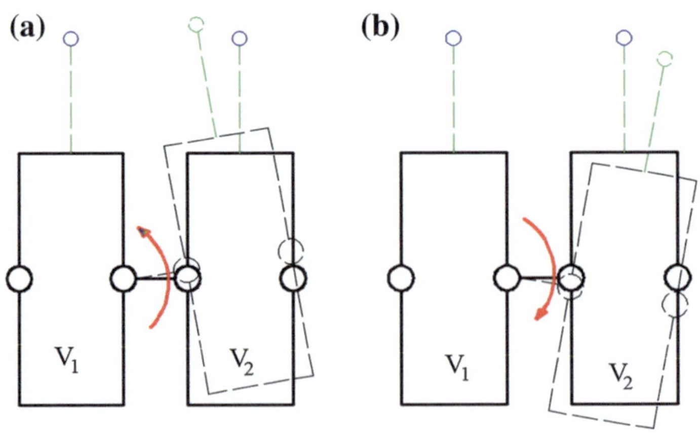

Fig. 2 Relative rotation of the vertebrae

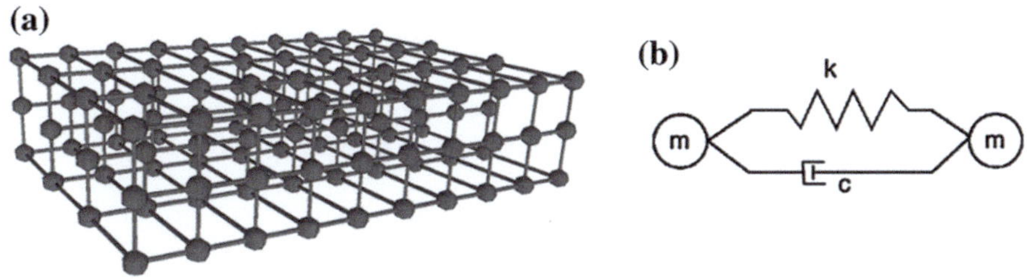

Fig. 3 Multi-point system

model is a collection of particles subject to a set of absolute and relative constraints and forces from external sources or springs and dampers. The biomechanical system is replaced by a set of mass points, equivalent from the inertial viewpoint with the original body, and a set of springs and dampers which will reproduce the elastic properties of the skin. The main benefit of MPS formulation is that it works with geometric data that is similar to FEM analysis (particles vs. nodes), which makes it more suitable for use in the study of flexible systems or multi-physics simulations.

The constraint equations (imposed motion and geometrical constraints) and dynamic equations constitute a set differential algebraic equation (DAE) in the coordinates of the mass points (q) and the Lagrange multipliers (λ):

$$\begin{bmatrix} [M] & [J]^T \\ J & 0 \end{bmatrix} \begin{bmatrix} \ddot{q} \\ \lambda \end{bmatrix} = \begin{bmatrix} Q_{ex} \\ \psi \end{bmatrix}. \tag{1}$$

where M is the mass matrix, J is the constraints Jacobian matrix, Q_{ex} the generalized external applied forces vector and ψ is the term obtained from the second time derivation of the constraint equations.

In this study we aimed to establish a methodology for correction of the measured displacement obtained from the tracking system. For this, we consider a portion of the spine which consists of the first four thoracic vertebrae (Fig. 4a). Outer tissues (skin) was modeled using multi-point system, using two layers of mass points.

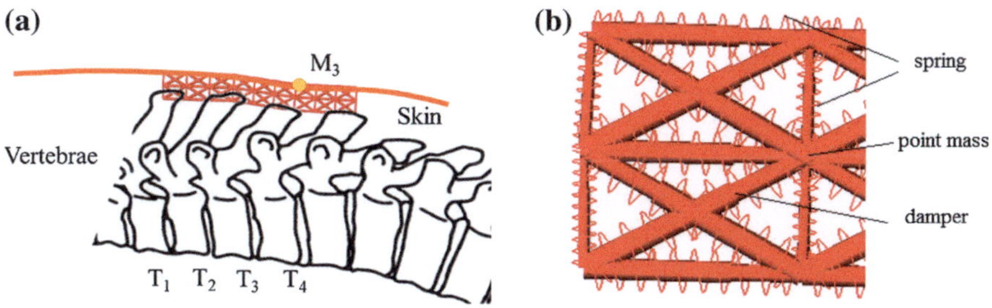

Fig. 4 The model of outer tissue linked on spine (**a**) and detail of multi-point model (**b**)

Assumptions are:

- dimensional values of the vertebrae and outer tissues are considered for an child;
- the spring factor k is calculated for the multi-pattern dimensions shown in Fig. 4b and based on Young's modulus E determined in [6, 13] and using Eq. (2):

$$k = E\frac{S}{l_0}. \tag{2}$$

  where S is the normal section surface and l_0 the initial length.
- the inner layer of the outer tissue is rigidly connected to the vertebrae;
- we consider one marker rigidly attached on the skin;
- we consider only elastic behaviour of the tissues.

In the following are presented some technical characteristics of the elements that compose the analyzed model. The bone tissue is one of the most rigid structure of the human body due to the mixture of inorganic (calcium and phosphate) and organic (collagen) components. The bone is an anisotropic material, its behavior will change depending on the direction of load application. In general, the bone can lead to large loads in the longitudinal direction, and a smaller loading value when it is applied to the surface of the bone. The bone is also viscoelastic, which means that it responds differently depending when it receives loads in different speeds: the bone responds more rigidly if the load acts quickly and the bone is not so rigid or strong when it receives the load slowly. The flexibility properties of the bone are provided by the concentration of collagen in the bone. The bone is at the same time a fragile material, its fragility degree depending on the mineral constituents given by the ability of compression [3].

The skin is the largest organ in a human being, representing 15–20 % of the human body weight. The mechanical characteristics of the skin are extremely complex and have not been satisfactorily simulated using conventional mathematical models. The ability to predict the human skin behavior and assessing changes in the mechanical properties of tissue are important information for modeling in various fields, which are currently based on experimental animal models.

Some studies have aimed to create an anisotropic predictive model built on hyperelastic properties of human skin and comparing it with the results obtained in the laboratory using Finite Element Method (FEM) [5].

Other research [13] reveals that three distinct types of mechanical behavior of the skin can be defined: immediate expansion when tension is applied, the subsequent expansion continues while the force is maintained and gradually thinning under local compression. Considering all the above in order, the first behavior is called elastic extension, the second which is irreversible and gradual is called viscous extension or viscous slip and the third phenomenon—viscous flow.

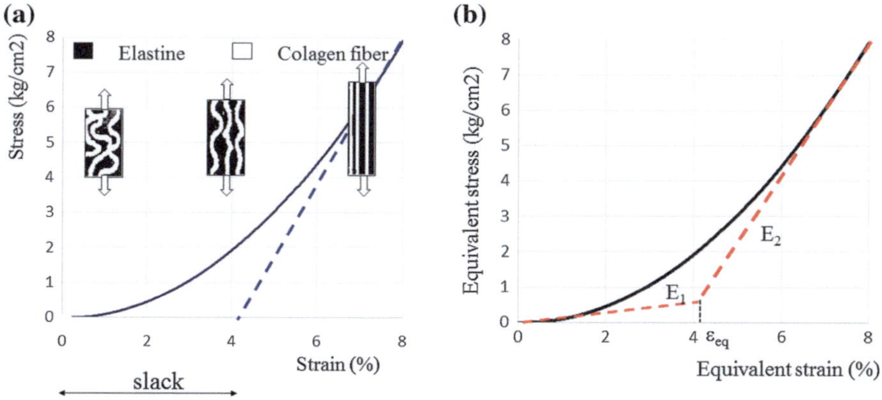

Fig. 5 Strain/stress behavior (adapted by [4, 12])

Looking at Fig. 5, where the skin behavior as a result of tensions is plotted, the first observation is that the skin can be easily stretched with a few percentages from the initial length, but then it requires much higher force values to stretch it further.

The graph in Fig. 5a can be transformed into a single formula, due to very different curvature between the first and last part, these two areas described separately by different equations.

Without using mathematics, there are two parameters which can be deduced from the graph: the average slope of the last area, which is quasi-linear (representing the Young's maximum elasticity modulus for this specimen) and the intersection of extending this zone to horizontal axis.

The average values for the human skin are in the range of $2\ldots10 \times 10^3$ N/cm^2 [6, 10, 13]. The elasticity modulus increases proportionally with the patient's age and is lower in women than in men. Through the extension of the last area of the graph and the intersection with horizontal axis it can be determined the residual elongation of the tissue tested, which can vary between 3 and 14 % [13].

Other researchers experimented stretch determinations in vitro on human skin, collected from female patients who underwent reconstructive plastic surgery. The data collected for stress/strain curve were used to fit the theoretical hyperelastic models (General Polynomial, low Polynomial and Ogden). Among these models, only the low Polynomial model proved to be stable, therefore it has been in an explicit finite element model [7].

Viscous slip is other mechanical properties of skin. To determine the viscous slip, the same equipment is used as in the case of elasticity measurement, the only difference being the time of application of the load. Research in the field shows that for a few seconds load, there is a rapid relaxation of the material in contrast with the demands of lesser value but long lasting, which causes elongation persisting for a few hours (Fig. 5). Viscous extensibility (u)—extension rate/unit of force applied, very slow process–e.g. a request for 10 N/cm^2 causes a slip of 0.05 %.

This process is irreversible. The viscous flow—it is a very little studied process. It is determined by measuring the modification of skin thickness after some type of demands pressure (compression) [13].

On the other hand, there are approaches of some researchers [1] measuring this property in vivo, on human patients. The equipment used is based on mechanical and optical measurements.

In practice, the three properties of the skin (elastic extension, viscous slip and viscous flow) cannot be separated, but in research activity we could take into account every phenomenon in part in order to obtain suggestive results [13].

To calculate the displacements of points on the outer tissue we used the MSC ADAMS® software.

In Fig. 6a the initial position of the multi-point system is presented. On the outer surface of the skin, we consider a marker M_3 (see Fig. 1, reflexive marker attached to the skin). The points P_1, P_2, P_3 and P_4 correspond to thoracic vertebrae T_1, T_2, T_3 and T_4. During the simulation, it is considered that these points remain in contact with the vertebrae and movements of these points are known, due to spine flexion with δ angle (Z-axis rotation angle in XZ plane).

The simulation was performed assuming that the segment P_1P_5 remains fixed; points P'_1 and P'_5 from Fig. 6b (final position of the multi-point system) are the same with P_1 and P_5 from Fig. 6a. It is assumed that during flexion of the spine, the relative position of the point M_3 to P_1 … P_4 has changed.

In order to determine the position of point M'_3 during the simulation, it was measured the length of $P'_4M'_3$ segment and the angle between segment $P'_4M'_3$ and X axis.

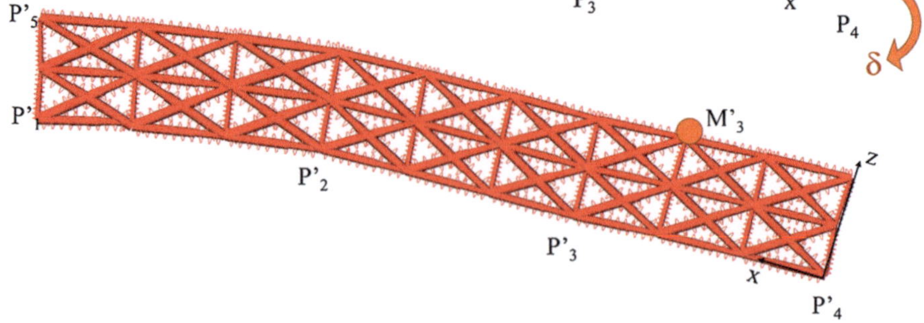

Fig. 6 Initial (**a**) and final (**b**) position of the multi-point system

The multi-point model will have dimensions close to the actual dimensions of the subject. Thus, the distances between the defined above points are: P_1P_2 = 21 mm, P_2P_3 = 24 mm and P_3P_4 = 26 mm. These dimensions were measured on reconstructed 3D model of human spine used in this research. The thickness of the tissue was 2 × 5 mm (P_1P_5 = 10 mm), similar to those of the human body.

The results obtained lead to the following considerations: during the flexion of the spine we can observe that it is a deformation of the tissue, which leads to a new position of the marker M_3 in the reference frame of the considered vertebra.

Variation of tissue deformation has a linear trend, which is explained by a constant factor k used. For these analyzes, the value of damping factor c has no influence over the results.

Another way of illustration of the results is presented below. In Fig. 8a a series consists of several vertebrae and the outer surface of the tissue (skin) is shown. Considering the first vertebra fixed, when the spine is flexed with δ angle (Fig. 8b), it can be seen that the outer tissues are subjected to tensile stresses, leading to a change in their thickness from h_0 to h. Also, in addition to changing the thickness of tissue, a lag (sliding) can be observed of the outer tissue against the rigid part (vertebrae).

Any point on the surface of the outer tissue will have a sliding (red line) point compared to the theoretical geometrical position (the blue line), corresponding to $\alpha_1 \ldots \alpha_n$ angles of flexion.

Knowing the coordinates of a point on the surface of the skin and knowing that this is a position relative to a vertebra, in conjunction with the value of correction of relative displacement of the point, we can say that it is possible to estimate the positions of the vertebrae in relation to external markers. The relative displacement of the markers can be obtained from the marker's coordinates acquired from the motion capture system, followed by the assessment of the spine's flexion from the results shown in Fig. 7. This can be very important in the primary diagnosis of spine disease using reflexive markers and a motion capture system.

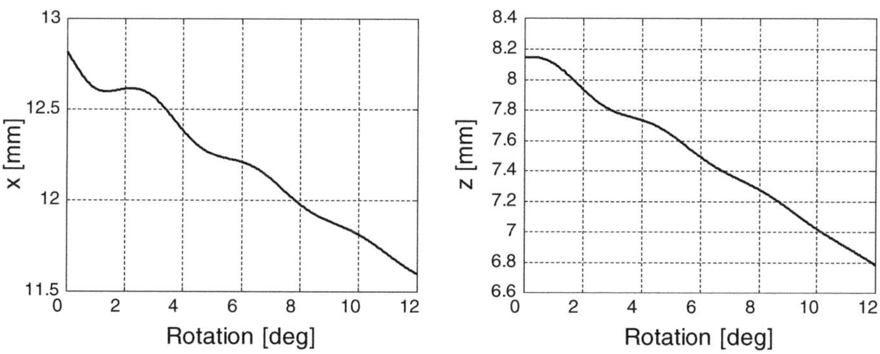

Fig. 7 Relative displacement of marker, x and z direction

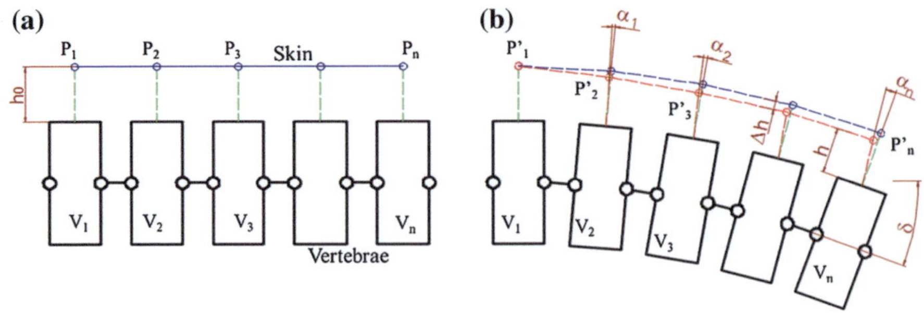

Fig. 8 The scheme illustration of skin deformation

4 Conclusions

It was considered a segment of tissue outside the human body in order to establish a possible inconsistency between the markers glued on the skin surface and the fixed markers. Not taking into account the size on the Z-axis. For analysis, it was built a 2D model of human skin, in the XZ plane, corresponding positions of thoracic vertebrae T_1 … T_4.

Points P_1 … P_4 are considered fixed on extremities of the vertebrae T_1 … T_4. On the outside of the model we consider a point M_3, corresponding of vertebra T_3. We considered that the segment P_1P_5 is fixed, and we watched the movement of point M_3 depending on the movement of points P_2 … P_4 and elastic characteristics of the built model (see Fig. 6).

The results show that the relative displacement of the point M_3 point follows an approximately linear trend due to constant factor k and because the damping factor c was not considered (see Fig. 7).

By analyzing the results, we can highlight some clear conclusions. First, we believe that the markers on the skin surface don't keep their positions on benchmarks represented by hard tissues (bones), but there will be a slip due to the elastic properties of the skin (Fig. 8b).

If there is a boundary condition that involves fixing segments analyzed at one extremity of the model, then the displacements values to the fixed benchmarks will be summed, and will get very high values on the extremity of the analyzed segment.

The results are approximately anticipated, considering the assumptions used. For the future, it is necessary to make the analysis taking into consideration the hyperelastic properties of the skin.

Acknowledgments This paper was realized within the Partnership Programme in priority domains—PN-II, which runs with the financial support of MEN-UEFISCDI, Project no. 227/2014, System for Diagnosis and Therapy of Spine Diseases (SPINE).

References

1. Boyer, G., Molimard, J., Ben Tkaya, M., Zahouani, H., Pericoi, M., Avril, S.: Assessment of the in-plane biomechanical properties of human skin using a finite element model updating approach combined with an optical full-field measurement on a new tensile device. J. Mech. Behav. Biomed. Mater. **27**, 273–282 (2013)
2. Corazza, S., Mundermann, L., Chaudhari, A.M., Demattio, T., Cobelli, C., Andriacchi, T.P.: A markerless motion capture system to study musculoskeletal biomechanics: visual hull and simulated annealing approach. Ann. Biomed. Eng. **34**(6), 1019–1029 (2006)
3. Dalla Pria Bankoff, A.: Biomechanical characteristics of the bone. In: Dr. Tarun Goswami (ed.) Biomechanical Characteristics of the Bone, Human Musculoskeletal Biomechanics, pp. 61–83. InTech (2012). ISBN: 978-953-307-638-6
4. de Sousa Crespo, J.: Human tissue hyperelastic analysis. Dissertation thesis, Technical University of Lisboa (2009)
5. Groves, R.B., Coulman, S.A., Birchall, J.C., Evans, S.L.: An anisotropic, hyperelastic model for skin: experimental measurements, finite element modelling and identification of parameters for human and murine skin. J. Mech. Behav. Biomed. Mater. **18**, 167–180 (2013)
6. Holt, B., Tripathi, A., Morgan, J.: Viscoelastic response of human skin to low magnitude physiologically relevant shear. J. Biomech. **41**(12), 2689–2695 (2008)
7. Lapeer, R.J., Gasson, P.D., Karri, V.: Simulating plastic surgery: from human skin tensile tests, through hyperelastic finite element models to real-time haptics. Prog. Biophys. Mol. Biol. **103**(2–3), 208–216 (2010)
8. Lu, T.-W., O'Connor, J.J.: Bone position estimation from skin marker coordinates using global optimisation with joint constraints. J. Biomech. **32**, 129–134 (1999)
9. Moltedo, M., and Sophie Sakka, S.: Improving skin artifacts compensation for knee flexion/extension and knee internal/external rotation. In: Proceedings of 2014 IEEE International Conference on Robotics and Automation (ICRA), Hong Kong, China. doi:10.1109/ICRA.2014.6907565, pp. 4825–4830 (2014)
10. Sanders, J.E., Goldstein, B.S., Leotta, D.F.: Skin response to mechanical stress: adaptation rather than breakdown—a review of the literature. J. Rehabil. Res. Dev. **32**(3), 13 (1995)
11. Sholukha, V., Bonnechere, B., Salvia, P., Moiseev, F., Rooze, M., Van Sint Jan, S.: Model-based approach for human kinematics reconstruction from markerless and marker-based motion analysis systems. J. Biomech. **46**(14), 2363–2371 (2013)
12. Talaba, D., Antonya, C.: The multi-particle system (MPS) model as a tool for simulation of mechanisms with rigid and elastic bodies. In: Multi-body Dynamics: Monitoring and Simulation Techniques III, Ed. Professional Engineering Publishing Ltd., pp. 111–119 (2004)
13. Tregear, R.T.: The mechanical properties of skin. J. Soc. Cosmet. Chem. **20**, 11 (1969)
14. Tsai, A.G., Musahl, V., Steckel, H., Bell, K.M., Zantop, T., Irrgang, J.J., Fu, F. H: Rotational knee laxity: reliability of a simple measurement device in vivo. BMC Musculoskelet. Disord. **9**, 35 (2008). PubMed PMID: 18366671. doi:10.1186/1471-2474-9-35
15. Wang, Y., Rahmatalla, S.: Human head-neck models in whole-body vibration: effect of posture. J. Biomech. **46**(4), 702–710 (2013)

Anthropomorphic Underactuated Hand with 15 Joints

E. Matheson, Y. Aoustin, E. Le Carpentier, A. Leon and J. Perrin

Abstract Underactuated robotic hands are becoming popular in complex robotic designs where mass and size are yet limited. Such designs require a tradeoff between versatility and simplicity. This is the case for prosthetic robotic hands, which need to imitate the human hand both in functionality and dimensions as closely as possible to achieve a natural feeling solution for the patient. This paper presents the initial mechanical analysis of the design of an anthropomorphic hand with 15 degrees of freedom using six electric motor actuators. A transmission system of cables and pulleys is used as the underactuated mechanism in order to propagate the motor torque over the three joints of each finger, and springs are used to provide the passive return actuation. The design has been validated according to its ability to stably grasp different cylindrical objects. The stability of the grasp has been judged according to the criterion of positive or zero contact forces being present at all points of contact between the hand and the object in a static case. A simulation of the grasping procedure where the contact forces are modeled over time has been developed in Matlab®. It has been shown that the design process requires iterative steps, as multiple factors

This work was performed while the first and fourth authors were with IRCCyN.

E. Matheson
ESA, ESTEC, Keperlaan 1, 2201 Noordwijk, AZ, The Netherlands
e-mail: Eloise.Matheson@esa.int

Y. Aoustin (✉) · E. Le Carpentier (✉)
L'UNAM, Institut de Recherche en Communications et Cybernétique de Nantes, UMR CNRS 6597, CNRS, Université de Nantes, 1 rue de la Noë, 44321 Nantes Cedex 3, France
e-mail: Yannick.Aoustin@irccyn.ec-nantes.fr

E. Le Carpentier
e-mail: Eric.Le-Carpentier@irccyn.ec-nantes.fr

A. Leon (✉) · J. Perrin (✉)
Alpes Instruments, 61 chemin du Vieux Chêne, 38240 Meylan, France
e-mail: contact@alpes-instruments.com

J. Perrin
e-mail: contact@alpes-instruments.com

P. Wenger et al. (eds.), *New Trends in Medical and Service Robots*,
Mechanisms and Machine Science 39, DOI 10.1007/978-3-319-30674-2_21

such as spring stiffness, pulley radii, and motor torques will affect the stability of grasping of the hand and its effectiveness as a prosthetic device.

Keywords Grasping · Anthropomorphic underactuated robotic hand · Contact effort · Stable grasps

1 Introduction

The imitation of the versatility of a human hand for dexterous manipulation and robust grasping is a challenge. However; the design of robotic hands for grasping has become a very active field in robotics to perform tasks for industrial applications, or to control a prosthesis. Among pioneer designs is [9], where a hand is controlled through signals from pressure sensitive transducers. A multifingered hand is proposed in [6] to investigate the basic concepts of manipulation theory, control system design and tactile sensing. In [7] authors study how hard it is necessary to squeeze an object to ensure a secure grasp, the required finger joint motions to manipulate an object, and the determination of the hand workspace.

Mechanism design requires a compromise between versatility and simplicity to obtain relevant practical systems; for a review see [2]. To achieve a lightweight hand with a similar size to a human hand, it is necessary to limit the number of actuators. Due to this requirement, the concept of underactuated mechanisms is gaining increasing popularity. Underactuated hands are able to overcome the gap between traditional industrial robotic grippers and advanced fully actuated hands, see [5] and [3]. The principle of underactuation in grasping is to use a mechanical system, with more degrees of freedom than actuators, which can adapt to the shape of the object automatically. Gosselin et al. [5] presents an anthropomorphic underactuated robotic hand with 15 degrees of freedom (DOF) and only one actuator, and its experimental validation. The main contributions of [3] is to theoretically analyse underactuated hand mechanisms, the distribution of forces and the stability of the grasping task. Catalano et al. [4] proposed an approach, called *adaptative synergy* and based on ideas coming from underactuated hand design, to control the underactuated device *Pisa/IIT softhand*. This approach provides a model of how synergies may generate and control the internal forces required to successfully hold an object. Despite theses remarkable advances, the problem of stability for any 3D object needs more numerical investigations. This paper aims to fill this gap.

An anthropomorphic underactuated robotic hand is presented and several numerical tests of grasping tasks. It has been designed by the French compagny *Alpes Instruments*. In future this robotic hand will play the role of the prothesis for our applications about the grasping tasks through a EMG control. It is arranged in four fingers and opposable thumb. Our main objective is to develop a global strategy to control a prosthetic hand through electromyographic (EMG) signals.

The paper is outlined as follows. Section 2 describes the mechanical design of the anthropomorphic underactuated robotic hand. Section 3 presents the geometric structure and its associated frame through the modified Denavit and Hartenberg notation. A static model of the contact forces is calculated in Sect. 4. Section 6 is devoted to the numerical tests to evaluate the stability of the grasping of different objects as function of their shape. Finally, conclusions and potential extensions of this work are presented in Sect. 9.

2 Mechanical Design

In this section the chosen options of the design are detailed. The design requirements for the prosthetic hand are as follows;

- Dimensions similar to a human hand,
- Weight similar to a human hand, and
- Able to successfully grasp objects that a human hand can easily lift.

The hand, shown in figures and Fig. 1a, consists of four fingers and one thumb which together exhibit 15 DOF actuated by six motors. The four fingers are identical and their abduction and adduction degrees of freedom have been omitted for all fingers in order to decrease the complexity of the mechanical design and to limit the hand weight. The total weight of one hand is 0.62 kg. The dimensions are based upon average values of a male human hand. All the digits are underactuated. Each finger has one DC electric motor form *Maxon* company as the actuator, which drives the first joint. A transmission system of pulleys and cables is used to transmit the torque to the succeeding joints. The cable wraps around each joint before being firmly anchored in the final phalanx. The thumb has two motors. The first controls the movement of

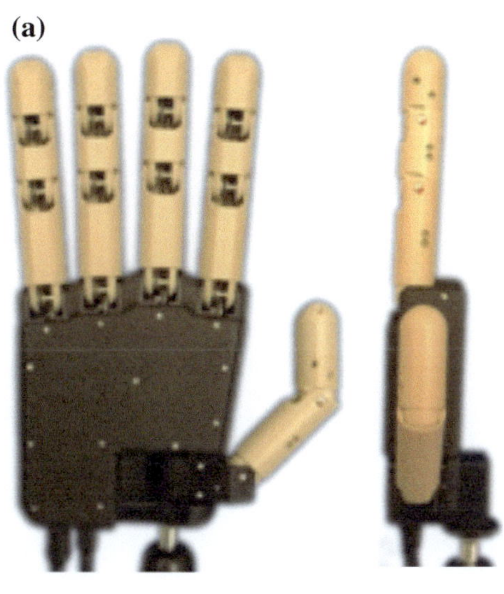

Fig. 1 CAD model of the hand in an extended position (**a**)

the thumb about the palm, and the second controls the flexion and extension of the following two joints. Movement of the motors creates flexion of the rotational joints, the return extension movement is provided by straight springs placed over each joint. When using a cable and pulley transmission system in an underactuated design it is necessary that the joint is able to move around the pulley without directly being pulled by the cable or spring. This introduces compliance into the design, meaning that one joint can be held or moved independently of the others when acted upon by an external force such as that from the object being grasped. The chosen DC motor is a 12 V Maxon combined with a planetary gearhead of ration 256:1. This motor includes a current sensor, which is useful to determine its delivered torque and an encoder sensor with a resolution of 32,768 points per revolution. The total weight of each motor is 25 g, and, when combined with the planetary gear head, is able to produce a continuous torque of 0.15 Nm.

3 Geometric Structure of the Anthropomorphic Underactuated Robotic Hand

Each finger on the thumb consists of three parallel revolute joints (see Fig. 2) to ensure the flexion and extension of each phalanx. The thumb also has three revolute joints. However; the first joint allows for the pronation/supination of the thumb about the palm and so is perpendicular to the following two joints. The 2nd and 3rd parallel joints of the thumb allow for flexion and extension of the phalanges.

Fig. 2 Tree structure of the joints in the hand with global base at the palm

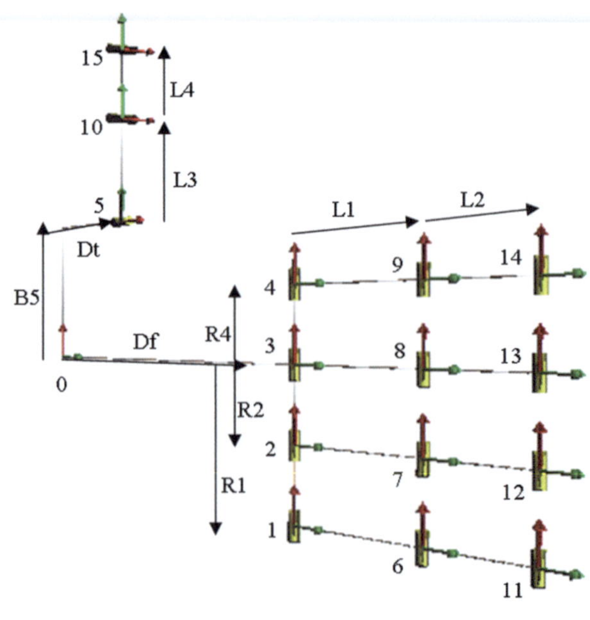

Initially each finger and the thumb of the hand are modeled as an independent serial chain. Each motor can be controlled independently, meaning that each finger and thumb can also be independently controlled.

A tree geometric structure is considered for the hand, composed of the palm, the four fingers and the thumb, see Fig. 2. The origin of the reference frame is located in the middle of the 'wrist' (bottom face of the palm) directly in line with the middle finger of the hand. All transformations are derived from this fixed origin.

The geometric and kinematic models have been developed using the modified Denavit and Hartenberg (D-H) notation first introduced by Khalil and Kleinfinger, see [8].

3.1 Direct Geometric Model

To determine the direct geometric and kinematic models it is necessary to know the joint values (position and velocity), which is only possible in a real robot if there is a sensory system able to achieve this. For this prosthesis, the only sensor present will be the motor encoders, and a current sensor in each motor. The readings of the current sensor will provide the estimated torques applied at the six active joints 1–5, 10, however; will not be able to give detailed information on the joint variables. Similarly, for the inverse geometric and kinematic models it is necessary to know the end effector position and velocity which cannot be determined in our system design. The fact that the design is underactuated further complicates the analysis. If no external forces are present, with the knowledge of the reference position of each finger and that all the joints are coupled it is possible to evaluate a position mapping of their tip as function of the information from the motor encoders. The direct geometric model is derived from the table of modified D-H parameters. Table 1 depicts the D-H parameters for the hand, where the 0 frame is the reference frame of the robot, and the digits are numbered from one (smallest finger) to five (the thumb), where,

- $a(j)$ denotes the frame antecedent to frame j,
- $\mu(j)$ indicates if the joint is active (motorized) ($\mu(j) = 1$) or passive ($\mu(j) = 0$),
- The parameters (a_j, γ_u, α_u, $d(u)$, $\theta(u)$, $r(u)$) determine the location of frame j with respect to its antecedent $a(j)$,
- $\sigma(j)$ specifies the type of joint j, 0 if revolute, 1 if translational and 2 if fixed.

Geometrical representations of the constants are shown in Fig. 2.

4 Contact Force Model

Birglen et al. in [3] introduce a static model of the contact forces for an underactuated hand through the theory of reciprocal screws, see [1] and [10]. Springs with pre-loading are used as passive actuators which provide the extension movement.

Table 1 Modified D-H parameters of tree structure hand

j	$a(j)$	$\mu(j)$	σ(j)	γ(u)	b(u)	α(u)	$d(u)$	$\theta(u)$	$r(u)$
1	0	1	0	0	0	0	Df	0	R1
2	0	1	0	0	0	0	Df	0	R2
3	0	1	0	0	0	0	Df	0	0
4	0	1	0	0	0	0	Df	0	R4
5	0	1	0	$\pi/2$	B5	$\pi/2$	0	$\pi/2$	R5
6	1	1	0	0	0	0	L1	$\theta 6$	0
7	2	1	0	0	0	0	L1	$\theta 7$	0
8	3	1	0	0	0	0	L1	$\theta 8$	0
9	4	1	0	0	0	0	L1	$\theta 9$	0
10	5	1	0	0	0	$\pi/2$	L3	$\theta 10$	0
11	6	1	0	0	0	0	L2	$\theta 11$	0
12	7	1	0	0	0	0	L2	$\theta 12$	0
13	8	1	0	0	0	0	L2	$\theta 13$	0
14	9	1	0	0	0	0	L2	$\theta 14$	0
15	10	1	0	0	0	0	L4	$\theta 15$	0

Notation from [8]

When external forces are present, for example when grasping an object, it is difficult to predict which joints will be blocked or actuated upon due to contact with the object. To present this model, for kth finger ($k = 1, \ldots, 4$) with three phalanges, let us consider:

$\Gamma(3 \times 1)$ - input torque vector (actuator and spring contribution)
ω_α - vector of joint velocities
$\dot{\theta}_i$ - joint velocity of ith phalanx
ξ_i - twist of ith contact point on ith phalanx
ζ_i - wrench of ith contact point on ith phalanx
o - reciprocal product between a twist $\xi_i^\top = [\omega_i^\top \; v_i^\top]$
and a wrench $\zeta_i^\top = [f_i^\top \; \tau_i^\top]$ $is f_i^\top v_i^\top + \omega_i^\top \tau_i^\top$
K_i - stiffness of spring at joint θ_i
ω_i - angular velocity vector of ith phalanx
v_i - linear velocity vector at ith contact point
f_{ti} - tangential force vector at ith contact point
f_i - normal force vector
τ_i - torque vector applied by ith phalanx

The model is based on the fact that the contact forces over all the phalanges of an underactuated finger can be determined by correlating the input and output virtual powers of the system. The model assumptions are:

- One contact point per phalanx,
- Contact force is in the plane perpendicular to the extension/flexion movement,
- Only revolute joints are present.

Furthermore for the numerical tests in Sect. 5 the movements of the thumb and the four fingers are considered taking place in the plan. Considering the balance quality of the virtual power we,

$$\begin{aligned} \Gamma^{\mathsf{T}} \omega_\alpha &= \sum_{i=1}^{3} \xi_i \; o \; \zeta_i, \\ &= \sum_{i=1}^{3} v_i^x f_{ti} + v_i^y f_i + \omega_i \tau_i, \end{aligned} \tag{1}$$

with

$$\xi_i = \begin{bmatrix} \omega_i \\ v_i^x \\ v_i^y \\ 0 \end{bmatrix}, \; \zeta_i = \begin{bmatrix} f_{ti} \\ f_i \\ 0 \\ \tau_i \end{bmatrix}, \; \boldsymbol{\Gamma} = \begin{bmatrix} \Gamma_a - K_1 \Delta\theta_1 \\ \Gamma_2 = -K_2 \Delta\theta_2 \\ \Gamma_3 = -K_3 \Delta\theta_3 \end{bmatrix}, \; \omega_\alpha = \begin{bmatrix} \dot\theta_1 \\ \dot\theta_2 \\ \dot\theta_3 \end{bmatrix}.$$

The case of the thumb is similar, except that there are two actuators and two phalanges. At ith contact the limit of equilibrium is assumed to be on the edge of the friction cone, which is characterized through the static coefficient μ_i^{static} defined such that:

$$f_{ti} = \pm \mu_i^{static} f_i \tag{2}$$

From this notation a coefficient μ_i, which is not necessary equal to μ_i^{static} is introduced such as $f_{ti} = \mu_i f_i$ for each ith contact point.

Similarly for τ_i, we can write $\tau_i = \eta_i f_i$. These coefficients η_i are usually small and will hereafter be zero in the case of punctual contacts. However these coefficient are useful to describe contacts with friction and with phalanges that have a non-negligible thicken, see [3]. Let r_{ki} be as the vector from joint origin O_k to the ith contact point such that:

$$\begin{bmatrix} v_i^x \\ v_i^y \\ 0 \end{bmatrix} = \omega_i \times r_{ki} \tag{3}$$

Through Eqs. (1), (2), and (3), we can deduce the following relation:

$$\xi_i \; o \; \zeta_i = f_i \left(\sum_{k=1}^{i} \dot\theta_k r_{ki}^{\mathsf{T}} x_i - \mu_i \sum_{k-1}^{i} \dot\theta_k r_{ki}^{\mathsf{T}} y_i + \eta_i \sum_{k=1}^{i} \dot\theta_k \right) \tag{4}$$

x_i and y_i being unit vectors respectively tangential and orthogonal to the ith phalanx. Correspondingly;

$$\Gamma^{\top}\omega_{\alpha} = \mathbf{f}^{\top}(\mathbf{J}\dot{\theta}) = \mathbf{f}^{\top}(\mathbf{J}\mathbf{T}\omega_{\alpha}) \tag{5}$$

with;

$$\mathbf{J} = \mathbf{J}_1 - \begin{bmatrix} \mu_1 & 0 & 0 \\ 0 & \mu_2 & 0 \\ 0 & 0 & \mu_3 \end{bmatrix} \mathbf{J}_2 + \begin{bmatrix} \eta_1 & 0 & 0 \\ 0 & \eta_2 & 0 \\ 0 & 0 & \eta_3 \end{bmatrix} \mathbf{J}_3$$

$$= \begin{bmatrix} k_1 + \eta_1 & 0 & 0 \\ r_{12}^{\top}(x_2 - \mu_2 y_2) + \eta_2 & k_2 + \eta_2 & 0 \\ r_{13}^{\top}(x_3 - \mu_3 y_3) + \eta_3 & r_{23}^{\top}(x_3 - \mu_3 y_3) + \eta_3 & k_3 + \eta_3 \end{bmatrix}$$

where;

$$\mathbf{f}^{\top} = [f_1, f_2, f_3]^{\top},$$

k_i = distance between ith joint and the ith contact point,

$$r_{ii}^{\top} x_i = k_i,$$

$$r_{ij}^{\top} x_j = k_j + \sum_{k=i}^{j-1} L_k \cos\left(\sum_{m=k+1}^{j} \theta_m\right), \; i < j,$$

$$r_{ii}^{\top} y_i = 0,$$

$$r_{ij}^{\top} y_j = -\sum_{k=i}^{j-1} L_k \sin\left(\sum_{m=k+1}^{j} \theta_m\right), \; i < j,$$

L_i = length of ith phalanx

These formulas are illustrated through Fig. 3, which depicts a punctual contact between the third phalanx and a spherical object.

Matrix **J** is dependent on the location of the contacts on the phalanges, the relative orientation of the phalanges and the friction and inertia coefficients, while **T** is dependent on the transmission method used to transmit the actuation of the motor. Matrix **T** relates vector ω_{α} to the time derivatives of the phalanx joint coordinates.

$$\dot{\theta} = \mathbf{T}\omega_{\alpha} \tag{6}$$

Fig. 3 Punctual contact with a spherical object of the third phalanx of a finger

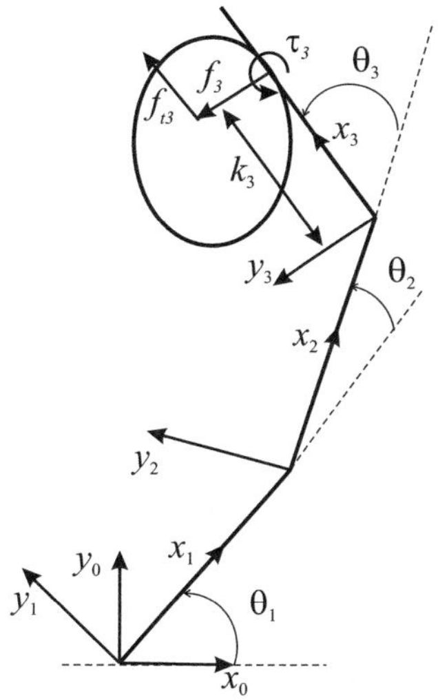

When using a transmission method of cables and pulleys for a three phalanx finger, the **T** matrix is as follows.

$$\mathbf{T} = \begin{bmatrix} 1 & \frac{-r_2}{r_1} & \frac{-r_2 r_4}{r_1 r_3} \\ 0 & 1 & 0 \\ 0 & 0 & 1 \end{bmatrix} \tag{7}$$

Here r_1 is the radius of the pulley located at the first joint, r_2 and r_3 are the radii of the pulleys located at the second joint and r_4 is the radius of the pulley at the third joint.

Finally the contact forces can be determined from:

$$\mathbf{f} = \mathbf{J}^{-\top}\mathbf{T}^{-\top}\boldsymbol{\Gamma} \tag{8}$$

It should be noted that the $\boldsymbol{\Gamma}$ vector here of joint torques is as function of the available torque from the motor that can be used in grasping i.e. the maximum possible torque that can be used for grasping is the total torque output from the motor minus the torque required to move the joints to the required position.

In [3] a grasp is defined as statically stable when all the contact forces are positive or zero. Any singularities in matrices **J** or **T** will result in undefined contact forces and potentially unstable grasps. When using a system of pulleys, cables and springs these singularity cases are avoided. Authors also noticed that if the ratio of pulley radii is 1:1 then when a contact force becomes negative, the grasp can never recover stability as a contact force will always remain negative. For this reason it is a better design practice to ensure that $\frac{r_{i+1}}{r_i} \leq 1$.

5 Simulation

A model and simulation of a grasping hand is developed and implemented in Matlab®. The direct geometric model developed in Sect. 3.1 is used to determine the coupled motion of the fingers and the thumb as the digits are moved through their possible extremes of motion (full extension to full flexion of joint 1 of each digit). At each step in the trajectory, the contact forces on each phalanx are determined from the model developed in Sect. 4.

The aim of the simulation is to see if a stable grasp can be achieved by the under-actuated hand on a target object. If all the contact forces applied to the object are zero or positive, then the grasp is statically stable. In order to determine if the grasp is stable over time, it is necessary to estimate the net wrench applied by the hand onto the object. Then to move the object with an effort of the hand by some distance in the direction of the net wrench, and determine the contact forces of the digits in the new position. It is possible to tune the results of the grasp stability by changing parameters of the model including the spring stiffness values, the radii of the pulleys and/or the lengths of the phalanges.

5.1 *Program Overview*

Figure 4 shows the main functions in the Matlab® program and the program flow. The numerical values that define the models of the fingers and the thumb referenced in Table 1, are shown in Tables 2 and 3.

In the implementation of the contact force model, because the contact is assumed punctual the coefficients η_i are set as zero. Friction effects at the contact point are also neglected and so all μ_i values are set as zero.

Once the mechanical model of the hand has been defined the simulation step is initiated. The transformations of all the joint frames with respect to the base frame are determined using the direct geometric model of the hand, and the coupled trajectory of each digit based on the transmission system of pulleys and cables is defined. The hand follows the coupled motion trajectory until there is either impact with the object

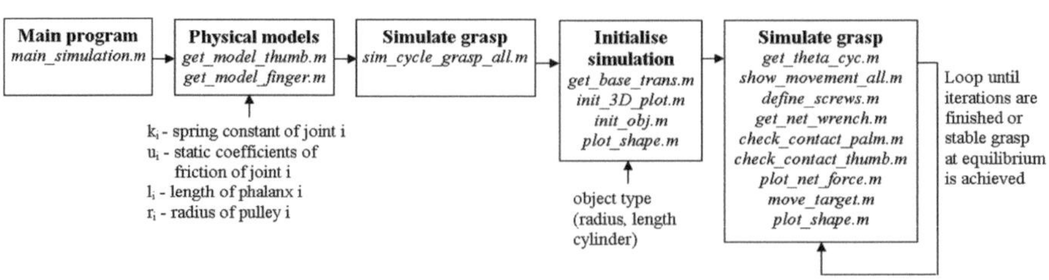

Fig. 4 Program function flow for the simulation developed in Matlab®.

Table 2 Numerical model values used for each finger

Variable	Value	Unit	Description
L1	0.05	m	Phalanx 1 length
L2	0.03	m	Phalanx 2 length
L5	0.024	m	Phalanx 3 length
K_1	0.0	Nm/rad	Joint 2 spring constant (torsion)
K_2	0.04	Nm/rad	Joint 2 spring constant (torsion)
K_3	0.03	Nm/rad	Joint 3 spring constant (torsion)
r_1	0.004	m	Joint 1—pulley 1 radius
r_2	0.0035	m	Joint 2—pulley 2 radius
r_3	0.0035	m	Joint 2—pulley 3 radius
r_4	0.003	m	Joint 3—pulley 4 radius
Df	0.1	m	Distance from base to MCP joint of each finger (*x* dir'n)
R1	−0.04	m	Distance from base to MCP finger 1 (*z* dir'n)
R2	−0.02	m	Distance from base to MCP finger 2 (*z* dir'n)
R4	0.02	m	Distance from base to MCP finger 4 (*z* dir'n)

Table 3 Numerical model values used for the thumb

Variable	Value	Unit	Description
L3	0.02	m	Phalanx 1 length
L4	0.03	m	Phalanx 2 length
K_1	0.0	Nm/rad	Joint 1 spring constant (torsion)
K_2	0.03	Nm/rad	Joint 2 spring constant (torsion)
r_1	0.004	m	Joint 1—pulley 1 radius
r_2	0.0025	m	Joint 2—pulley 2 radius
max t	0.15	Nm	Maximum torque exerted by active joint
B5	0.03	m	Distance from base to MCP thumb (*z* dir'n)
R5	0.03	m	Distance from base to MCP thumb (*x* dir'n)

to be grasped or joint 1 is fully flexed and the digit cannot close further. Contact with the object occurs when the axis of the phalanx (effectively the phalanx skeletal bone plus the radius of the phalanx) is tangential to the cylinder surface. Once all the digits have been moved, the contact forces are determined and the net wrench on the object is found. It should be noted that all wrenches are with respect to the global base frame of the hand located in the middle of the wrist directly underneath the middle finger. In order to determine the net wrench, the screw of each contact force is determined and retrospectively applied to the global frame. This is determined using the formula from [8], which defines the screw transformation, **S** from frame *j* with respect to frame *i* as;

$$ {}^{i}\mathbf{S}_{j} = \begin{bmatrix} {}^{i}\mathbf{R}_{j} & {}^{i}\hat{\mathbf{P}}_{j} \\ \mathbf{0} & {}^{i}\mathbf{R}_{j} \end{bmatrix} $$

where **R** is the rotation matrix and $\hat{\mathbf{P}}$ is the skew symmetric translation matrix. Conversely, the screw transformation from frame *i* with respect to frame *j* is;

$$ {}^{j}\mathbf{S}_{i} = \begin{bmatrix} {}^{j}\mathbf{R}_{i} & -{}^{j}\mathbf{R}_{i}^{i}\hat{\mathbf{P}}_{j} \\ \mathbf{0} & {}^{j}\mathbf{R}_{i} \end{bmatrix} $$

In this simulation the wrench, **W** at a frame i is defined as the forces in *x*, *y*, and *z* in the local frame, and the moments in *x*, *y* and *z* in the local frame. That is;

$$ {}^{i}\mathbf{W}_{i} = \left[f_x f_y f_z \; m_x \; m_y m_z \right]^{\mathrm{T}} $$

The wrench in frame i that includes the wrench applied in the succeeding frame j is determined with this equation;

$$ {}^{i}\mathbf{W}_{i} = {}^{i}\mathbf{W}_{i} + {}^{j}\mathbf{S}_{i}^{\mathrm{T}\,j}\mathbf{W}_{j} $$

Once the net wrench on the center of mass of the cylinder (defined to be in the middle of the homogenous cylinder) is found, then the object is moved by an increment (0.01 m) in this direction. Checks are made to see if the object impacts with the palm. The palm is treated as a rigid body, and if contact occurs then any force that the object may experience into or along the palm is cancelled by an equal and opposite reaction force from the palm. If the thumb is fully extended and the object is impacting the thumb, then the thumb is also treated as a rigid body that will resist any force the object exerts on the thumb. In this way, the net force acting into or along the palm, or into the thumb are treated as zero.

The simulation is finished when the object experiences a net force of zero, or the iterations are complete. At this point, the grasp is considered stable if all the contact forces are non-zero. If there are negative contact forces present, then the object may still slide from the grasp - incurring a change of position of the fingers that may still be able to grasp the object, or they may lose contact and eject the object.

5.2 Target Objects

Different types of objects to be grasped were developed. These were all cylindrical in nature, though with different radii. A cylindrical object was modeled as it approximates many objects in the real world that a human may want to grasp. Examples of these are a door knob, a glass or a handrail. Four objects were developed in Matlab®. In the program the object size and location can be modified. The cylinder can either be homogeneous (or equal radii along its length), or non-homogeneous (different radii along different sections).

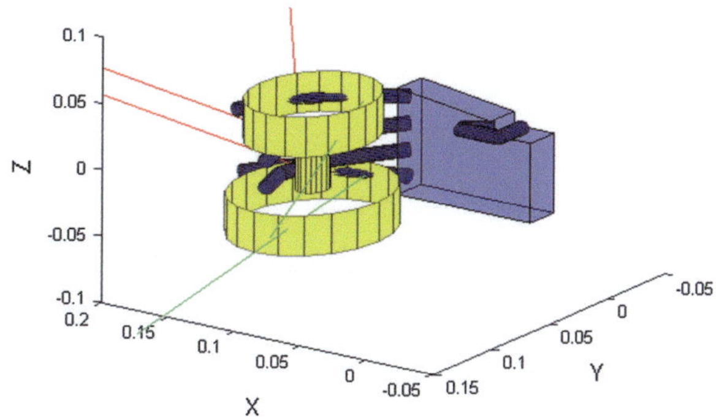

Fig. 5 Target object—non-homogeneous cylinder, isometric view

Table 4 Target object—contact force values (*N*)

Phalanx	Finger 1	Finger 2	Finger 3	Finger 4	Thumb
1	62.7021	–	–	66.3722	–
2	−58.8017	−59.6835	−59.6835	−59.1324	–

5.3 Contact Force Validation

For the implementation of the simulation tool, each digit is treated as a separately controllable serial chain, or independent chain of a tree structured robot. This has been done in order to be able to choose which fingers can take part in a grasping action, and to see that depending on the orientation of the joints, each digit can produce different maximum contact forces on the target object. With a non-homogeneous cylindrical object we can see Fig. 5, that each finger has a different orientation, and so different maximum contact forces are defined for each finger.

The thumb does not take part in this grasping action. A positive contact force, depicted with a green line in Fig. 5 means that the phalanx pushes against the object. A negative contact force, depicted with a red line in Fig. 5, means that the phalanx will experience a sliding/slipping motion. The program outputs which phalanges are in contact with the object and what value the contact forces have. The results for this scenario are shown in Table 4.

5.4 Program Validation

In order to validate if the program works as expected an object is defined with mass and an external force of gravity, $g = 9.81$ m/s, is applied on the center of mass (CoM) of the homogeneous cylinder. Gravity is defined in the positive global x frame, meaning that it acts along the palm towards the fingers. If the fingers were fully extended, they would point in the direction that gravity is acting. This is done in order for the greatest possible contact forces (those applied by four parallel fingers) to resist the effect of gravity.

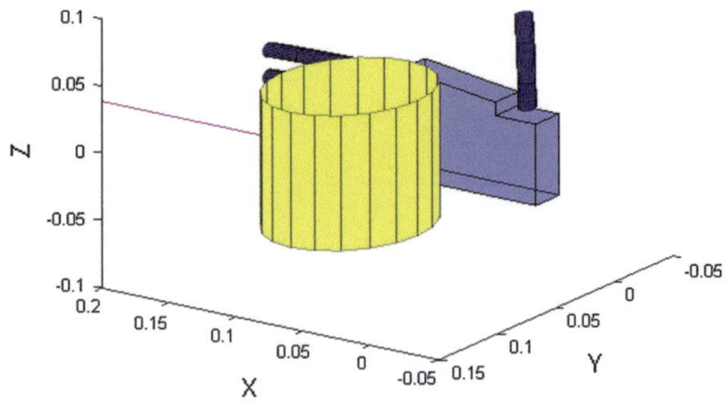

Fig. 6 Object with external force of gravity

A cylinder was defined with a mass of 7 kg. Without any contact forces from the hand, it is expected that the net force experienced at the object's CoM would be $f_x = mg = 68.67$ N. In Fig. 6 the net force vector is shown in purple line. It is pointing in the direction of gravity (positive global x axis) as expected as there are no contact forces from the hand onto the object. This result is validated by the simulation as no contact forces were obtained for any fingers/thumb and the net force on the object was 68.67 N, acting purely in the linear x-axis.

6 Simulation Results

One key factor is the success of the stability grasping is the initial placement of the hand around the object. Ideally the object should be located close to the palm near the base of the fingers in order to maximise the chance of the underactuated hand being able to grasp it. It is difficult to predict the behavior of the hand when acted upon by the external forces of the object, however; an estimation can be made with this program.

6.1 Grasping Stability Results

The movement of the object is governed by the net force, and not the net moment, on the object. Future improvements to the simulation would be to include the influence of the net moment as this could cause the object to twist in the hand. Contact forces are shown in green if they are positive and red if they are negative. The net force applied to the COM of the object is shown in purple. At each iteration the object is shifted a small amount (approximately 0.01 m) in the direction of the net force. The phalanges adjust to this shift by repositioning their contact points around the target object, simulating the movement that would occur as the object applied an external force on the underactuated hand. A non-zero net force on the hand means that the object is not at rest, and the grasping task is not complete.

Table 5 Case 1: Simulated results of final contact forces (N) and net wrench (Nm) on the object

Phalanx	Finger 1	Finger 2	Finger 3	Finger 4	Thumb
1	14.9848	14.9848	14.9848	14.9848	–
2	–	–	–	–	–
3	7.446	7.446	7.446	7.446	6.8617
Fx	Fy	Fz	Mx	My	Mz
−15.3281	0	0	0	0	15.5533

Table 6 Case 1: Simulated grasping sequence SUCCESS

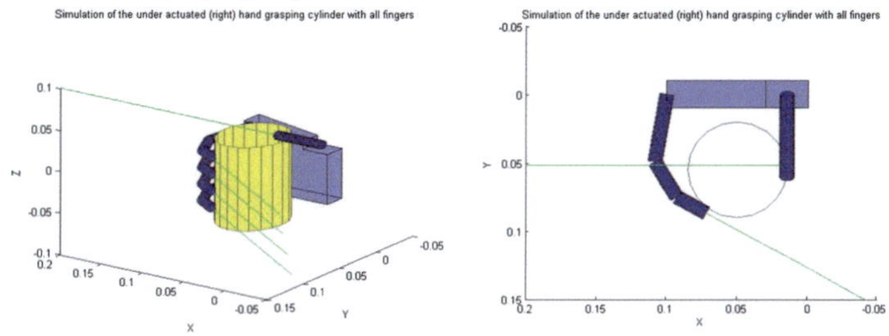

The initial contact only occurs at the third phalanx of each digit

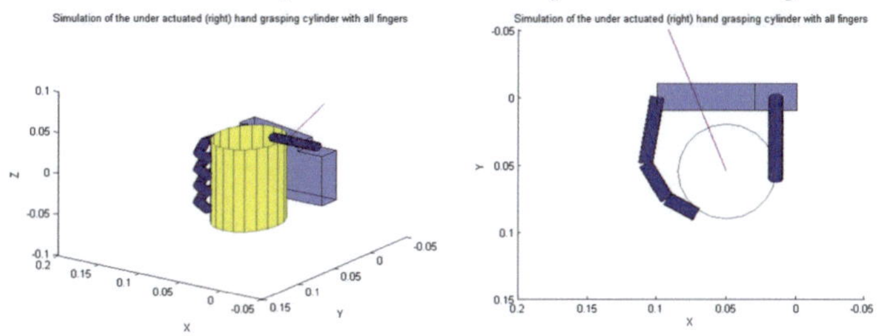

The net force is in the direction of the palm

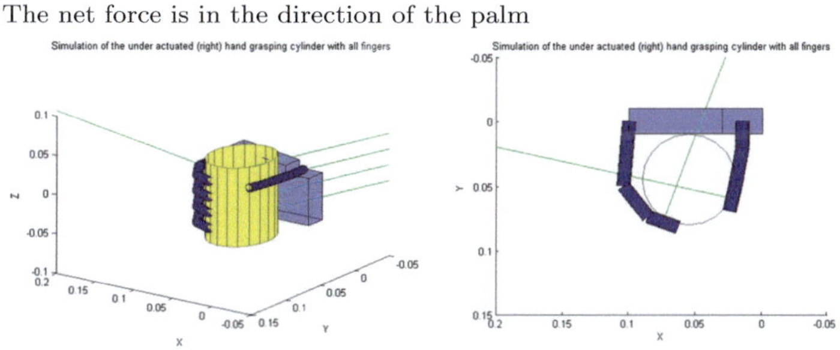

Contact occurs at phalanx 3 of the fingers, thumb and the palm.
All contact forces are positive.

6.2 Case 1: Successful Full Hand Grasp

The object chosen is a homogeneous cylinder of radius 0.05 m and mass 4.6 kg. This weight was found to be approximately the maximum mass that the hand could support, as heavier masses always resulted in ejection.

Table 6 shows the sequence of steps for the hand to grasp the cylindrical object. For this simulation, the grasp is stable and at equilibrium, implying that the hand can successfully grasp the object. In the final sequence, the contact force results are shown below in Table 5.

6.3 Case 2: Unsuccessful Full Hand Grasp

It is interesting to study objects, particularly in cases where an ejection occurs and the grasp is not stable. The object used in this simulation was a homogeneous cylinder with a mass of 5 kg and a radius of 0.05 m. For this simulation, the initial position of the object was such that the thumb could not reach it, and the collective effort of the fingers was not enough to overcome the gravity force. As a result, the hand was not able to grasp the object and ejection occurred (Table 7).

Table 7 Case 2: Simulated grasping sequence EJECTION

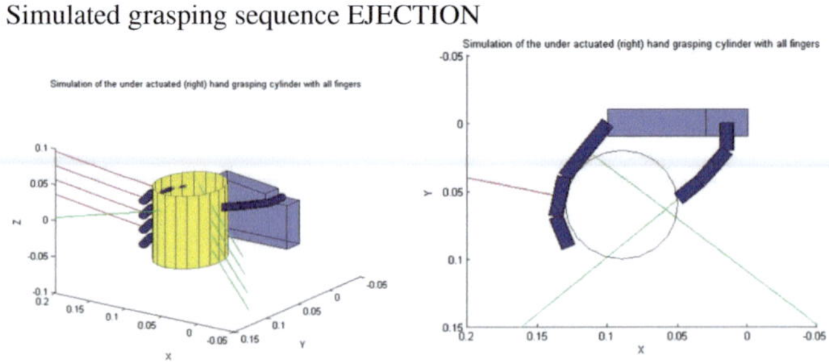

Finger phalanges 1 and 2 and thumb tip are in contact.

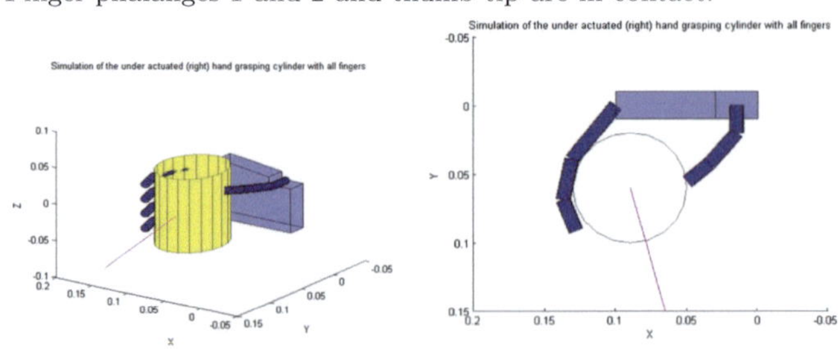

The net contact force moves the object away from the thumb

Table 8 Values of pulley radii used in simulations

	Finger				Thumb	
	r_1	r_2	r_3	r_4	r_1	r_2
Simulation 1	0.004	0.0035	0.0035	0.003	0.004	0.0025
Simulation 2	0.001	0.002	0.003	0.004	0.001	0.004

7 Results of Changing Pulley Radii

It is possible to tune the grasping effectiveness of the hand by changing mechanical model parameters such as the pulley radii and the springs used. The results shown previously have used the most optimal values found in this simulation, which are detailed in Sect. 5.1. The radii should decrease in size towards the fingertip in order that the greatest force is applied at the MCP joint, and smaller forces are applied at joints further away from the palm. If the pulley radii are the same, then force can be well transferred, however; if a negative contact force appears, and no springs are included in the model, then it will always remain negative [3] which has implications for the grasping ability of the hand. The best results are achieved when the pulley radii decreases towards the fingertip.

Table 9 summarizes the results when the pulley radii decrease towards the fingertip and when the pulley radii increase towards the fingertip. The values of the pulley radii used in these two scenarios defined in Table 8. For the same object, we see that grasping is successful when the pulley radii decrease towards the fingertip, and is unsuccessful when the radii increase towards the fingertip.

8 Results of Changing Spring Stiffness

The chosen spring stiffness can also have a large effect on the ability of the hand to grasp an object. The spring stiffness determines the amount of resistive torque that the transmitted motor torque must first overcome before the non-active joint can be rotated. Higher spring stiffness result in lower contact forces being produced in the same orientation. The higher the spring stiffness values, the lower the amount of mass that can be supported by the hand. However, the springs must be stiff enough to provide the extension force, to effectively open the digits. The amount of force this extension requires is dependent on the mass of the hand itself, and the friction within the system. Testing is best carried out on the physical prototype of the hand, and once the minimal spring stiffness value that can successfully extend the hand is defined, then these values can be used in the simulation to determine the maximum contact forces that the hand can produce, hence the maximum mass the hand can support.

Table 9 Implications of pulley radii on contact forces

SIMULATION 1: Pulley radii decrease towards the fingertip

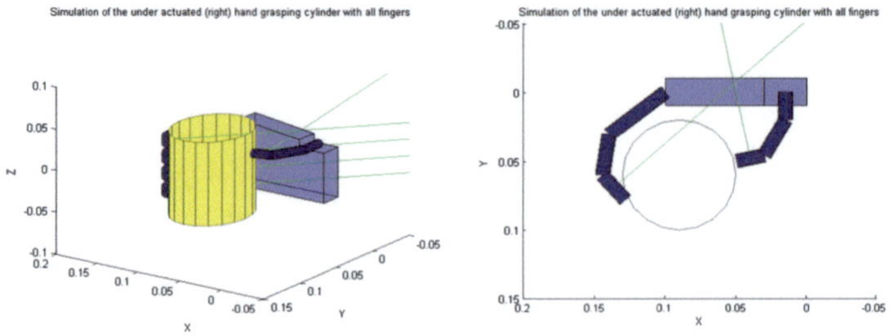

Positive contact forces (green line) when the fingers initially come in contact with the object (case 1 in previous section)

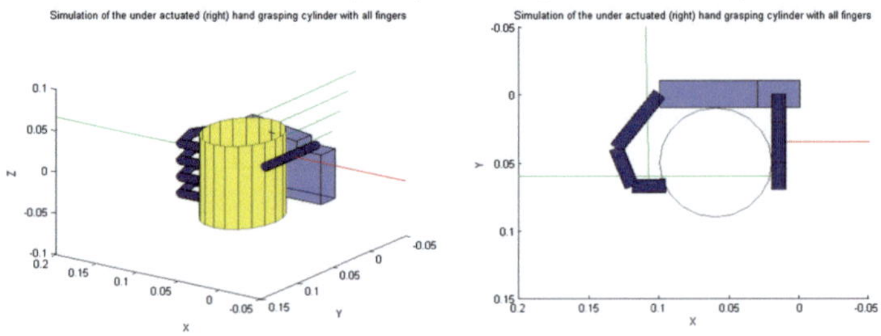

Final, stable grasp is achieved by the hand

SIMULATION 2: Pulley radii increase towards the fingertip

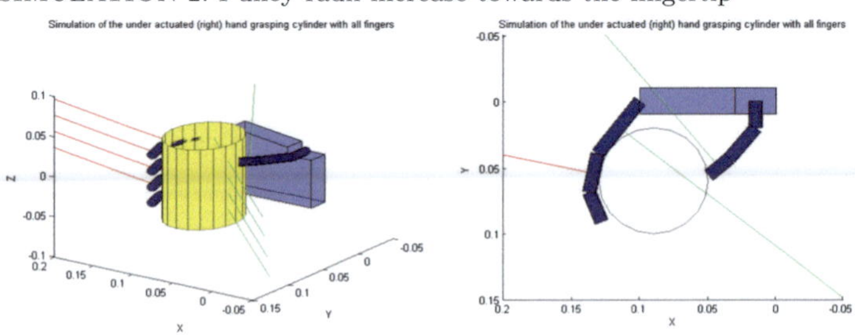

Negative and positive contact forces when the fingers initially come in contact with the object

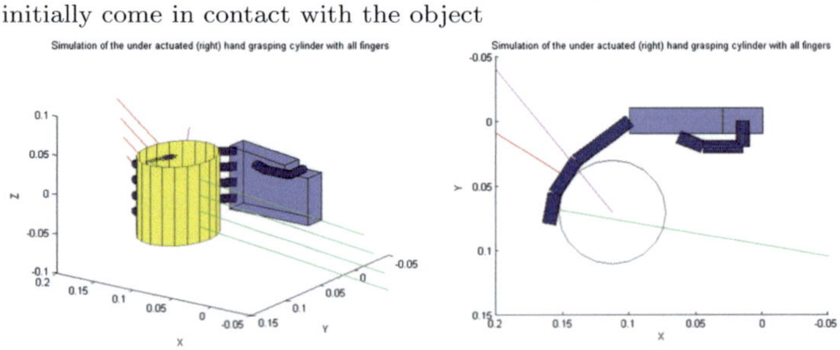

The hand is unable to grasp the object, ejection will occur.

9 Conclusion

Using underactuated mechanical systems is a valuable method of reducing weight, cost, power requirements and the size of the device while maintaining its usefulness and maneuverability. However; they are not well understood regarding the best methods of design, particularly when analyzing grasping stability and effectiveness. This paper has addressed the analysis of an underactuated prosthetic hand regarding its ability to stably grasp objects. Birglen's model of contact forces has been seen to be a well presented methodology of determining contact forces for specific underactuated mechanisms. Being able to define a hand based on the hand Jacobian $\mathbf{J}$ and transmission matrix $\mathbf{T}$, allow the analysis to be easily updated for new designs.

The ratio of these pulley radii will determine the transmission of torque from the active joint to the passive joints, and should be chosen so that the last joint is fully flexed when the first joint is is fully flexed, thereby maximizing the workspace of the digit. The springs used should be strong enough to provide the return, extension movement, but not so stiff to avoid high torques.

Acknowledgments This work is supported by Région des Pays de la Loire, CNRS and Erasmus Mundus program.

References

1. Ball, R.S.: A Treatise on the Theory of Screws. Cambridge University Press, Cambridge (1900)
2. Bicchi, A., Kumar, V.: Robotic grasping and contact: A review. In: Proceedings of International Conference on Robotics and Automation, vol. 1, pp. 348–353 (2000)
3. Birglen, L., Gosselin, C., Laliberté, T.: Underactuated Robotic Hands. Springer, Berlin (2008)
4. Catalano, M.G., Grioli, G., Farnioli, E., Serio, A., Piazza, C., Bicchi, A.: Adaptive synergies for the design and control of the Pisa/IIT SoftHand. Int. J. Robot. Res. **33**(5), 768–782 (2014)
5. Gosselin, C., Pelletier, F., Laliberté, T.: An anthropomorphic underactuated robotic hand with DOFs and a single actuator. In: Proceedings of International Conference on Robotics and Automation, vol. 2, pp. 1520–1532 (2008)
6. Imai, Y., Namiki, A., Hashimoto, K., Ishikawa, M.: Design of the Utah/MIT Dextrous Hand. In: Proceedings of International Conference on Robotics and Automation, vol. 2, pp. 1520–1532 (1986)
7. Kerr, J., Roth, B.: Analysis of multifingered hands. Int. J. Robot. Res. **4**(4), 3–17 (1986)
8. Khalil, W., Kleinfinger, J.: A new geometric notation for open and closed-loop robots. In: Proceedings of International Conference on Robotics and Automation, vol. 3, pp. 1174–1179 (1986)
9. Tomovic, R., Boni, G.: An adaptive artificial hand. Trans. Autom. Control **7**(3), 3–10 (1962)
10. Waldron, K.J.: The constraint analysis of mechanisms. J. Mech. **1**(2), 101–114 (1966)

Effects of the Rolling Mechanism of the Stance Foot on the Generalized Inverted Pendulum Definition

Sylvain Devie and Sophie Sakka

Abstract This paper addresses the way the rolling mechanism of the human foot influences the Generalized Inverted Pendulum (GIP) model during normal walking. A test on 6 subjects was performed, and two ways of modelling were used: the first one uses the filtered data of the Center of pressure (CoP) trajectory to rebuild the human inverted pendulum; the second one linearizes the CoP trajectory with time, which is equivalent to ignoring the effects of the rolling mechanism of the foot. The results show that the linearized model leads to an observable clear area of convergence of the dynamics support lines showing a neat inverted pendulum, while the non-linearized forces to make the distinction between the three sub-phases of single support: damping, stabilizing, propelling.

Keywords GIP · Normal gait · Walking · Human beings · Rolling mechanism · Center of pressure

1 Introduction

Generating trajectories for walking gaits for bipedal structures with rigid feet, like humanoid robots, is a challenge especially when vertical equilibrium is at stake. When such rigid structure is aimed at imitating a soft, complex and compliant natural system like a human being, a common mechanical model should be proposed. Humanoid walking is traditionally based on Resolved Momentum Control [6], Kart-Table and Inverted pendulum (IP) models [5]. On the other side, human walking

---

S. Devie (✉)
Ecole normale superieure of Rennes, Rennes, France
e-mail: sylvain.devie@ens-rennes.fr; Sylvain.Devie@irccyn.ec-nantes.fr

S. Sakka (✉)
University of Poitiers, Poitiers, France
e-mail: Sophie.Sakka@irccyn.ec-nantes.fr

S. Devie · S. Sakka
Research Institute for Communications and Cybernetics of Nantes,
Nantes, France

P. Wenger et al. (eds.), *New Trends in Medical and Service Robots*,
Mechanisms and Machine Science 39, DOI 10.1007/978-3-319-30674-2_22

gait observation mainly provides with human joint angles trajectories obtained from kinematics measurements. As the kinematics and dynamics of these two structures is very different, the human joint angles trajectories cannot be directly implemented for the humanoid robots and provide with the same result.

A way of connecting the natural and artificial systems may be found using more general reference points like CoM or CoP [10], Generalized pivot [11], Virtual Pivot Point [8] or the concept of virtual pendulum [7, 12]. Basics may be found in the IP representation. Indeed, some authors proposed such "simplified" representation for human beings. Historically, and taking inspiration from robotics, discontinuous models were proposed (compass gait or single support representation in the sagittal plane). Then appeared the first continuous IP model in 3D, proposing a fixed pivot point located at ground level and in the middle of the single support, similarly to robotics gait generation [14, 15]. But this model would widely overestimate the human center of mass trajectory amplitude, and as a consequence need much more energy when performing normal walking [3]. An analysis of these observations showed that a fixed pivot point at ground level, together with a constant rod length, would be equivalent to neglecting the rolling mechanism of the feet, a major component of the low energy cost of human walking [2].

The next IP model proposed in the literature (*Extended inverted pendulum*, EIP) would then attempt to take this remark into consideration [4]: The IP pivot point would be moving during the single support phase, its location being superposed to the measured Center of pressure trajectory. The corresponding energy consumption would get much closer to reality, as the CoP displacement would reduce the vertical amplitude of the CoM. The EIP model requires the dynamics measurement of human walking, which makes it more complex to set. As a consequence, a study proposed a third 3D continuous IP model called *Generalized inverted pendulum* (GIP) to consider a fixed pivot point but under the ground level [11]. This approach was inspired by the passive walking researchers who designed curved feet mechanism to lower walking energy consumption of their machines [9]. A method was proposed to locate the subject pivot point based on kinematics and dynamics measurements of the first and last instant of the single support.

This paper aims at better understanding the effects of the rolling mechanism of the foot during single support on the GIP definition. After heel strike, the foot is rolling around the heel which results in a fixed CoP in the sagittal plane. Before toes off, the foot is rolling around the toes which again results in a fixed CoP. In the middle, the CoP tracks a quasi-linear trajectory going fast from heel to toes. Because of these three sub-phases, the location of the pivot is made difficult. We will then study the impact of rigid feet (such as the ones of the humanoid robots), which will minimize the two previously mentioned rolling phases, in comparison to compliant human feet, by linearising the CoP trajectory with time: at each time step, the CoP displacement is constant during the whole single support phase. We will compare the obtained GIP with the reference one. Section 2 describes the GIP model and the three sub-phases of the single support in the sagittal plane. Section 3 will report the experimental data and post-treatment, and show the obtained results when using a CoP linear trajectory. Section 4 will analyse the results.

2 Model and Walking Phases

This section first introduces the Generalized Inverted Pendulum. Then, the three subphases of the single support (SS) of normal walking are presented. These two tools will allow explaining why the humanoid walking gait cannot be the same as the human walking gait.

2.1 *Inverted Pendulum Model*

The *Generalised inverted pendulum model* (GIP) was first introduced by Sakka et al. [11] in 2010. It permits the modelling of human walking from an external point of view. Its originality, in comparison with other existing IPs, is that the rolling mechanism of the foot is considered: the IP pivot is not on the ground level, but under it.

The GIP approximates the human body as an inverted pendulum: a punctual mass fixed to one extremity of a massless rod of constant length, which other end rotates around a fixed pivot point. The punctual mass correspond to the *Center of Mass* (CoM). The rod is built using a line linking the CoM and the *Center of Pressure* (CoP) at each time step. These lines are called *dynamics support lines*, and they show an area of convergence under the ground level, which allows defining the pendulum pivot point (PP) [11]. This model respects the following assumptions.

- The gait is in steady state: there is no variation of CoM walking speed or trajectory amplitude during observation;
- The walking is symmetric: similar motion is performed by left and right legs;
- The system is conservative; Painlevé first integral is valid.

Based on the descriptions and definitions in [11]and according to Fig. 1, let us propose a systematic calculation of the instantaneous pivot point (IPP) at each time step t_i. Let P_0 be the IPP. It is defined as the intersection point of two consecutive support lines. These lines may not cross in 3D, so let us consider that P_0 is the midpoint of the shortest distance separating two consecutive support lines. It is then located on a line perpendicular to both support lines. Let $\mathbf{v}$ denotes the unit vector in the direction of the common perpendicular between the two consecutive support lines, let C_k and P_k denote respectively the CoM and CoP at time t_k. Then

$$\mathbf{v_i} = \frac{\mathbf{C_iP_i} \times \mathbf{C_{i+1}P_{i+1}}}{\| \mathbf{C_iP_i} \times \mathbf{C_{i+1}P_{i+1}} \|} \tag{1}$$

Let M_k be the orthogonal projection of P_0^k on C_kP_k at time t_k, and O_0 the center of the reference frame. Then the vector $\mathbf{P_iP_{i+1}}$ may be decomposed as follows:

$$\mathbf{P_iP_{i+1}} = \mathbf{P_iM_i} + \mathbf{M_iM_{i+1}} + \mathbf{M_{i+1}P_{i+1}} \tag{2}$$

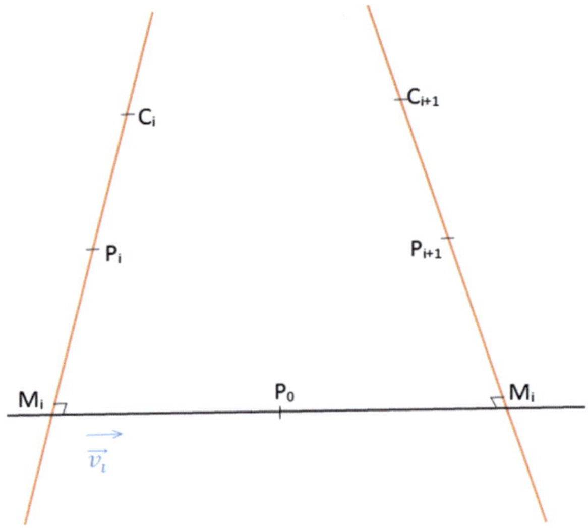

Fig. 1 Used model for the calculation of the closer point P_0 between two support lines (*red*) connecting the CoM C_i, C_{i+1} to the CoP P_i, P_{i+1}. The common perpendicular is defined by the intersection points M_i, M_{i+1} and it direction $\mathbf{v}$

Introducing $\lambda = (\lambda_1, \lambda_2, \lambda_3)$ such that

$$\mathbf{M_iM_{i+1}} = \lambda_1 \mathbf{v} \tag{3}$$

$$\mathbf{P_iM_i} = \lambda_2 \mathbf{C_iP_i} \tag{4}$$

$$\mathbf{M_{i+1}P_{i+1}} = \lambda_3 \mathbf{C_{i+1}P_{i+1}} \tag{5}$$

Eq. 2 can be solved easily as the linear system (6).

$$\lambda = \left(\mathbf{v}, \mathbf{C_iP_i}, \mathbf{C_{i+1}P_{i+1}} \right)^{-1} \mathbf{P_iP_{i+1}} \tag{6}$$

2.2 *Definition of the Sub-phases*

The human walking gait is a succession of single support (SS) and double support (DS) phases. We will focus here only on the SS phases. A SS phase can be decomposed into three sub-phases [13] corresponding to a rolling mechanism along the heel, a linear tranfert with flat foot and a rolling mechanism along the toes. We will here point out the different behaviors of the CoM, CoP and IPP which allow separating the three subphases. Let us first consider Fig. 2 that represents the x (frontal) and y (lateral) evolution of the CoP with time during SS according to measurement from one actor. The three subphases may be observed on the x component with time, depending on the slope of the curve:

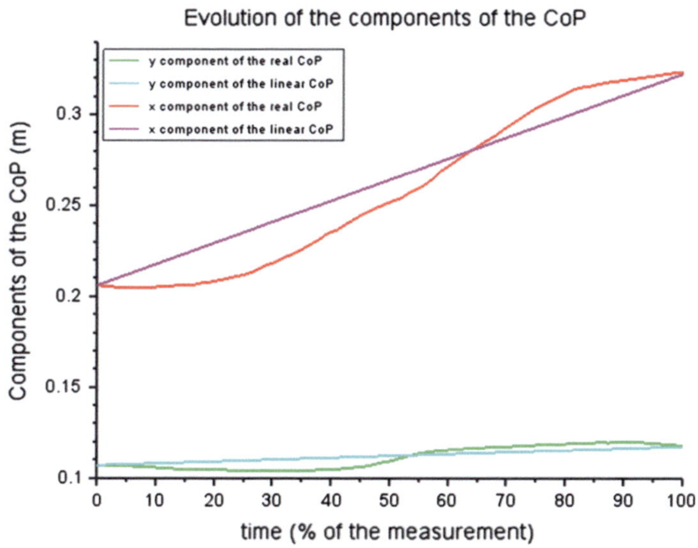

Fig. 2 Frontal (x) and lateral (y) components of the CoP [m] with respect to time (% of SS) for real and linearised trajectories of the CoP

- The first sub-phase is a rolling phase, between 0 and 25 %. It corresponds to a rotation of the foot around the lateral axis at the heel. During this phase, the human body amortizes the extra weight due to the take-off of the other foot. Just before this rolling phase, the CoP was defined in the support pattern between the two feet. So, at the beginning of this phase, the fictitious moment point (FZMP), defined by Borovac [1] is located outside the foot. The new support pattern matches to the footprint on the ground. So, during this phase, the CoP is defined on the heel and do not evolve too much.
- The second sub-phase is a linear phase, between 25 and 80 %. The CoP moves linearly with time from heel to toes. The walking gait is dynamically stable and the human body is in control of its equilibrium. The CoP is equal to the ZMP.
- The third sub-phase is a rolling phase, between 80 and 100 %. It corresponds to the rotation of the foot around the lateral axis at the toes. During this phase, the heel takes off of the ground and the support pattern become smaller, the human body is not dynamically stable and falls down until the other foot touches the ground. In this case, the FZMP is calculated outside the foot and there is a horizontal torque on the CoP, which stays close to the toes.

The effects of these three subphases may be observed with many measured variables during walking. We will see in what follows that the GIP also faces their influence, and how *walking without rolling* may simplify the generated GIP.

3 Rolling Mechanism and Generalized Inverted Pendulum (GIP)

3.1 Data and Post-treatment

6 subjects performed normal walking at comfortable speed. Whole body kinematics (motion capture) and dynamics (force plates) data were acquired, and post-treated similarly to [11].

The CoP trajectory was directly obtained from dynamics data. The CoM trajectory was calculated using a decomposition of the body into 16 rigid segments. The homogeneous transformation matrices T_j^k between two segments j and k were extracted and at each time step, the position of the CoM C with respect to the reference pole O is obtained as follows.

$$\begin{bmatrix} OC \\ 1 \end{bmatrix}_{\mathscr{R}_0} = \frac{1}{M} \sum_{i=1}^{16} m_i T_i^{i+1} \begin{bmatrix} O_i C_i \\ 1 \end{bmatrix}_{\mathscr{R}_i} \tag{7}$$

where $\mathscr{R}_0$ denotes the reference frame and $\mathscr{R}_i$ the local frame attached of segment i (pole O_i); C_i is the center of mass of the body i whose mass is denoted by m_i.

At each time step, the instantaneous dynamics support lines were built linking synchronized CoM and CoP positions.

3.2 GIP and Rolling Mechanism

Figure 3 shows the evolution of the IPP in the sagittal plane for one subject. The direction of advancement is from left to right. The Blue line at the top denotes the CoM trajectory, the green line is the CoP trajectory (ground level). At each time step, CoP and CoM where linked to build the instantaneous support line. All the support lines for SS are represented in red. The black squares represent the closest distance between two consecutive support lines, previously defined as the instantaneous pivot point. The trajectory tracked by these points shows a characteristic "V"-shape (see Sect. 4).

The first rolling subphase holds from 0 to 25 % of SS. During this phase, the IPP dives from ground level to around 50 % of CoM height into the ground, tracking a curved line. This tendency is reversed in the second rolling subphase, during which the IPP goes back from −50 % to ground level. The trajectory tracks a straight line in this last case.

The linear subphase is characterized by a quick going back-up from −50 to −100 %.

3.3 GIP Without Rolling Mechanism

Let us now linearize the CoP trajectory $OP(t)$ with time. This action is equivalent to suppressing the two rolling subphases of ssp. The CoP data are treated as follows:

$$\mathbf{OP}(t) = \mathbf{OP}(t_i) + \frac{\mathbf{OP}(t_f) - \mathbf{OP}(t_i)}{t_f - t_i}(t - t_i) \tag{8}$$

where t_i and t_f are the initial and final instants of ssp, respectively. The effect of this calculation is illustrated in Fig. 2, which shows for one subject the measured trajectory of the CoP in the horizontal plane, and is linear match.

The effect of the CoP trajectory linearization is illustrated in Fig. 4. The two rolling subphases having disappeared, a convergence area of the dynamics support lines can be clearly identified. As a consequence, only in this case can a global pivot point of SS be extracted.

4 Analysis and Discussion

Comparing Figs. 3 and 4, one can see that the linearization of the CoP trajectory leads to the clear appearance of an inverted pendulum during SS. Some characteristics are common to all the observed subjects, while some are related to each subject characteristics. We will here point out the common characteristics.

The first observation when comparing the two models, is the "V"-shape of the IPP trajectory. The linearization did not remove this characteristic, just changed the scale and shape of it. The IPP trajectory is given for the six subjects, in Fig. 5a using measured CoP and Fig. 5b using linearized CoP trajectory.

Considering first Fig. 5a: for all subjects,

- the starting point of the trajectories occur between 0.32 and 0.63 % of SS. The later the start, the more horizontal in the forward direction is the V-shape. Moreover, with an early start, the first branch of the V-shape is curved and the branch is straight, while this tendency is reversed for later starts.
- the tip of the V-shape occurs around −1.3 CoM height.
- the ending points of the IPP trajectory all happen at ground level, at around 0.55 % of SS;
- except for the red subject, the starting points of the first branch of the V-shapes are under the ending points of the second branch.

The starting point of the IPP trajectory depends on how important was the impact velocity at heel strike. This particularity is directly linked to the length of the previous step and defines the future behavior to control the walking velocity and balance. It is always difficult for all subjects to strike exactly in the same way. But we can

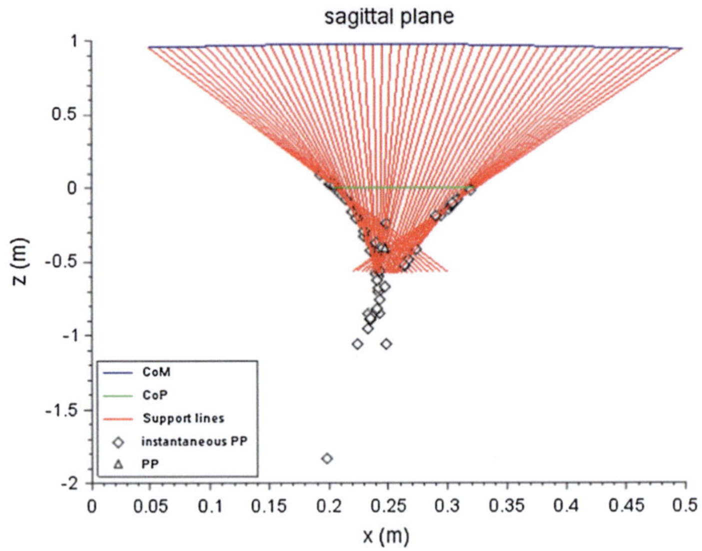

Fig. 3 Evolution of the CoM, the CoP and the IPP during SS for one subject, in the sagittal plane. The "V"-shape of the IPP trajectory is characteristic

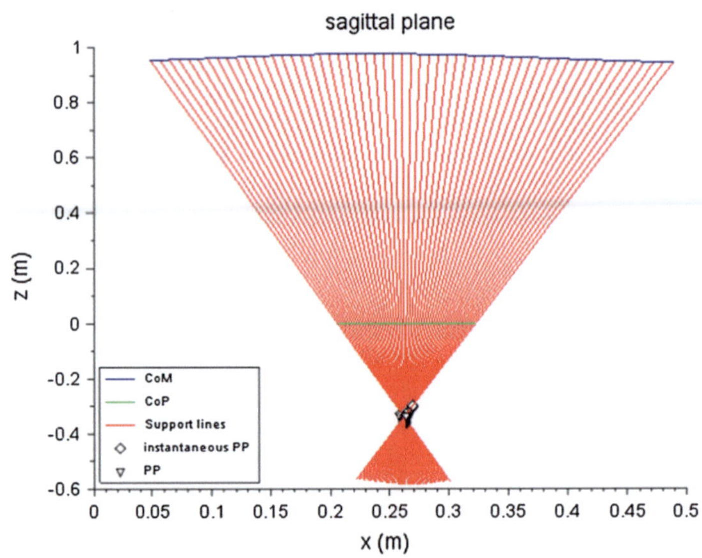

Fig. 4 Evolution of the CoM, linearized CoP and IPP during one SS in the sagittal plane, for one subject

observe that all the subjects finish SS in the same configuration, from the IPP similar behaviors. At this ending instant, trajectory, velocity and balance are controled.

Let us now focus on the V-shapes of Fig. 5b. Numerous observations can be made in comparison to the previous ones.

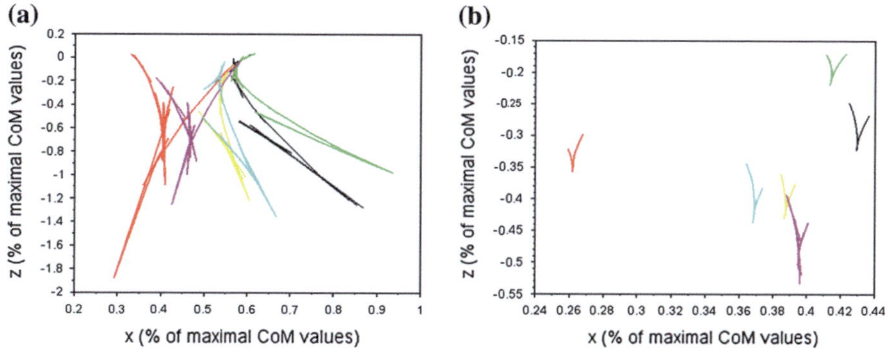

Fig. 5 Evolution of the IPP trajectory for the six subjects. **a** Using real CoP trajectory. **b** Using linear CoP trajectory

- the V-shapes occur much earlier, at around 40 % of SS (except for the red subject, at 26 %);
- the V-shapes are located under ground level, occuring in the range −20 to −50 % of CoM height;
- the tips of the V-shapes are now pointing down vertically. As a consequence, all the V-shapes look similar;
- the V-shape is now characterized by its position in x and z, instead of its starting point and tip orientation;
- the size of the V-shape is around 20 times smaller, at around 7 % of CoM height;
- except for the red subject, the starting point of the first branch of the V-shape is above the ending point of the second branch.

Two of the biggest problems in GIP model are 1) its sensitivity to disturbances and 2) normalization. Indeed, for the second point, this approach considers that interactive forces with the environment should not be neglected in the analysis of walking, such as when considering either CoM or CoP trajectories separately. What is observed here is the coordination between these two key points of human dynamics, and the model offers information on the nature of walking that other studies may not lead to. When separate, it is easy to normalize the CoM trajectory alone, or the CoP trajectory alone, and extract separate behavioral statistics on a given population. When grouped, the normalization of the CoM trajectories (for example) does not lead to a fine normalization of the CoP trajectories and reciprocely. This explains why a big difference between the subjects could be observed in the position of the IPP trajectories in Fig. 5.

We have nevertheless normalized each trajectory (CoM and CoP) separately, which is equivalent to considering that all the subjects have positioned their support foot in the same way relatively to their CoM. Figure 6 illustrates the result of this normalization, using a linear trajectory of the CoP. The CoM and CoP trajectories can be seen in blue and green, respectively, and the localization of the IPP trajectories are represented by their average point (see [11] for calculation details).

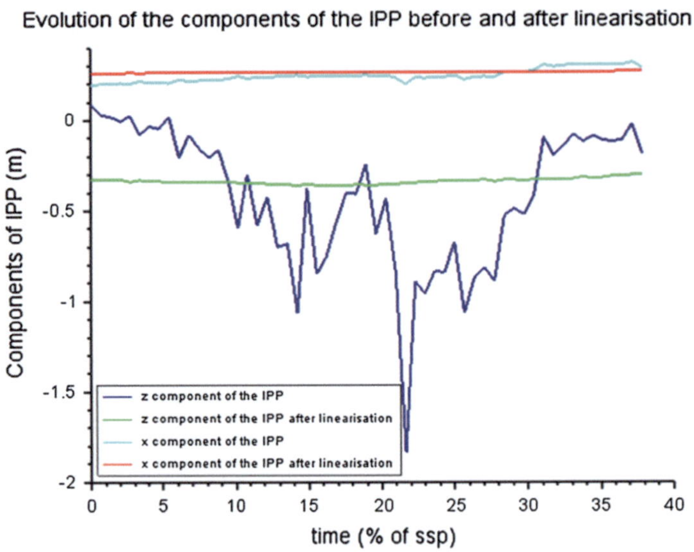

Fig. 6 Normalized positions of PP for 6 subjects

In this situation, the PP for all the subjects are located in an area, denoted by the light blue ellipse in Fig. 6, occuring at 45 % of SS. The only characteristic that varies according to the subject is the depth of the PP, which occurs in the range from −23 to −45 % of maximal CoM height. We believe this characteristic completely depend on the subject morphology and way of coordinating his/her movements, but more subjects are necessary to confirm as well as to fix the population range.

Figure 6 also shows the localization of two average PP, calculated according to Sakka et al. [11]: an average PP taking all the IPPs into consideration, and a PP only considering the first and last support lines. As pointed [11] observing only one subject, these two points remain very close for all our subjects, with a maximal 3 mm distance in the worst case. This means that all the calculation on the IPP trajectories may be simplified to using only the first and last dynamics support lines, when only the position of the PP is required.

5 Conclusions

In this paper, we have extended the analysis of the GIP model proposed by Sakka et al. in [11]. Six subjects were observed performing normal walking at comfortable velocity. Two situations were considered, either using measured data of the CoP trajectories or linearizing the CoP trajectory with time between the first and last instant of SS. In the first situation, the three subphases of SS could be identified, with two rolling (heel/toes) and one linear subphases. In this case, the PP of walking could not be extracted, as the IPP trajectory is too wide, forming a V-shape. In the second situation, the PP could be clearly identified, either by making an average position from all the IPP positions, or by using the extremal CoM and CoP positions of SS.

The GIP model not only considers CoM and CoP behaviors, but adds a knowledge on the coordination between these two points. It is sensitive to disturbances (disbalance, asymmetry of walking, and so on) but simple to set and leads to additional observations of normal gait. This model allows a better understanding on how balance is managed during human walking.

It is necessary, in the next step, to study a wider population in order to fully understand which characteristics of the GIP are common and which depend on a subject morphology or walking specificity.

References

1. Borovac, B., Vukobratovic, M.: Zero-moment point thirty five years of its life. Int. J. Humanoid Robot. **1**, 157–173 (2004)
2. Hayot, C., Sakka, S., Lacouture, P.: Kinematic and dynamic analysis of gait determinants theory. Comput. Methods Biomech. Biomed. Eng. **14**(sup1), 153–154 (2011)
3. Hayot, C., Sakka, S., Lacouture, P.: Assessing the respective effects of the gait determinants on the vertical trajectory of the center of mass using the compass gait representation. Gait Posture (2010)
4. Hayot, C., Sakka, S., Lacouture, P.: Contribution of the six major gait determinants on the vertical center of mass trajectory and the vertical ground reaction force. Hum. Mov. Sci. **32**(2), 279–289 (2013)
5. Kajita, S., Hirukawa, H., Harada, K., Kazuhito, Y.: De la modlisation la gration du mouvement. Introduction la commande des robots humanodes. Springer, France (2009)
6. Kajita, S., Kanehiro, F., Kaneko, K., Fujiwara, K., Harada, K., Yokoi, K., Hirukawa, H.: Resolved momentum control: humanoid motion planning based on the linear and angular momentum. In: IEEE/RSJ International Conference on Intelligent Robots and Systems, pp. 1644–1650 (2003)
7. Maufroy, C., Maus, H.M., Seyfarth, A.: Simplified control of upright walking by exploring asymmetric gaits induced by leg damping. In: 2011 IEEE International Conference on Robotics and Biomimetics, pp. 491–496, Dec 2011
8. Maus, H.M., Lipfert, S.W., Gross, M., Rummel, J., Seyfarth, A.: Upright human gait did not provide a major mechanical challenge for our ancestors. Nat. Commun. **1** (2010)
9. McGeer, T.: Passive dynamic walking. Int. J. Robot. Res. **9**(2), 62–82 (1990)
10. Popovic, M.B., Goswami, A., Herr, H.: Ground reference points in legged locomotion: definitions, biological trajectories and control implications. Int. J. Robot. Res. **24**(12), 1013–1032 (2005)
11. Sakka, S., Hayot, C., Lacouture, P.: A generalized 3D inverted pendulum model to represent human normal walking. In: IEEE-RAS International Conference on Humanoid Robots (Humanoids) (2010)
12. Sharbafi, M.A., Maufroy, C., Maus, H.M., Seyfarth, A., Ahmadabadi, M.N., Yazdanpanah, M.J.: Controllers for robust hopping with upright trunk based on the Virtual Pendulum concept. In: 2012 IEEE/RSJ International Conference on Intelligent Robots and Systems, pp. 2222–2227, Oct 2012
13. Viel, E.: La marche humaine, la course et le saut. Biomcanique, explorations, normes et dysfonctionnements. Elsevier Masson (2000)

14. Zijlstra, W.: Assessment of spatio-temporal parameters during unconstrained walking. Eur. J. Appl. Physiol. **92**, 39–44 (2004)
15. Zijlstra, W., Hof, A.L.: Displacement of the pelvis during human walking: experimental data and model predictions. Gait Posture **6**(3), 249–262 (1997)

Index

P. Wenger et al. (eds.), *New Trends in Medical and Service Robots*,
Mechanisms and Machine Science 39, DOI 10.1007/978-3-319-30674-2

MIX
Papier aus verantwortungsvollen Quellen
Paper from responsible sources
FSC® C105338

If you have any concerns about our products,
you can contact us on
ProductSafety@springernature.com

In case Publisher is established outside the EU,
the EU authorized representative is:
Springer Nature Customer Service Center GmbH
Europaplatz 3, 69115 Heidelberg, Germany

Printed by Libri Plureos GmbH
in Hamburg, Germany